Transforming Home Care

Quality, Cost, and Data Management

Donna Ambler Peters, RN, PhD, FAAN
Senior Product Consultant
Delta Health Systems
Altoona, Pennsylvania

Tad McKeon, MBA, CPA, CQM
Principal Consultant
McKeon and Associates
Jeffersonville, Pennsylvania

AN ASPEN PUBLICATION®
Aspen Publishers, Inc.
Gaithersburg, Maryland
1998

The authors have made every effort to ensure the accuracy of the information herein. However, appropriate information sources should be consulted, especially for new or unfamiliar procedures. It is the responsibility of every practitioner to evaluate the appropriateness of a particular opinion in the context of actual clinical situations and with due considerations to new developments. Authors, editors, and the publisher cannot be held responsible for any typographical or other errors found in this book.

Peters, Donna Ambler.
Transforming home care:
quality, cost, and data management/
Donna Ambler Peters, Tad McKeon.
p. cm.
Includes bibliographical references and index.
ISBN 0-8342-1072-X
1. Home care services—Quality control.
2. Home care services—Cost effectiveness.
3. Database management. 4. Home care services—Databases.
I. McKeon, Tad. II. Title.
RA 645.3.P48 1998
362.1'4—dc21
98-15281
CIP

About Aspen Publishers • For more than 35 years, Aspen has been a leading professional publisher in a variety of disciplines. Aspen's vast information resources are available in both print and electronic formats. We are committed to providing the highest quality information available in the most appropriate format for our customers. Visit Aspen's Internet site for more information resources, directories, articles, and a searchable version of Aspen's full catalog, including the most recent publications: **http://www.aspenpub.com**
Aspen Publishers, Inc. • The hallmark of quality in publishing
Member of the worldwide Wolters Kluwer group.

Editorial Services: Jane Colilla
Library of Congress Catalog Card Number: 98-15281
ISBN: 0-8342-1072-X

Printed in the United States of America

1 2 3 4 5

To Gary,
my life partner and best friend,
who inspires me to reach for the stars.

—Donna Ambler Peters

To Leslie and Victoria,
my sources of inspiration
and well-being.

—Tad McKeon

TABLE OF CONTENTS

FIGURES, TABLES, AND EXHIBITS

FOREWORDS

It is with pleasure that I recommend *Transforming Home Care* to anyone with interest in the home care community.

This new book by Donna Peters and Tad McKeon does an excellent job of preparing readers to deal with the dynamic and changing future of the home care industry.

It should be obvious to all Americans that home care will continue to be the heart of health care in America going into the twenty-first century. The good news is that more people are living longer. The bad news is that we are surviving with multiple disabilities. These disabilities will require the intervention of nurses, therapists, and home care aides to keep people at home in independence with the alternative being placement in an institution at many times the expense.

New technology is also pushing the need for home care services, as is cost effectiveness and changes in demographic patterns. The portion of the national health care dollar that is paid into home care will continue to increase from an average of about 10 percent today to as much as 40 percent or more of the health care dollar in the year 2020. Home care will be more important to the nation as the huge baby boom generation begins to move into their retirement years.

Given the increasingly important role of home care in American health care, individuals who are currently involved in the industry and those who are seeking to become involved will have a great need for resources such as this new book. The book provides an excellent exposition of the key issues that home care corporations must confront if they are going to continue to be relevant and successful in providing the highest quality of health care services to the increasingly large population that will be using these services.

—*Val J. Halamandaris*
President
National Association for Home Care
Washington, DC

". . . We're not in Kansas anymore . . ."

Writing an introduction to change is somewhat like trying to catch water in a sieve! The harder you try, the more you have slipping through the holes. Ensuring future success is part of a process where you identify each step that needs to be taken as you begin the journey toward the "Land of Oz," or toward establishing the goals that you've set. Unfortunately, unlike our friends over the rainbow, the pathway isn't a big yellow brick road, but we do have signs to help guide us to where we need to be.

Envision your agency in five years. Can you identify the issues that you must be addressing to reach your goals? Does your organizational culture support a mission and values required to achieve goals and to create an environment to meet the challenges that your agency faces?

Being involved with the home health industry for the last 20 years, I know there are many opportunities to succeed in meeting the challenges that home health is facing. This is a very exciting time to step outside of the box, not only to learn from where we've been, but to be the pioneers for the next decade.

The authors have captured organizational concepts that have been used effectively in companies and have focused on the importance of incorporating these concepts into a model for change. They guide you through important considerations to prepare for this "big change" including process thinking and managing the quality triad of cost, quality, and service. The total quality management movement has helped businesses to reshape their operations and direct their activities toward cost containment and developing a high customer focus. Successful companies are those that are customer driven and don't underestimate the importance of the organizational culture. Home health can learn from other industries that have implemented strategies to meet the challenges to keep them viable and competitive in the coming years.

Additional key factors include challenging existing paradigms and exploring new ways of providing care. Building blocks of creative management such as leadership, managing costs, and identifying best clinical practice for positive outcomes will strategically position your agency for future growth and success. Remember, it takes brains, courage, *and* heart to face and conquer the new challenges of the coming years!

—*Kathleen Dodd*
President and CEO
The Corridor Group, Inc.
Overland Park, Kansas

PREFACE

"The times they are a-changing" is a phrase that has been used since the beginning of time. It is perhaps a cliché, but it is also a truism, especially in today's world of home health care with the influence of managed care, new regulations, new payment methodologies, and new technologies. Anyone involved in the industry can attest to the magnitude and the rapidity of the movement, but not everyone in home care understands all that's changing with the times.

This book is a journey through those times. It is both a personal and professional pilgrimage offering insight into the expansion of the home health industry and the development of persons working in home care. It is a book about where home care has been, and what we in home care are facing now. It offers both concepts and how-to's. It is a book about growth and about perspective. The process of writing this book confirmed for us, the authors, both the value and necessity of incorporating these fundamental beliefs and actions into agency operations.

The intent of the book is to give you, the reader, a perspective on the evolving home care industry and how you, the provider, the clinician, the educator, the supervisor, the administrator, or the interested party, fit into these unsettled times. It is our belief that if you can understand the changing concepts, you can then make informed choices about how to deal with what is going on, rather than just taking a stab in the dark or waiting to see what others do. Making proactive, informed choices can lead to a transformation of home care, rather than just a transition from one time to another.

With that in mind, we have divided the book into an introduction and four sections. The introduction sets the stage by defining the concept of paradigms and some key principles that operate within a shifting paradigm. We felt this introduction important since the word paradigm has been used extensively in this decade, but has not been well understood.

The first section of the book presents the three major concepts that are key to managing a home care agency successfully: quality, cost, and data management.

Each of these concepts is discussed from the perspective of how it has always been used (the old paradigm). This old paradigm is then contrasted with the key elements of each concept in today's paradigm.

The second section describes the tools necessary to survive within these chaotic times. These tools encompass both the abstract and the concrete. For example, some of the tools are philosophical approaches, such as involving the customer, dealing with the environment, and defining organizational values. Other tools are more specific, such as developing mission and vision statements, using outcomes, OASIS, standards, guidelines, clinical pathways, and activity-based cost management.

The third section integrates the survival tools into management and clinical methodologies that support success. The key to success is making a difference in the health of our customers while staying financially solvent. Critical to making this difference is providing a service that is both meaningful and that meets a need. So, this section identifies the foundation for determining success—data, and how to manage them so they tell you what you need to know to measure performance. It defines the critical steps in managing agency systems so they can be made more efficient and/or effective. It describes the process for keeping care meaningful, and it discloses the means to keep stakeholders aligned with the defined outcomes of the agency systems.

Finally, there is a capstone chapter that pulls together all the key concepts in the book to provide a plan for agency transformation. Key themes include customer-focused care, a learning environment, the alignment of mission vision and values, information accessibility, benchmarking, and an intrinsic perspective. You will see each of these mentioned many times throughout the chapters, from different viewpoints. There is no one right way to approach transformation. The way to do it is the way that is meaningful to your organization. Therefore, the richness of the material in this book comes from the various viewpoints for you to choose from.

There are several ways to absorb the information contained in this text. One is to start at the beginning and read straight through. Another is to look up items you want to learn more about, such as outcomes, pathways, or cost accounting, and go to those specific segments. A third way is to read the capstone first and then go back and read the sections that address the integrated elements more fully. No matter which way you choose, we hope you will benefit as much from reading it as we did from writing it.

We of course could not have done it alone. We attribute the richness of the approach to the respect we have for each other's discipline, one of us being a clinician, the other of a financial persuasion. We also acknowledge the many hours that Linda J. Burns labored over our early manuscripts, ably assisting us in developing and clarifying the documentation of our ideas. We hope you enjoy the fruits of our journey.

INTRODUCTION

In 1992, the U.S. system of health care—actually sickness care—cost $817 billion, an average cost of $3,200 for every man, woman, and child in the country.[1] In actuality, it is not a system at all, but a series of fragmented episodes of care that are vicious in their cycles of wastefulness. For example, the higher the cost of insurance, the fewer the number of people insured. The fewer insured, the more the insured are charged to cover the uninsured and the cost of insurance goes up.[2] Managed care is thought to be a solution for these rising costs and ways of providing health care.

Managed care organizations view home care as a more desirable, less costly alternative to hospitalization. The home care industry has grown from a $12.1 billion business in 1995 to one projected at $18.8 billion by the year 2000. Home care services are expected to continue to increase three- to fourfold as a percentage of health care expenditures.[3] In order to be successful, home care programs must rethink some key business practices that have been the foundation of their operations under the Medicare program.

In doing so, it is important for agencies to realize that the fundamental change that is taking place is greater than just the move to managed care. There is a basic reformatting of our society and a changing of values. This change started several decades ago, and is not yet fully evolved. It began as certain dilemmas appeared that challenged the validity of our existing worldview. The dilemma that ultimately forced the change in worldview was the emergence of systems theory around the time of World War II. A system is defined as a whole that consists of two or more parts. Each part affects the behavior of the whole. The prevailing worldview said that to understand something, one must take it apart (analysis), but when you take a system apart, the system loses all of its essential properties. Thus, another type of thinking was required (synthesis) in order to understand systems, and the shift from the Machine Age and its way of thinking to the Systems Age began.[4] This change in ages is referred to as a paradigm shift and is important to acknowledge in order both to understand and to manage many of the changes taking place in our health care arena.

PARADIGMS

The word *paradigm* comes from the Greek word *paradeigma,* which Webster's defines as a model or pattern and is used to explain fundamental change. A paradigm shift is the movement to a new model, which means new boundaries, new problems, and new ways of solving those problems.

A paradigm shift is a powerful process, and understanding some of the underlying dynamics can assist in understanding the intricacies of the process. The following are some illustrations:

1. New paradigms (models) put everyone practicing the old paradigm at risk. The better people are at practicing the current paradigm, the more they are invested in it, and the more difficult it is to be motivated to change because they will lose that investment.[5] For example, if people are currently solving problems using the old way of thinking and are making money, they can, and are likely to, continue to work the old way. Others, not so invested, however, may be looking for a less expensive way to solve the same problems. At some point in time those using the old way will no longer be able to keep up because the cost per problem solved becomes too high (time and/or money). They are then forced into looking into a new way. Unfortunately, waiting until the crisis hits decreases the likelihood of success. Far better to change while there is still money and time (i.e., begin the search for new rules while the old rules are still successful).[6]

   This scenario is happening for many with the advent of managed care. Some are delaying the entry into a managed care model until they learn more about it, or until managed care becomes more active in their region, or until regulations are changed, or whatever. A *managed care model* is a health care system, and yet we try to solve many of the problems it brings using approaches from our traditional health care system, which was not a system at all but a series of events pasted together based on mechanistic, or fragmented, views of the world.

2. When people change their paradigms they are empowered by the new rules to perceive things in the world they were unable to perceive before; thus, what may be perfectly visible and obvious to persons in one paradigm may be literally invisible to persons in a different paradigm. What is defined as impossible today, therefore, is impossible only in the context of present paradigms.[7] This is important to remember as we look into a managed care model from our traditional care point of view.

3. There is almost always more than one right answer.[8] The universe is multidimensional with indeterminate ways of looking at it, and each way will result in a different picture.[9] Much of our thinking up to now has been that there is a right way and a wrong way of doing things. When we do things the right way we have quality. We need to remember that with indeterminate ways of looking at things, we can have an indeterminate number of views of quality.

4. You don't have to create a paradigm shift to gain its benefits.[10] From a managed care perspective this means that even though we might not be able to create the principles of the model itself, we still have much to gain by buying into and using the model.

5. Agencies are forests of paradigms, both administrative and clinical, each with their own boundaries and rules for success. There are paradigms at several different levels.
   * the larger health care system or macro level
   * the agency as a system itself including patient-focused care processes, support processes, subprocesses, and teams
   * the individual caregiver's practice

   All of these levels operate as their own model or paradigm using their own view of the world. One of the challenges to managers and administrators is to provide everyone with an understanding of all the worldviews of those with whom they interact. This job is made more difficult because one's mind always tries to make new realities fit into old ways. So strong is this tendency that one's mind will actually reshape and distort reality in order to get it to conform to what is known. Therefore, in considering a new paradigm, one must slowly place aside one's existing viewpoint and move into a place of "I don't know." Unfortunately, this place is neither easy nor comfortable. The choice becomes: (1) does one transform the old way with all its comfort and reliability into a new revitalized but unsure way, or (2) does one remain limited but certain? Unfortunately, the second choice, although more comfortable, places one's future in the hands of others such as Medicare and leaves one without further empowerment and/or resources to succeed.

The purpose of this book is to offer assistance in transitioning into this new worldview. Its mission is to offer different perspectives on quality, cost, and the management of data. Quality has always been an elusive concept and becomes more confusing as we add new dimensions such as a more involved consumer and a managed care provider/payer. Managers, professionals, and consumers all demand data on quality in order to defend what they value. This is no easy task, as can be seen by the poor way it has been done up to now. Some of the steps include developing data-driven performance measurement systems and integrating cost and quality. In addition, one must learn to think broadly and systematically, which is a process in itself, something like learning a new language—it doesn't happen overnight. There is no one formula dictated by the accumulation of data, but rather a flexible set of options that are based on the specific circumstances at any one moment in time. Our intent is to put some of the issues of this new worldview or model in some type of perspective to provide you, the reader, with a guide or map for exploring this new land of managed care.

NOTES

1. D. Meadows, Health System Needs Radical Surgery, *The Systems Thinker* 4, no. 4 (1993): 4.
2. Meadows, Health System Needs Radical Surgery, 4.
3. E.M. Stern and G.S. Tidd, Health Care Reform's Effect on Home Care: Strategies For Survival, *Medical Interface,* May 1994: 85–90.
4. R. Ackoff, The Interactive Planning Model (Paper presented at the educational conference for Strengthening Hospital Nursing Program, Gainesville, FL, October 1989).
5. J.A. Barker, *Discovering the Future: The Business of Paradigms*, 3rd ed. (St. Paul, MN: ILI Press, 1989).
6. Barker, *Discovering the Future.*
7. Barker, *Discovering the Future.*
8. Barker, *Discovering the Future.*
9. Ackoff, The Interactive Planning Model.
10. Barker, *Discovering the Future.*

PART I

The Concepts of Quality, Cost, and Data Management

CHAPTER 1

The Eternal Question of Quality

Quality. What is it? An essential characteristic? A desired attribute? A comparative rank? A worldview philosophy? Like a sunbeam, quality is hard to grasp, although attempts to define and describe it have consumed hundreds of journal articles and books and hours upon hours of classroom time.

Avedis Donabedian, the founder of the field of health care quality assurance as a recognizable discipline, has written that quality is largely a social construct that represents our concepts and values of health, our expectations of the provider-client relationship, and our viewpoints about the role of the health care system.[1] The congressional committee charged with designing a strategy for Medicare quality reviews and quality assurance has written that quality is "the degree to which health services for individuals and populations increase the likelihood of desired health outcomes and are consistent with current professional knowledge."[2 (p.21)] Industry encourages the consumer to define quality by the "I know it when I see it" standard.[3 (p.18)]

These definitions, however, raise the question of measurement; for example, how does one measure "the degree to which health services ... increase ... desired health outcomes"? The classic way of approaching the measurement of quality was offered more than 30 years ago by Donabedian in his formulation of the components of structure, process, and outcome.[4] *Structures* are the resources used to deliver care, such as the credentials of the health care professionals and the administrative policies of home health care agencies. *Process* means the care itself, such as the use of the nursing process, or the actual interventions performed. *Outcomes* are the results of the care, such as the relief of pain or the healing of a wound.

Source: This chapter is adapted from D.A. Peters, Measuring Quality: Inspection or Opportunity? *Holistic Nursing Practice*, vol. 5, no. 3, pp. 1–7, © 1991, Aspen Publishers, Inc.

Even with Donabedian's approach, however, numerous papers have been written and hours of classroom time have been spent on defining good structures, sound processes, and suitable outcomes, along with approaches to their measurement. Hundreds more papers have sought appropriate links among the three components, usually guided by the notion that outcomes are the target of the measurement and that structures and processes are only important to the extent that they are known to be connected to certain outcomes.[5]

All of these definitions and debates about quality include an element of personalization (for example, value of health, desired health outcome), thus alluding to the fact that the perception of quality is embedded in the human experience. Therefore, understanding quality, and subsequently, measuring and improving quality are fundamentally based on one's worldview or paradigm.[6] A worldview that recognizes humans as holistic and integrated with their environment will enable a fuller understanding of human experiences, such as the perception of quality, than is possible with a mechanistic worldview.[7] One worldview, however, builds on the other. For a richer understanding of the differences in the mechanistic and systems worldviews and their associated impacts on quality measurement and improvement, both are discussed. Exhibit 1–1 offers a summary comparison of the two worldviews of quality in respect to the recipient of care, illness, an organization, the environment, quality itself, and data measurement.

This chapter addresses many aspects of quality in the shifting paradigm:

- quality as inspection
- quality as opportunity
- measuring quality
- the bridge to quality as opportunity
- quality in the changing health care environment
- challenges faced by home care in improving quality

QUALITY AS INSPECTION: THE OLD PARADIGM

Quality as inspection offers the mechanistic worldview—a view that still pervades much of our thinking about quality (see Exhibit 1–1). The mechanistic worldview focuses on parts, or is reductionistic, and is based on three fundamental beliefs.

1. It is possible to have complete understanding of the universe.
2. The world can be understood through analysis (breaking things down to their most basic level), and therefore every experience and everything is reducible to individual parts.

Exhibit 1–1 Comparing Worldviews of Quality

Areas That Influence Quality	Mechanistic: Quality as Inspection	Systems: Quality as Opportunity
Recipient of care	Patient; incidental to quality inspection of technical care	Patient; Client; Consumer; Person; crucial in determining outcomes
Illness	A technical problem to be fixed by an expert	A challenge to be approached by partner
Organization	Hierarchy	Collaboration/teams/ community
	Power/change at the top	Many interacting centers of power/change
	Division of labor/functional fragmentation—quality has its own person/ group	Multifunctional/integration —quality is everyone's business
	Manage the quality inspection	Tolerate mistakes and allow room for innovation
Environment	Blame and justification	Responsibility and accountability
	Control	Trust
	Employees are passive units and are underutilized	Employees are cocreators and are assets to be invested in
	Reward system is individually focused	Reward system is group focused
	Training and education is haphazard	Learning is key to promoting continuous improvement
Quality	Absence of negatives	Positive
	Inspect things	Improve systems/ relationships
	Imply one right way	Many ways of doing things "right"
	Quality assurance	Quality improvement
	Meeting regulations	Philosophy/way of life
	Extrinsic (comes from outside rules/inspectors)	Intrinsic (defined by the agency)
	Reactive (catch mistakes after they occur)	Concurrent
Data measurement	For punishment/blame	For learning/improving
	Subjective analyzers	Use of statistical tools

3. All relationships can be described through simple cause and effect scenarios.

Cause and effect thinking led to some fundamental doctrines that permeated our thinking for almost 400 years.

- To explain a phenomenon, one need only to find the cause.
- The environment is not needed to explain something, so events could be looked at in a vacuum.
- Everything that occurs is the effect of an earlier cause—nothing ever happens by chance.[8]

In this model, a traditional organization emphasizes bureaucracy, narrowly defined job descriptions, policies and procedures (rules to be followed), and distinct departments. The organizational structure is vertical; power is vested at the top and spread thinner through descending layers of hierarchy, and the front-line workers at the bottom have the least amount of power of all.[9] One of the ways this is played out in home care is by having supervisors, or those with the power (knowledge), constantly check the work of the caregivers, or front-line workers, to be sure it complies with standards (for example, this patient meets the criteria for admission; Medicare form 485s are properly filled out). Quality is therefore defined and ensured through inspection by these experts. This *quality as inspection* is defined by Berwick as the theory of bad apples: Good quality is the absence of negatives, or no harmful outcomes.[10] Furthermore, good quality is approached with a passive longing, constantly focusing on the negative or "bad" quality and its producers, and trying to eliminate them. In other words, find the bad apples and remove them.

The "bad apples" are thought to be deficient workers (professionals). Thus, the causes of poor quality are the caregivers: their incompetence, insufficient caution, or poor intention. Therefore it makes sense to have tools such as peer review to find the bad apples and either have them change their ways or get rid of them. If, on the other hand, the caregivers are people of professional excellence, then the quality will be good. Interestingly enough, however, even with these beliefs, little attention is given to the knowledge development of the professional and/or professional judgment. When budgets are cut, continuing education for staff is always among the first to go. Furthermore, within agencies few resources are allocated to orient, mentor, and groom new staff. This is especially true for part-time and contract staff. No wonder maintaining quality is so difficult!

Although the recipient of health care, the patient is not deemed an important part of the worldview of quality by inspection. Instead, the focus is more on the technical delivery of care and the competence of the clinicians, because those things can be inspected. Patient satisfaction is important only to the extent that it influences compliance with the patient's plan of care and thus reduces the chances of a negative or harmful outcome.

The environment that predominates in this model is one of managing the quality inspection. The overseers of quality see employees as passive units that have to be motivated with rewards and penalties using warnings such as, "If you don't do your care plans we won't pass accreditation and you'll lose your job." It is also an environment of control.

Quality is in the hands of the inspectors or the quality assurance specialist and is extrinsic to the caregivers and even the agency itself. Thus, individual caregivers do not feel responsible for quality. Trying to improve quality in this environment involves catching the mistakes after they occur, which is accomplished by more inspection—more people inspecting more things in greater detail. One form this takes in home care is having quality assurance or supervisory persons checking charts for proper payer documentation to make sure wording "follows the rules." The more people inspecting the same item, however, the more blurred the lines of responsibility, and the mindset of staff becomes one of "If I make a mistake (document incorrectly) someone else will catch it (so why bother to learn all the rules)." Experience has shown that the number of mistakes actually expands to fill the inspection capacity of the system.[11] There are no inherent rewards for feeling personally responsible for quality. Thus, using inspection to define quality makes quality a boring, if not negative, activity and somebody else's problem.

QUALITY AS OPPORTUNITY: THE NEW PARADIGM

In contrast, *quality as opportunity* offers a more holistic, systems point of view (see Exhibit 1–1). With this model, parts are acknowledged but have meaning only within the context of the whole. Ackoff calls this doctrine expansionism, which "maintains that all objects, events, and experiences of them are parts of larger wholes. It does not deny that they have parts but focuses on the wholes of which they are part."[12 (p.12)] Providing quality service depends in part on how well various elements function together in a service system. These elements include the people who perform the service, the equipment that supports this performance, and the physical environment in which the services are performed.[13] In addition, since the effectiveness of the parts is a function of the relationship of the parts, quality must also consider the relationships.

Recognizing and understanding the interrelationships that exist in agencies and the implication that individual actions have on an agency's mission is central to systems thinking.[14] Systems thinking is central to quality management. It averts the suboptimization that can occur when quality focuses on a fragment of the process rather than the whole process. The reality of this is often heard in the employee comment, "It's not my job." Although the language involved in systems thinking is new, the concept is quite intuitive. To assist with the reader's understanding of new language, a glossary of terms has been provided at the end of the book. Figure 1–1 shows the components of a system.

Figure 1–1 could be considered a model for a home health agency in its most basic form. Within this home health agency there are many processes that occur. Each of the processes consists of activities, and each of the activities is made up of steps, tasks, actions, and interventions that can be extremely challenging to measure. The inputs into this home health agency are resources in the form of staff, management, and capital. Processes are determined through strategic planning. Information for strategic planning comes from feedback on the outputs from the customers. The activities within the processes are carried out by staff as part of day-to-day operations. Processes in home care can be divided into two categories: (1) patient-focused care processes, and (2) support processes such as information systems, human resources, financial management, marketing, and quality improvement. The core process is the central component of the patient-focused care process. The core process consists of activities that are central to the delivery of nursing care, such as reassessment, instruction, direct hands-on care, and coordination. Process output ultimately goes to the customer, although the output from one process may feed into another process. For example, the process of care provision is divided into three components: upstream, core, and downstream. One output from the upstream process is a completed referral form. That form becomes one of the inputs to the core process of care provision. Customers can be classified as either internal or external. Internal customers are staff members or management. External customers include the community at large, patients, patients' families, physicians, payers, regulatory bodies, the community, board members, and shareholders.

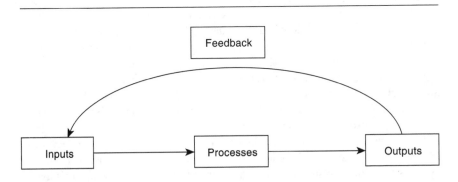

Figure 1–1 System Components

Once the interconnectiveness of systems is understood, it becomes clearer how widespread are the effects of decisions and activities. Questions begin to get asked, such as:

- What is the aim of our work?
- Who are our customers and what do they need?
- What results are we expecting and how do they compare with our customer needs?
- How will we go about obtaining these results?
- How may the environment affect how things will turn out?
- What information do we need to get the results we want?
- What materials and equipment do we need?
- How do we go about improving the process of servicing our customers?[15]

In this model, quality is more than just the absence of negatives; it is seen as something powerful in its own right because the focus is on noticing opportunities for improvement. Mistakes are not viewed as being caused by lack of motivation or lack of effort on the part of workers, but rather as a result of problems in the system, including poor job design, failure of leadership, an unclear purpose, complexity, or poor communication.[16] This model of quality has been presented as the Theory of Continuous Improvement by various American theorists, including W. Edwards Deming and Joseph M. Juran. The worker is viewed as doing the best he or she can. There is respect for workers, and the workers are viewed as trying hard, acting in good faith, and not willfully failing to do what they know is correct.[17] Quality is seen as an intrinsic value within the organization and within workers that they can take with them wherever they go, whether it be to a different position or a different organization.

The recipient of care is also given respect and attention. It is recognized that the client's first interest is not in the technical quality of care (was the procedure done correctly?) because that level of quality is assumed, but rather in the outcome of the care (did I get what I wanted?). Clients play an important role in defining quality care by determining what values should be associated with different outcomes.[18] For example, in a cardiovascular accident (CVA) patient, the outcome may be that the client is independently mobile within the home. For some clients, that may mean learning to walk up and down stairs, whereas for others it may mean being able to transfer to a wheelchair and using it to get around.

Smart agencies compile a community profile that describes the people, environment, health status, and health resources, in order to individualize health planning activities for the community. This community could be a geographical area or the lives covered by a managed care contract. In either case, each community has patterns of functioning that either contribute to or detract from its state of health. In order to effect change one must

1. Identify cultural differences in relationship to consumer interests, strengths, concerns, and motivations
2. Analyze the processes through which community beliefs, values, and attitudes are transmitted
3. Recognize the community dynamics in order to influence the direction of health programs and activities[19]

Other consumers an agency must consider include physicians, suppliers, referring institutions, and payers. Each of these consumers is also given respect and attention.

Viewing quality as opportunity fosters an environment that thrives on teamwork. Staff are seen both as internal consumers and active participants, interacting with their environment rather than reacting to it. The former practice of control from the top is replaced by an atmosphere of trust. Workers evaluate and continuously improve the quality of their work. People share skills and lessons they have learned. They try experiments together and offer suggestions for reducing waste, work, and complexity. As this type of environment is fostered, a sense of community develops. An organization acting as a community is a learning organization that brings out the best in people, is responsive to change, and is receptive to challenges. People become aware of what they are a part of and where they fit in. The intuitive knowledge about the system and how to improve it begins to come forth. This knowledge is more valuable for making things better than many of the tools (e.g., process flow diagrams, control charts) that are gaining popularity.

Qualities that are associated with a community environment include authentic communication, respectful inclusion, acceptance, honesty, listening, and a safe feeling.[20] Quality becomes everyone's job but management's responsibility and, because most quality problems are built into the system, quality is improved by improving the system. This requires an empowered worker with the ability to be a decision maker in the delivery of services. The most direct way to facilitate this is for people to see for themselves that they do matter. You cannot simply tell people that they are important and should make more decisions; they have to discover it for themselves. Thus, the first task for the manager is to recognize and assimilate the concept of the inherent potential in each individual in order for that individual to realize his or her greatness.[21]

This type of leadership is called "servant" leadership by some.[22] These leaders serve their workers by inspiring and enabling them to achieve. These leaders believe in the capacity of people to achieve and thus give their workers the tools and freedom to perform. Because they believe in their workers they invest much of their personal energy and time coaching and teaching, challenging and inspiring, and perhaps most of all listening to what their workers have to say. This improved communication alone reduces misunderstandings and improves quality.

MEASURING QUALITY

The two paradigms, quality as inspection and quality as opportunity, are logically incompatible, but both types of quality require measurement. Thus, different approaches to measurement are required depending on the worldview to which one subscribes. One difference, for example, is that quality as inspection is generally retrospective in nature. Everyone is familiar with chart reviews that look at care well after it has been rendered, and frequently after the patient has been discharged. This type of quality requires tools with an excellent measuring ability, high sensitivity, and specificity so that those who are "deficient" do not escape and those who are innocent are not made victims.[23]

In contrast, under quality as opportunity, measurements are more concurrent or close in time to the rendering of care. Quality tools are used by the workers themselves, not for punishment but for learning, so the specificity is not as important as the intent. Quality improvement does have many specialized tools to help the workers on their journey. There are tools to learn about processes and to assist in discovering possible causes of problems. Examples include process flow diagrams, brainstorming, and cause-effect diagrams. There are also tools mainly to collect data such as data collection forms, surveys, and nominal group technique. There are statistical techniques to test theories and display information such as Pareto diagrams, histograms, scatterplots, and control charts. Finally, there are graphs and charts used to monitor a process after a remedy has been applied.[24]

Because the data produced in the quality improvement process are for learning and not for punishment they tend to be less threatening. The data focus not on the staff and who performs well or poorly, but on the systems or processes of care and what works and what does not work. Thus data can be aggregated centrally to help caregivers learn from each other rather than having them fear retribution. This is a serious need because some of the quality problems arising in today's health care system result from treatment decisions and interventions that are based largely on individual practitioner observations and experiences rather than on any vast body of clinical experience. Thus there is a wide variation depending on the extent of any one practitioner's scope of experience and knowledge.

The aggregation of these data determines the level of performance. Performance refers to results. Looking at it from a systems perspective, results occur through the offering of services, the output of patient-focused care processes and support processes, and the performance of activities within those processes. Using a football metaphor, a process could be an offensive drive. An activity within that process is the throwing of a pass. Activity output would be the number of completed passes. Process output would be the number of touchdowns per scoring drive. Therefore, completed passes and touchdowns are examples of performance results.

Performance excellence is a term that exemplifies the meaning of continuous improvement measurement. In the preceding example, performance excellence would be a quarterback whose percentage of completed passes increases with every game he plays. Although this is an impossible scenario to continue, it demonstrates the point. At a certain point, that quarterback's average would be the best in the football league. This demonstrates *best of class*. Eventually, that quarterback may even beat all previous records (benchmarks).

Performance excellence begins with measuring what is important to the customer and then implementing continuous improvement activities and comparing the results with internal growth targets, industry standards, and world-class results. It is a lifelong and evolutionary process.

Another difference in measurement created by differing worldviews has to do with the establishment of standards. Under quality as inspection, standards are crucial because they are required by inspectors to determine what is an acceptable threshold. Unfortunately, establishing and defining standards are usually left to the inspectors or regulators. Standards are developed to define a minimum rather than an optimum level of acceptable performance. When in use, the minimal becomes the optimal, and standards end up defining adequacy rather than excellence.[25] This process is exemplified in both our professional and institutional licensing standards. In nursing, for example, our license (registered nurse) standard is considered so minimal that we have devised a complex, confusing system of defining excellence through certification. Furthermore, standards become technically obsolete, retarding rather than promoting effective health care delivery, unless they are frequently changed.[26] Changing standards is problematic; it is expensive and no one is sure who should do it—federal or state regulators, private accreditors, or perhaps insurance companies or managed care organizations. Finally, the proliferation of standards by all these regulators, licensers, and professionals has left workers legally liable for practicing in compliance with more (and sometimes conflicting) standards than they can remember. Under the quality as opportunity paradigm, the implications are that standards are basic and that the authority to reach and exceed the standards is owned by those who act on them.

To date, much of the measurement of quality in home health care has been through the worldview of quality by inspection. Quality is viewed as an event (such as a peer review meeting or audit), not an ongoing process that is part of everyone's position. Agencies continue to abdicate to others, including regulators, insurers, and accreditors, the power for setting standards. For example, the Joint Commission on Accreditation of Healthcare Organizations (Joint Commission) has set and monitored standards of excellence for care in the hospital setting since 1951. It recently announced its ORYX Initiative, the requirement to include the measurement of outcomes within a home care agency's quality assurance program. Agencies must select a performance measurement system from among the system vendors that have been accepted by the Joint Commission and then select at least two clinical measures by December 31, 1998. The goal is to establish a data-driven continuous accreditation process to

1. Help agencies improve their processes
2. Provide comparisons
3. Develop new accreditation standards

The performance measurement data will not be used directly for accreditation decisions but will be used to enhance the accreditation process, such as determining when to survey, what areas to look at, and the context for evaluation standards. Already agencies are clamoring to find out what outcomes the Joint Commision deems acceptable and to begin using them rather than deciding for themselves what outcomes are meaningful for their client case mix and helpful in determining the value of their services.

Perhaps it is time to look at quality differently. If quality were measured under the worldview of quality as opportunity, home care agencies would have the advantage of examining the services they render to clients for the purpose of improving them, for learning how to perform them better. The caregivers would be valued for the unique contributions they each make, and the focus would be more on "how to change the system(s)" instead of "you have to do/be better." Quality would be guided by consumer input, and home care's contribution would be more highly valued because it would be more in concert with the consumer's needs. Perhaps it is time for us to redefine quality as opportunity, for in the end quality really does hold an element of personalization; it depends on the human spirit itself and how individuals treat themselves and others. Without a personal commitment to quality and respect for oneself and others, there will never be a means to achieve quality. There will never be enough financial resources, organizational stratagem, or measurable standards to safeguard quality any other way. Each of us must care enough to make it happen.

THE KEY TO THE PARADIGM SHIFT

Shifting from quality as inspection to quality as opportunity is a challenging undertaking and requires a bridge to get from one to the other. Dveirin and

Adams[27] define that bridge as empowerment—the means by which employees can contribute their intelligence, knowledge, and experience utilizing *full-circle thinking*. These authors compare full-circle thinking, or thinking that enables one to reflect on and modify one's actions and to learn from one's past experience, with *arc thinking,* which does not follow the implications of one's actions around to the end consequences. Arc thinking is only a section of the circle and so thinking stops at a certain point of the circle rather than coming all the way around to where one started and being able to learn from comparing the ending to the beginning. Empowered workers follow their actions all the way around the circle; nonempowered workers complete only an arc segment, and someone else completes the circle. Thus nonempowered workers never are able to compare the ending consequences of their actions with their beginning activities.

Creation of an empowering environment is the responsibility of the leaders of the organization. Nine leadership actions that promote such an environment follow:

1. *Mission and vision.* Mission and vision are of such importance that a chapter is devoted to these concepts later in the book. (See Chapter 5.) Suffice it to say that they drive the entire system. Without mission and vision, there is no way for employees to prioritize their activities and needs.
2. *Authority and permission to use it.* Employees' judgment and capabilities must be respected by granting a scope of authority that is sufficient for what is expected of them. Furthermore, employees must be trusted to execute that authority without having to ask or gain approval for every action.
3. *Control over resources.* Each employee needs a clearly defined level of resource control commensurate with his or her authority. For example, a nurse should have a defined amount of supplies per month or per year or per case that she or he has the ability to write off or give to clients at her or his discretion.
4. *Access to information.* Empowered employees are totally "in the know" on everything that affects their work or mission. This includes direct information on long-term plans, technical information, feedback on quality issues, and feedback on their performance.
5. *Access to continuous learning opportunities.* Continuous learning is distinct from training and education. Although training and education opportunities are required for empowerment, continuous learning is implicit in empowerment. Education and training refer to the transmission of the known and are "done to" people; continuous learning is an interaction with the unknown that people initiate themselves for their own reasons.
6. *Trust and respect.* Most adults are inherently mature and able to manage their own affairs. Therefore, given the resources, training, authority, information, respect, and a clear mission and vision, they can be trusted to do a good job.

7. *Avenues of influence.* There needs to be a way for the organization to learn what employees require to do their job; conversely, employees need evidence that the organization utilizes and benefits from their input. In systems terminology what this defines is a feedback loop. Employees feed back to the organization what is required for them to do their job (e.g., equipment, time, education). The organization feeds back to the employees the results of their labor (e.g., awards, complimentary letters, outcome reports).

8. *Meaningful incentives.* In addition to rate of pay, bonuses, and other recognition that may be dependent on accomplishments, there are other aspects to meaningful incentives. A basic incentive to do what was best for the organization used to be job security, although with today's marketplace, that may no longer be true. Instead, an organization can offer opportunities to enhance employee skills and develop their credentials, making them more marketable and simultaneously benefiting the organization.

9. *Clear boundaries.* Processes need to be in place to negotiate boundaries to one's area of influence. Within the established boundaries an employee has the authority to manage her or his time and resources, and make decisions for carrying out what is expected.[28]

THE MACRO LEVEL OF QUALITY

The new model of quality considers the larger environment of which a system is a part. Therefore it is natural that questions should arise about the larger health care delivery system and the level of quality that is being defined in that macro level of care. What is perceived is a disintegration of the traditional approach to health care. The reasons given are usually rising costs and serious quality problems; but there are also our changing values as one enters this new paradigm. As far back as the 1980s, wellness was becoming more of the paradigm as the health care system began its evolution. In addition, the changing values shifted the way illness was viewed. For example, instead of focusing on reducing the length of stay for hip replacement patients, we may concentrate on whether or not hip replacement is the right thing to do. Exhibit 1–2 shows some of the other paradigm shifts in the health care delivery system.

The question then arises: What will quality look like in the new health care system? That answer is not fully determined, although it will deal with continually improving and aligning systems using outcomes as a guide. It will include measures to decrease cost and utilization, but it will also ask more difficult questions such as, Was that intervention the right thing to do? For example, a quality improvement team may look at reducing the number of visits required for home infusion and set up some creative methods for teaching and supporting

Exhibit 1–2 Shifts in the Health Care Delivery Ssytem

Mechanistic View	Evolving Systems View
• Manage illness	• Manage health/prevention
• Manage episode of care for an individual/family	• Manage health status of a population
• Functional orientation	• Outcome orientation
• Provider-centered care/autocratic	• Consumer-centered care/self-management
• Optimize the performance of caregivers	• Optimize the performance of the system
• Hospital at the center of the system	• Continuum of care/services
• Manage an organization	• Manage a network of services
• Local systems/fragmentation	• Regional/national systems
• Independence	• Interdependence
• High technology	• Reconsideration of human values
• Anecdotal data from isolated events	• Intense use of systematic information
• Complaint/symptom driven	• Evidence-based
• Biomedicine: objectivism, determinism	• Whole healing: dynamism, holism, purposefulness

infusion services at home. This same quality improvement team may also ask whether home infusion was the best course of action or whether it would have been more appropriate to send someone to the home to sit and feed the client sufficient quantities of food by mouth, regardless of ease or cost of the service.

PROMOTING AGENCY QUALITY

Understanding the purpose and direction of the macro, or containing, system is important for understanding the subsystems including the home health agency, its many care processes and support processes, and the individuals working within. In fact, all the systems are interrelated and, therefore, what affects one will affect all. There is a reinforcing process that develops as these systems become aligned— the results created by one become more consistent with the purpose of another, which leads to a deeper understanding of that purpose and more commitment to the overall direction and in turn an even deeper alignment. Therefore one way to promote quality is to evaluate how well your agency fits into its environment.

Health care workers too are more aware of what they are a part of, what their actions really help to accomplish, and therefore where they "fit in."[29] One thing an administrator can do to promote quality is to evaluate how well the systems of the agency give the workers what they need. Probably the most important thing an administrator can do to promote quality is to place authority and accountability at the level of the customer contact; give workers the necessary tools, and then evaluate how well they do for learning purposes and feedback. What people need is a chance to discover for themselves. The real act of discovery is seeing the same old thing with new eyes since how one thinks and acts is all associated with how one views the world.

CHALLENGES

As a new view of reality is created there will be challenges. We will discover how our current worldview affects the way we perceive and respond to problems. The old paradigm with its reductionistic viewpoint will continue to slip back in, largely unnoticed. Furthermore, the better quantitative measures used for solving problems will actually come from the people using the old paradigm because they have hundreds, even thousands, of problems solved using their rules while people using the new rules/paradigm will have only a few solved. Thus, those people who choose to be among the early changers often do it as an act of faith rather than factual proof because there is never enough proof to be convincing in the early stages. Early joiners must have courage, intuitive judgment (ability to make good decisions with incomplete information), and a commitment to the long term, since the evolution of a new paradigm takes years.[30] What this means is that it will be easier for people to continue to give care and measure quality as they have under fee-for-service and implement improvements for outcomes within an episode of care rather than take on the managed care arena, which has no firm rules for measuring costs or quality. How *do* you measure prevention (an event that never happened) anyhow? The challenge is not to succumb to the easy path or the way things used to be.

Another challenge is learning systems thinking. It has been likened to learning a new language. It doesn't happen overnight, and there are different levels of proficiency involved. For example, let's look at reengineering. Reengineering has been seen as an exhilarating new trend that administrators have adopted, tried to implement without understanding its impact on the organization as a whole, seen stall, and discarded as a failed change program. Because of its misuse, reengineering has become a tainted term that represents restructuring and downsizing. In actuality, it creates new processes (systems) within an organization and requires a level of mastery in system thinking and system tools. Reengineering requires the ability to think, map, analyze, and act at the systems level. One of the pitfalls in implementing a reengineering effort is focusing only on the business processes and ignoring the human aspects of change. A true systems thinker who understands the importance of relationships and interactive systems would never dream of undertaking a major reengineering effort without delving into the culture and underlying beliefs that created the existing system.[31]

One way an administrator can become more systems-oriented is to utilize the framework of the Malcolm Baldrige Award criteria. The seven categories that make up the criteria for this quality award are a good description of an organizational system. Actually, it is the first six categories that represent an organization's system: leadership, strategic planning, customer and market focus, information and analysis, human resource development and management, and process management. The seventh category—business results—represents the collective outcomes of all efforts within that organization. The Malcolm Baldrige criteria are currently expanding into the health care/home care arena.

Besides changing our approach to solving problems to a more systematic way of thinking and changing our measurements to quantify different activities/concepts, there are other changes that will be equally, if not more, challenging. We need to change our leadership style to be less controlling and more serving; we need to treat employees differently so that their view of and method of relating to the agency changes; we need to establish a more trusting, empowering environment (no easy task!); and we need to facilitate a change in the way employees think about each other. Again, this is no easy task. For example, employees are often as guilty as they claim their supervisors are in parsimoniously giving out praise or thanks to their peers. During a group session of nurses that was held as part of a change implementation project, each nurse was asked to say something nice about the person next to her. It took much coaxing on the part of the facilitator before they were able to do it. Excuses ran rampant and included the "fact" that they already knew each other well and how they felt about each other was "understood." The truth was they were uncomfortable saying something nice or having something nice said about them; it would have been easier and more familiar to complain.

What is quality? Quality is a multifaceted diamond that shines brightly when polished but dulls quickly when it is not attended to. Quality requires a persistent awareness of all that matters—systems, human and financial resources, the environment, data. Quality is organization; quality is management; and most of all, quality is improved outcomes for customers.

CONCLUSION

This chapter gave an overview of quality. It compared quality in mechanistic and systems worldviews, and described the shifts in paradigms. It discussed the environment and measurement of quality in the shifting paradigms, and the bridge between the two. It described the changing macro system, or health care system with which home care must align in order to maintain quality, and discussed the modifications and challenges home care faces as it attempts to improve quality.

NOTES

1. A. Donabedian, Quality Assessment and Assurance: Unity of Purpose, Diversity of Means, *Inquiry* 25, no. 1 (1988): 173–192.
2. K. Lohr, ed., *Medicare: A Strategy for Quality Assurance* (Washington, DC: National Academy Press, 1990), 21.
3. J. Guaspari, *I Know It When I See It* (New York: American Management Association, 1985), 18.
4. A. Donabedian, Evaluating the Quality of Medical Care, Part 2, *Milbank Memorial Fund Quarterly: Health and Society* 44 (July 1966): 166–203.
5. D.M. Berwick et al., *Curing Health Care* (San Francisco: Jossey-Bass Publishers, 1990), 11.
6. J. Fawcett, *Analysis and Evaluation of Conceptual Models of Nursing,* 2d ed. (Philadelphia: F.A. Davis, 1984).
7. J.H. Larrabee, Emerging Model of Quality, *Image* 28, no. 4 (1996): 353–358.
8. R. Ackoff, Interactive Planning Model (Paper presented at the educational conference for Strengthening Hospital Nursing Program, Gainesville, FL, October 1989).
9. T. Broersma, In Search of the Future, *Training and Development* 49, no. 1 (1995): 38–43.
10. D. Berwick, Continuous Improvement as an Ideal in Health Care, *New England Journal of Medicine* 320 (1989): 53–56.
11. Guaspari, *I Know It When I See It*, 45.
12. R. Ackoff, *Redesigning the Future: A Systems Approach to Societal Problems* (New York: John Wiley & Sons, 1974), 12.
13. L.L. Berry et al., Improving Service Quality in America: Lessons Learned, *Academy of Management Executive* 8, no. 2 (1994): 32–44.
14. D.H. Gustafson, The Total Costs of Illness: A Metric for Health Care Reform, *Hospital and Health Services Administration* 40, no. 1 (1995): 154–171.
15. D.H. Gustafson, The Total Costs of Illness, 154–171.
16. Berwick, Continuous Improvement, 53–56; Guaspari, *I Know It When I See It*, 66.
17. Berwick, Continuous Improvement, 53–56.
18. P. Cleary and B. McNeil, Patient Satisfaction as an Indicator of Quality Care, *Inquiry* 25 no. 1 (1988): 25–36.
19. S. Clemen-Stone et al., *Comprehensive Community Health Nursing* (New York: Mosby, 1995), 429–459.
20. G. Zlevor, Creating a New Workplace: Making a Commitment to Community, *The Systems Thinker* 5, no. 7 (1994): 1–4.
21. P. Senge, Systems Thinking, *Executive Excellence* 13, no. 1 (1996): 15–16.

22. Berry et al., Improving Service Quality, 32–44.

23. Berwick, Continuous Improvement, 53–56.

24. Berwick et al., *Curing Health Care.*

25. B.C. Vladeck, Quality Assurance through External Controls, *Inquiry* 25, no. 1 (1988): 100–107.

26. Vladeck, Quality Assurance, 100–107.

27. G.F. Dveirin and K.L. Adams, Empowering Health Care Improvement: An Operational Model, *Joint Commission Journal on Quality Improvement* 19, no. 7 (1993): 222–232.

28. Dveirin and Adams, Empowering Health Care Improvement, 222–232.

29. Gustafson, The Total Costs of Illness, 154–171.

30. J.A. Barker, *Discovering the Future: The Business of Paradigms*, 3d ed. (St. Paul, MN: ILI Press, 1989).

31. V. Allee, Tools for Reengineering, *Executive Excellence* 12, no. 2 (1995): 17–18.

CHAPTER 2

How Much Does It Cost?

Since the inception of the Medicare program in the 1960s cost has had two meanings. The first meaning crosses all businesses and all industries and is a tool for valuation. Cost in this context provides a common unit of measure, the dollar, for describing outlays of (1) cash or (2) the accrual of expenses. Cash outlays include payroll expense of staff and their benefits, or costs associated with the rental of office space and the acquisition of supplies. The accruing of expenses provides a methodology to record the costs in the month that they were incurred even though they may not be paid until a subsequent month. Therefore, the combination of these two approaches provides a tool to identify total expenditures for a given time period and provides the basis for financial reporting.

The second meaning of cost does not cross industries. This meaning is peculiar to government-sponsored programs and deals with a concept related to reimbursement for cost incurred by a provider within the Medicare program. In the context of home health, cost is an element of a reimbursement methodology that has shaped the management philosophies and development of organizational structures since the inception of the Medicare program.

Cost in both of the above definitions has been used to manage home health organizations for years. Agencies monitored operations through the use of profit and loss statements. Profit and loss statements identified how much money they made or lost for a given year. This tool was developed to meet the needs of external users, such as banks, shareholders, and regulatory agencies. When presented in a consistent format, profit and loss statements could easily be interpreted and provided the basis for decision making.

Decisions around the reimbursement of cost helped to form organizational structures, management philosophies, and compensation packages, and to create a Medicare paradigm. In essence, the federal government provided agencies with a risk-free safety net to design their organizations as long as they followed the pre-prospective reimbursement formula of the lower of cost, charges, or the limits.

The Medicare paradigm became one of learning how to maximize returns while operating within the rules of the Medicare system.

A problem exists, however. The problem is that the paradigm has changed with respect to cost, as it has to quality. The old paradigm had very little business risk. The new paradigm has significant business risk.

This chapter addresses

- the old cost reimbursement paradigm
- the new financial leadership paradigm
- a systems approach to cost accounting
- an introduction to activity-based cost management (ABCM)

CHANGING PARADIGMS

There are many events external to an agency's daily operations that are reshaping the health care delivery system. A primary catalyst, at a societal level, is that individuals are living longer than at any other period in our nation's history.[1] Along with an increase in the average life expectancy is an increase in the amount of health care–related services that are consumed by aging Americans. Resource consumption consists of two elements, (1) volume and (2) cost per unit. Volume is the direct result of the number of tests, office or home visits, and the frequency of intervention. From a home health perspective, a change in federal regulations, as reflected in the *Medicare Health Insurance Manual*, Section 11 (HIM-11), expanded home health coverage and subsequently contributed to increases in the volume of services being provided to beneficiaries.[2] Cost per unit is the result of the location of the intervention (home or hospital), technology associated with the test or procedure, and the cost of all individuals who are involved in either a direct or indirect capacity.

In the 1980s two events occurred that were harbingers of what was to come for home health providers. Hospitals, which had been cost reimbursed for years, became prospectively paid based upon diagnosis-related groups (DRGs). This actually was beneficial for home health. Hospitals had incentives to get patients out of the door sooner. This caused a paradigm shift for hospital administrators— from length of stay maximization (keep beds filled) to managing clinical care within DRG formulas.

The second event in the 1980s was the introduction of managed care organizations (MCOs). MCOs had an economic incentive to reshape the entire delivery system. The principle is simple. If the cost of providing health care to members is less than the fees received for health insurance, then the MCO is profitable. This is a basic tenet of any business that does not have a safety net. MCOs' approach has been to spread the business risk to those individuals who are in a position to make or break the concept—the physicians. Physicians are in a position to reduce business risk by controlling utilization (for example, how often patients are seen and/or what treatment/medications/tests are rendered). Said differently, reduced utilization of medical services lessens the outlay of health care dollars and improves organizational profitability.

In the 1990s both of these events began to have applicability for home health providers. The federal government realized that in order to control the health care costs of an aging population it needed to adopt a prospective payment formula for home care that created risk for providers and limited the government's liability for volume of services. Fortunately for providers, the federal government did not have data to make a quick transition into a risk-based payment methodology such as episodic payments. An interim payment system (IPS), however, was implemented with the president's Balanced Budget Act of 1997.

The IPS is a temporary payment system to be in effect until the Health Care Financing Administration (HCFA) can design a more permanent episodic or prospective payment system. Essentially the IPS establishes a cap—an aggregate per beneficiary limit for every home care agency. This cap is based on 75 percent of an agency's cost and utilization experience for either 1993 or 1994, depending on the financial year, and 25 percent regional experience. At the last minute, the law was changed to reduce the calculation by another 2 percent. Furthermore, if an episodic payment system is not in place by 1999, rates will be reduced by another 15 percent. The IPS shifts some of the financial risks from HCFA to the agencies. If an agency provides services over the cap, it will not be reimbursed even if the services meet the Medicare coverage criteria. In addition, since not all regions of the country have the same per patient costs, IPS initially rewards those agencies that have the higher figures. For example, in Massachusetts, the average per patient cost for 1994 was $4,328, in Texas it was $5,977, and in Louisiana it was $6,700.[3] Those agencies in Louisiana will have a higher figure to use for the 25 percent regional experience.

Also in the 1990s, managed care extended its focus beyond the physician to all providers in the health care delivery system. From a home health perspective, this means that patients who were once free flowing from hospitals and other referral sources are being directed to providers who have negotiated with MCOs. Those providers who do not have contracts and have had referral streams altered are faced with the realities of making hard business decisions. Loss of volume can create problems with the existing cost reimbursement system because of an organizational structure that has been developed assuming fixed referral streams and increasing patient loads. On the other hand, those agencies that landed the managed care contracts may have different problems. Typically, managed care contracts have two elements that have the potential to negatively impact provider operations. One is severely discounting per visit rates, and the second is authorizing a smaller number of visits on a per patient basis. Both of these situations can force business decisions regarding staffing patterns, overhead, and organizational structure.

The impending prospective payment system and the proliferation of MCOs are creating a paradigm shift for home health providers. No longer can it be business as usual if providers expect their revenues to exceed costs. No longer will the models that were in effect to develop management systems in the old paradigm be sufficient to manage in the new paradigm. Thus, this creates a wonderful opportunity to develop systems for the new paradigm that are customer focused and values driven.

COST REIMBURSEMENT: THE OLD PARADIGM

The old paradigm was created by a system that taught nursing students that more was better, a reimbursement system that rewarded inefficiency, and a leadership that honored outdated approaches to personnel management. Some of the old paradigm's roots can be traced back to the early 1900s when Frederick Taylor developed his theories of scientific management.[4] The results of his theories have led to the development of top-heavy organizations, specialized tasks, and a belief that all decisions should be made at the top. Other factors that have influenced organizational structure have been the use of hierarchical organization structures similar to military hierarchies and the adoption of McGregor's Theory X, which basically states that all workers are unmotivated, lazy, and cannot be trusted.[5] These principles have been part of the organizational culture that has led to the development of highly complex and inefficient bureaucracies.

The enabling force behind the design of inefficient home care organizations has been the Medicare reimbursement system. As stated above, the design of a payment system that reimburses for costs incurred in the provision of patient care provides a safety net to providers, but it also promotes inefficiency and a proliferation of methodologies that would be extremely unprofitable in any business without a safety net. The nursing education system supported this clinically by incorporating these principles of reimbursement into their student curricula. In a cost-reimbursed world, more care was viewed as better, and thought to be synonymous with quality. This paradigm also supported the concept of visit maximization. From an organizational perspective this was akin to "hitting" the lottery. As visit volume increased, agencies had more opportunities to add staff, purchase equipment, design substantial pension plans, and increase staff salaries on a regular basis. From an administrative perspective organizations could be designed with layers of personnel. If a problem existed, the solution was to hire another individual or add a new manager to supervise the group of employees where the problem lay. The vast majority of these decisions were influenced by the relationship of agency costs to the Medicare cost limits and the agency's payer mix. This provided some help to administrators in adopting a budget-neutral war cry when defending their need to add additional personnel for symptom management.

The boundaries of rules and regulations created by the Medicare paradigm were instrumental in the development of accounting systems and measurement approaches. Accounting systems were designed to meet the needs of cost reporting and external compliance. Therefore, system development concentrated on capturing costs by reimbursable and nonreimbursable cost centers. Within the reimbursable framework, costs were further differentiated between direct and indirect costs by discipline, and administrative costs.

The cost reporting methodology provided HCFA with a relatively simple tool to determine cost reimbursement levels. From an agency perspective, all accounting systems were designed to facilitate the capturing of costs to feed the cost report. Therefore, the format for analysis typically replicated the cost reporting format. This approach identified administrative costs and then assigned them using the cost reporting methodology of accumulated cost by discipline. This costing methodology is arbitrary, but because it is easy to apply, it was commonly accepted and used.

The degree of acceptance of this arbitrary methodology is dependent upon whether you are the analyst or accountant who had responsibility for reporting, or the departmental manager who has responsibilities for operations. From the analyst's or accountant's perspective, the costing methodology may seem logical (i.e., consistent with external requirements) and may seem a measure of how organizational reimbursement will be affected. On the other hand, the departmental manager, more often than not, will question the assignment of administrative or overhead cost. Every time reports are produced, the age-old question of who should bear the cost of overhead is raised. This question will surface because a departmental manager has accountability for all costs incurred by his or her department.

The other element of the old paradigm that compounds the costing issue is the construct of departments, incentive systems, organizational culture, and long-term viability. Departments were developed to facilitate the management of similar job functions or activities. Costs, however, are charged on a departmental basis that may have no relationship to the activities that are performed within a specific department. Incentive systems were developed that reward one individual for bringing in new business but do not honor those who perform the work and satisfy the customers. This organizational culture will contribute to the creation of dysfunctional organizations. Dysfunctional organizations can be created because of professional bias.[6] For instance, if an agency is owned by a nurse, there is the potential that all decisions could be clinically driven and not in balance with financial realities. This would rarely create a long-term viability problem in a cost-reimbursed world because survival is not threatened when "big brother" is picking up the tab. In a cost-reimbursed world, there is no business risk, and thus an urgency does not exist to align organizational values with vision and mission, to design incentive systems toward a common cause, and to develop the management tools that will facilitate change for those who are interested in long-term survival.

Furthermore, in a cost-reimbursed world, the use of an arbitrary method for cost analysis is not detrimental. However, as the safety net begins to lower, and managed care continues to play a greater role in the delivery of health services, costing systems and management approaches will need to change. Inherent in the concept of costing systems is a global approach to management in the new paradigm. Management will need to adopt a customer focus, design a performance measurement system that looks at the agency in a holistic fashion, and begin to develop a management reporting system that provides relevant data (both financial as well as clinical) for the proactive management of the entire organization.

FINANCIAL LEADERSHIP: THE NEW PARADIGM

The old paradigm was characterized by free-flowing referrals, a reimbursement system that provided a safety net, and a "more is better" attitude. The new paradigm focuses on doing more with less; providing appropriate levels of care; developing long-term relationships with customers, suppliers, and staff; sharing financial risk; and transitioning to a place where management can understand, shape, and provide guidance to teams of individuals with multiple, and often differing, perspectives. The goal within the new paradigm is to channel organizational and financial resources toward the achievement of quantifiable, vision-driven strategies. In this context, organizational efforts include all processes, activities, and interactions among staff members, management, and suppliers within the organization.

The chief financial officer (CFO) has historically been the driving force behind cost management within the agency. His or her responsibilities were primarily driven by the external, compliance-oriented regulatory environment. The external regulatory environment requires the filing of taxes, the production of financial statements in accordance with Generally Accepted Accounting Principles (GAAP), and cost reporting. Subsequently, emphasis was placed on the deployment of tasks to meet these requirements. Therefore, it was quite natural that the same tasks would be used to perform analysis and provide information to management.

Unfortunately, the tasks that were deployed produced information after the fact. That is to say, information produced in a monthly financial statement was distributed several weeks after the month had ended. Also, the value to managers was negligible because of the information that was provided. Traditional financial reporting identifies the amount of money that has been spent by category. This does little to assist managers in assessing how their staff are performing, whether customers are satisfied with service, or whether there is improvement in clinical indicators such as activities of daily living (ADLs) function or medical condition.

Financial leadership within the new paradigm will require the development of systems that provide managers with meaningful indicators of organizational progress toward strategic objectives. This shift in perspective will require financial leaders to de-emphasize day-to-day, regulatory-driven accounting tasks whose products are financial and cost reports. In their place, financial leaders will need to adopt an external perspective, one that looks beyond financial indicators to include performance measures and indicators that are relevant to their peers. Expressed differently, financial leaders will need to adopt a service orientation and understand what is needed by clinical, operational, and administrative managers and teams to accomplish organizational goals. Within this context, financial leaders should begin to develop prospective assessment systems and balanced performance measurement perspectives and to become a partner in the pursuit of common objectives instead of the organizational police officer.

Figure 2–1 illustrates this point. If agencies are truly interested in long-term survival and viability, then the financial leaders within the agency will need to shift their perspective and approach to the management of cost. As financial leaders begin to transition away from the traditional paradigm of financial and cost reporting, they have an opportunity to provide value to their organization through the development of *off–balance sheet* reporting systems that are linked to strategy, continuous improvement objectives, and customer results.

Balance sheet reporting is the reporting of tangible assets, such as receivables or equipment. Off–balance sheet reporting concerns intangibles, such as the skill level of staff, staff satisfaction, process-oriented measurement, and the achievement of strategic objectives. Paying attention to both on– and off–balance sheet indicators provides an opportunity to look at an organization holistically. Beyond reporting, financial leadership can become a change agent or driving force in an agency's continuous improvement efforts by providing cost quantification of improvements, training, project prioritization, performance measure development, and strategic management.

Ultimately, cost will become one of many agency indicators. The emphasis will shift from the management of expenditures to understanding whether the resources consumed by the agency have created value for the customers served.

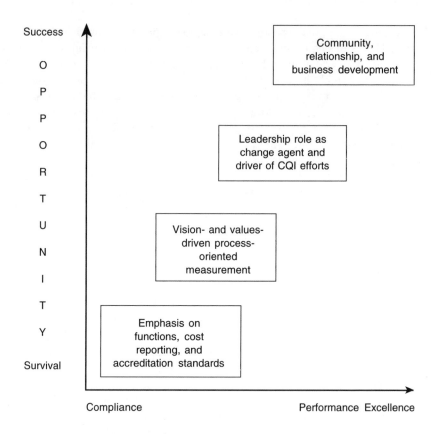

Figure 2–1 The Shifting Perspective of Financial Leadership

Then the cost paradigm will shift from monitoring expenditures to understanding process output and the relationship of output to capacity, cycle time, and satisfaction. Concurrently, financial leadership will realize that organizational viability will never occur through cost management, but instead by generating new sources of revenue, expanding existing opportunities for revenue, and building relationships in the community for the development of new services as needs are identified.

The new operating paradigm will need to rethink many of the old operating philosophies. No longer is home health outside of the purview of the primary delivery system. In the old days, once patients were discharged from the hospital, they were forgotten, and service was provided by one of the local home health agencies. Those were the days of free-flowing referrals. Once the patient was admitted to an agency, nursing was in control of the patient's plan of care. Now, referrals are being redirected away from free-standing agencies to agencies that are part of a larger health system or who have contractual relationships with the patient's insurance carrier. No longer is the design of a patient's plan of care left solely to the discretion of the agency's nurses; instead, nursing autonomy has been diminished by the existence of external care managers who control utilization and manage treatment protocols.

Care managers are the outgrowth of MCOs being required to effectively manage the cost of the care delivery process while providing high-quality services and satisfying consumers. Care managers are merely a symptom of a larger movement. The larger movement is viewing the delivery of health care services as a system. The concept of a system views all providers as a piece of a larger process. By consolidating the processes within the system and eliminating frag-mentation, there will be an opportunity to reduce business risk, enhance organiza-tional outcomes, and decrease cost.

The issues before home health providers are analogous to the health system as a whole. Providers will need to understand their role as either a customer or a supplier in the larger process. Within this paradigm there will be a need to evaluate intraorganizational paradigms for consistency in applications to the objectives of the organization as a whole. This consistency includes the development of costing and measurement systems that focus on the needs of customers regardless of where they are in the health care delivery system.

In essence, home health providers will need to view their organizations as systems within systems. From the larger perspective the health care delivery system is like the body. This body is made up of several smaller systems that enable the larger system to work. Each of the smaller systems consists of specific processes related to its role in the larger system. It is the challenge within the new paradigm to measure these processes and identify how they are impacting their element of the larger continuum. Eventually, these independent measures will become interdependent in an attempt to demonstrate systemwide quality.[7]

Before interdependent measures become commonplace, the new paradigm will witness organizational structures becoming flatter (eliminating layers of person-nel) as they attempt to become more flexible and cost-efficient. Quality will become a pervasive concept that encompasses both clinical and administrative processes, and cost will be one of the primary tools to demonstrate the multi-dimensional aspects of quality.

Organizations consume resources (time and money) in order to provide value to customers. If management wants to manage the provision of value to custom-ers, it needs to manage the underlying activities that consume resources. Manage-ment needs to link the consumption of resources to the various processes within an agency, and to correlate the results of clinical outcomes, customer satisfaction surveys, and quality improvement projects. This is not possible within traditional accounting systems.

Traditional accounting systems within home health have been designed to meet cost reporting requirements and the needs of external users. They have not been designed for proactive management of an organization. Proactive management is severely limited by financial statements designed to report total expenditures by category. For instance, a monthly financial statement may indicate that $200,000 was paid out in administrative salaries. Nowhere in a traditional financial statement is there any mention of what activities were performed to consume $200,000. Proactive management occurs through understanding the relationship between activities and the consumption of cost. Activity analysis provides a vehicle to link cost to outcomes, quality improvement efforts, and organizational vision. Understanding the relationship among the events that cause an activity to occur will provide a mechanism for streamlining organizations without jeopardizing the pursuit of organizational values.

Traditional financial reporting may still be required in the new paradigm to meet the needs of external users. In addition to the external users of financial statements, the internal customers of the financial statements will need to be considered. Internal customers represent an agency's management. Managers will need to understand what drives cost, how cost relates to the goals of the organization, and what impact cost has on operational decisions. Cost, time, quality, and satisfaction are all indicators of organizational outcomes. It is through developing an understanding of the relationships, patterns, and elements of the outcome equation that it is possible to continually improve elements of the outcome.

Survival in the new paradigm will require thinking of the agency as a system. Within the system there are multiple processes that have been developed to serve the customer. In order to better serve the customer, the agency should consider developing an ABCM system to measure cost and link cost to outcomes and continuous quality improvement initiatives. One thing is clear within this new paradigm: organizational learning and growth will come from learning from actual experiences. Learning, however, is the initial step. The integration of learning and action is required to remain viable within the new paradigm. Certainly, when the safety net of cost reimbursement is removed, agencies that do not continually acquire knowledge, improve organizational processes, demonstrate continuous improvement in organizational outcomes, and exceed customer expectations will slowly disappear from the evolving health care delivery system.

In the new paradigm cost is no longer a back office function. Everyone in the agency has a responsibility for resource consumption. Understanding resource consumption provides a vehicle to quantify efforts on behalf of customers and identify opportunities for improvement. This translates into a language that every executive understands, the dollar.

A SYSTEMS APPROACH TO COST ACCOUNTING AND OPERATIONAL MANAGEMENT

Traditional accounting systems are based upon a simple cause and effect formula. In its simplest applications, if one unit of profit is added and costs remain the same, then profit will increase by one unit. Conversely, if one unit of expense is reduced and revenues remain the same, then profit will increase by one unit. The roots of this linear equation go back to the sixteenth century.

> The scientific community that gave us this world view has, of course, adopted a new position in the 20th century. This story is well known. Quantum physicists and evolutionary biologists, among others, now believe that reality is not best described as a universe of eternally unchanging objects that interact with each other only through the influence of external forces. Rather, reality is best described as a web of interconnected relationships that give rise to an eternally changing and evolving universe of objects that are perceived only partially with the five limited senses. In that "systemic" view of the world, nothing is merely the sum of its parts; parts have meaning only in reference to a greater whole in which everything is related to everything else.[8] (p.16)

Stated differently, "You think because you understand one you must understand two, because one and one makes two. But you must also understand 'and'."[9]

The concept of systems is extremely important in the new paradigm. ABCM provides a language to understand the interdependent relationships within an agency. Unlike traditional accounting systems that were designed to identify total expenditures, the language of an ABCM system enables managers to understand the activities that were responsible for total expenditures.

The power of ABCM evolves from its ability to quantify the cost of activities across processes. From a systems perspective, every organization, or system, is made up of processes. Processes cross the entire organization and are not contained within departmental or functional structures. Processes are a series of activities linked together to accomplish a goal. Each process is made up of three primary components as illustrated in Figure 2–2.

Using the concepts of ABCM it is possible to quantify the cost of processes, to evaluate the relationship between cost and process performance measures, and to evaluate how the entire process can be improved. Improvement can take many

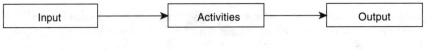

Figure 2–2 Process Components

forms. Improvement can be an increase in customer satisfaction, a reduction in the amount of time it takes to complete a process, or increased effectiveness of the process. Moreover, this simple design of process components provides the underlying foundation for systems thinking.

A further refinement of the concept of systems is illustrated in Figure 2–3. This figure illustrates the continuous quality improvement continuum as it relates to processes. Improvement occurs through listening to the customer, measuring results, and then using results as a feedback mechanism to improve input, the process, and process output. Improvement also occurs through addressing the controllable factors that affect outcomes. For instance, based upon input from customers, customer satisfaction is dependent upon cost and timeliness and responsiveness of service provision. Then, ABCM provides a methodology for quantifying process input by assigning a cost to the activities that occur within a process. When linked with customer satisfaction indicators and measurements of cycle time, a powerful relationship exists to quantify process improvement as it relates to customer satisfaction. Furthermore, if there are several subprocesses within a process, it is possible to determine the cost of each segment of the larger

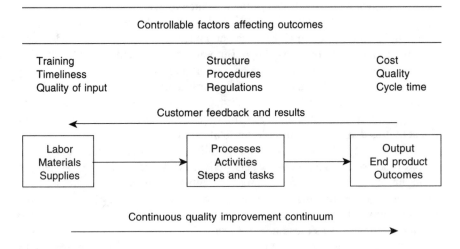

Figure 2–3 Refinement of the Interrelatedness of ABCM, Quality, and Processes

process. ABCM can also look at the relationships between process inputs and outcomes. If in the preceding example, the goal is to reduce cost and cycle time associated with service delivery, then an increase in training may be needed for employees and suppliers to accomplish the goal of improving these two outcomes. The activity cost of training, a controllable factor, can then be monitored in relationship to changes in outcomes.

One of the primary challenges to this type of approach is not to fall into the same mindset accountants developed using traditional accounting systems. Many accountants became invested in the budget and variance reports. This approach to financial management became a tool to say, "I got you," because expenditures exceeded budget. ABCM has a costing component. The costing component provides a tool to arrive at a clearer understanding of cost by product line, program, or division. Understanding costs by product line, for example, will enable managers to bid on contracts with higher levels of confidence.

The costing component to ABCM is called activity-based cost accounting. Essentially it amounts to attaching a dollar figure (a cost) to each of the activities for a given process. Activity cost is calculated by summarizing wages, benefits, and supplies. Wages, benefits, and supplies represent inputs, or said differently, they are the resources that are consumed by activities. Staff perform activities. Staff are paid to perform activities on behalf of the agency. Performing activities requires an individual's time, for which he or she is paid, and includes benefits and any supplies used while performing an activity.

Activity cost is determined by accumulating resources (wages, benefits, and supplies) for an individual, team, or work unit. Cost is assigned to activities using a mathematical algorithm. The mathematical algorithm is based upon an accumulation of time spent on each activity. The algorithm allows activity cost to be assigned to each respective activity.

In the example in Table 2–1, total inputs were $40,750. They consist of wages, benefits, and supply cost for an entire month. During the month, time was tracked. Sixty percent of all work-related time is associated with hands-on care, 25 percent with travel, and 15 percent with documentation. Understanding the time associated with each activity provides the basis to derive a mathematical algorithm for calculating activity cost. Hands-on care received 60 percent of total resource (input) cost to determine an activity cost for hands-on care of $24,450. Travel received 25 percent and documentation received 15 percent of the $40,750 to determine their respective activity costs.

If time spent performing the above activities was split evenly, each activity would receive one-third of the $40,750, or $13,582 per activity. A traditional costing system would have arrived at this result. An activity-based costing system does not assume that all activities are weighted evenly; it forces the weighting

Table 2–1 An Example of Activity-Based Cost Accounting

	Resources	Time Spent for Each Activity		Activity Cost
Wages	$35,000	60%	Hands-on care	$24,450
Benefits	5,250	25%	Travel	10,188
Supplies	500	15%	Documentation	6,112
	$40,750	100%		$40,750

through the use of drivers. In this example, time is the driver that creates a bridge between resource cost (expenditures for process inputs) and the costing of activities.

Activity-based cost accounting and ABCM will provide tremendous value to agency managers. There is a risk, however, with any accounting application that is viewed solely as an accounting application. Nonfinancial managers will resist providing information if it will be used against them. If ABCM is used as a tool to facilitate understanding among managers and quantify process costs, then the application becomes very powerful. The bottom line is to be clear about the intent or purpose of the ABCM system, to help all staff understand the value that implementation of an ABCM system can provide, and to ensure the tool is used to accomplish the larger mission of the agency, instead of being used as a club.

ABCM'S RELEVANCE TO THE NEW PARADIGM

ABCM is not a cure-all, a magic bullet, or the sole answer to survival in the new paradigm. When used properly, however, ABCM is a tool that will assist management in understanding how resources are consumed. When used in relationship with continuous quality improvement efforts, ABCM will provide a mechanism to understand the multidimensional aspects of quality. It is impossible to overstate the importance of this tool from both a strategic and tactical perspective. From a strategic perspective, decisions can be made about pricing, pursuing or discontinuing product lines, and identifying opportunities to improve service delivery through technology. From a tactical perspective, ABCM's power increases as a management tool when it is linked to other performance measures such as quality, time, and stakeholder satisfaction.

Traditional financial reporting is narrow in its application and definition of resources. ABCM, on the other hand, has the ability to quantify off–balance sheet assets, such as the amount of value-adding activities that contribute to the achievement of organizational vision, the amount of resources dedicated to training and its relationship to employee satisfaction, and the quantification of the cost of quality. ABCM also can support a lean operating philosophy through the identification of activities that are redundant, outdated, or inefficient.

From a systems perspective, ABCM provides a methodology to identify and quantify all the processes within the organization. Identification and quantification of processes facilitate the determination of process performance measures. Performance measures enable the processes to be quantified and improved. Process measures also enable managers to shift away from a focus on individuals to a team approach based upon the concept of processes. In essence, ABCM has the potential to become a tool to help managers understand their organization's mental model. *Mental model* is the unpublished criteria or structure that governs the design of processes—it is the picture that employees have in their minds. Therefore, through understanding the mental model, there exists an opportunity to enhance or redesign the model to meet evolving customer needs and requirements.

CONCLUSION

This chapter provided an overview of the changing paradigm in home care with respect to the management of cost, the changing role of financial leadership, and the integration of processes. Systems thinking, a process orientation, and customer-focused strategies are not new concepts. These concepts, however, provide a new framework for assessing organizational components and their individual and combined contributions to the larger whole. It is toward this perspective that the concept of cost management will transition. The transition will move cost away from being the historical tool of the "financial police officer" to becoming an integral element of a multidimensional measurement perspective shared and understood by all, and used to assess organizational output from the customer's perspective.

NOTES

1. Health Care Financing Administration, *Health Care Financing Review*, 1996 Statistical Supplement, 20.

2. HCFA, *Health Care Financing Review*, Human Resources Administration: An Alternative Model, 77.

3. Issue Brief: *The Interim Payment System for Home Health: A Patient Care Crisis*, Home Health Care Association of Massachusetts, Fall 1997.

4. N. Metzger, *Handbook of Health Care Human Resources Management* (Rockville, MD: Aspen Publishers, 1990), 9.

5. Metzger, *Handbook of Health Care Human Resources Management*, 11.
6. E.H. Schein, Three Cultures of Management: The Key to Organizational Learning, *Sloan Management Review* 38, no. 1 (Fall 1996): 9–20.
7. P. Boland, The Role of Reengineering in Health Care Delivery, *Managed Care Quarterly* 4, no. 4 (1996): 1–11.
8. H.T. Johnson, Management Accounting in the 21st Century, *Journal of Cost Management* 9, no. 3 (Fall 1995): 15–19.
9. M. Wheatley, *Leadership and the New Science: Learning about Organizations from an Orderly Universe* (San Francisco, CA: Berrett-Koehler, 1992).

CHAPTER 3

Managing Thy Data

Nurses have collected and analyzed data for more than a century, in fact as far back as Florence Nightingale and her use of statistical graphics to depict needless deaths in the Crimean War.[1] Today, home care providers have access to quantities of data that far exceed their ability to use them in a meaningful or effective way. Their lack of ability in managing these data was exemplified in 1993 under a Small Business Innovation Research grant from the Health Care Financing Administration (HCFA) whereby a survey was conducted to determine, in part, the data collection practices of home care agencies.[2] Among the findings of the study are the following:

- Quality management is being driven by the needs of the regulatory bodies and reimbursement agencies, *not* the needs of the patient(s), and thus data systems focus on compliance issues rather than patient care issues.
- Data are collected in great quantity on the medical, functional, and social status of patients and on agency operations, but these data are rarely used to improve patient care and/or agency operations.
- Problems with data collection included amount of time spent (20 percent to 40 percent of time); cost; amount of inaccurate or lost data; and lack of usable data. Yet only 25 percent of agencies participating in the survey reported dissatisfaction with current methods.

As we move into managed care, this type of data collection and utilization will become extremely problematic. The essence of managed care is data: data to guide treatment decisions, data to select a course of treatment most likely to result in a quality outcome, data to track a patient's care and outcomes so these can be evaluated for learning and for being able to continue to choose the best method, and data to monitor and determine cost.

This chapter addresses data. Aspects to be discussed include

- domains and sources of data
- the old paradigm for managing data
- the new paradigm for managing data
- data management strategy
- data management as a process
- data management principles
- data management challenges

Actually, data alone are of no value. They are the elements that need to be summarized and displayed in a meaningful way to create information. Understanding the information provides knowledge. Inaccurate information can lead to incorrect knowledge and faulty decisions or choices, which in turn can lead to ineffective and/or poor quality care, legal and/or regulatory problems, and nonreimbursement and/or financial loss. Imprecise information is the result of problems with the underlying data, or lack thereof.

In home health care, most home care agencies are still unable to collect data, let alone glean information from that data. Agencies are also randomly collecting unneeded data "just in case" they are needed later. Instead, agencies need to (1) begin the formation of databases (stored collections of organized, interrelated data) and (2) focus their data collection activities to track data that inform them about the wants and needs of those they serve, the outcomes they generate, and the processes that generate the outcomes. The next step is to summarize these data to provide information for ongoing, rapid, small tests of change based on what is learned. This information is also used for

- determining quality of care
- understanding outcomes, efficiencies, utilization, costs
- responding to markets/payers that don't believe you
- demonstrating accountability
- deciding on new business opportunities

Finally, these data and information need to be assimilated through clinical reasoning to form an accurate knowledge base for quality care. Although nurses as a whole are highly intuitive, quality practice cannot rest solely on the use of intuition, because not all knowledge is immediately known to us. If we do not recognize an unknown as unknown, then we are not able to recognize how much we do not know in relation to what we know, and we endanger the health and well-being of our clients.[3]

Critical thinking is becoming recognized as the cognitive engine that drives the process of knowledge development. Knowledge learned through memorization or rote repetition results in role drive, a practice based on poorly learned concepts and theories.[4] Critical thinking, on the other hand, provides a solid knowledge base for practice. Critical thinking is a nonlinear process defined as a purposeful, self-regulatory judgment.[5] It is the ability to monitor our thoughts by focusing on critical points in the process and checking to see if we are really on target.[6] A critical thinker differentiates significant data from insignificant data and determines what missing information is essential for quality care. Questions that are asked include

- For this purpose, what else do I need to know?
- Why do I need to know it?
- What difference will it make in the care of the client?

DOMAINS AND SOURCES OF DATA

Home health care data are detailed, extensive, and complex, and the "devil is in the detail."[7 (p.2)] Data requirements will always evolve and change as an agency learns and grows, as regulatory and payer demands change, and as the art and science of caring and curing progresses. Data are used to describe patient and family demographics, environmental and safety issues, emotional and cognitive status, disease and injury, nutritional status, and personal health care management. Data also record recovery or stabilization of a patient over short- or long-term periods. They depict standards of care and health care guidelines. They itemize revenues and expenses. They cover multiple disciplines, complex employment contracts, intense regulatory requirements, multiple payer and coverage criteria, complicated authorization processes, demanding reimbursement methods, and laborious definitions of costs.

These data are transformed into policies, flowcharts, position descriptions, schedules, procedures, protocols, care plans, critical pathways, charts, invoices, paychecks, utilization reports, and financial statements—all the information necessary for making agency operational decisions. The data are also compared, emphasized, and analyzed for outcome and management information for individual and agency performance improvement.

Data are produced because of demand. Demand comes from internal and external agency customers in the form of patients and families, physicians and providers of care, other care provision sites (hospitals, clinics, nursing homes), suppliers, managed care organizations and payers, regulators/accrediting bodies, marketers, clinical operations, and corporate stakeholders. These customers want the data to maximize patient/community health, improve services, make money, evaluate patient outcomes, demonstrate the value of services, identify opportunities for improvement, and evaluate the performance of services. Interestingly enough, the sources of data demand are often the sources of data themselves. For example, a managed care organization may demand data about utilization, outcomes, and value of services. They are first, however, a source of data about their population such as age, sex, educational level, benefits, and other sites of care; and about their clinical demographics such as incidence of various diseases, previous referrals to home care, and history of costs of care to be delivered. These data are critical for an agency in determining the mix, duration, and costs of services that will be required. Other sources of data are local public health trend reports, community environmental reports, surveys, quality improvement projects, and agency source documents such as patient charts and financial documents.

All of an agency's structure, processes, and outcomes also are domains for data. Structure includes policies, flowcharts, employee data, and case mix. Processes include all key agency systems that support care and the process of care itself. Outcomes can be financial (utilization/costs), quality oriented (physiologic/ functional/quality of life), and satisfaction oriented.

Internal and External Information Needs

It is impossible to decide what data to collect until you know how they fit into the greater picture. Therefore, which data are extracted from each of the domains depends on the agency's information requirements. Information needs can be divided into internal and external. Internal can be subdivided into operational and management requirements. Each of these divisions can overlap and will be examined further.

Internal Information Requirements

Operational Information. Operational information is used to direct the day-to-day agency operations and answers questions such as:

- What patients is Nurse A seeing today?
- Who comprises the caregiving team for the Jones family?
- Which patients have recertifications due by the end of the month?
- How many accounts receivable are past due over 90 days? What is the dollar amount?

Operational information tends to be narrowly focused within an agency. It usually has short timelines and is relatively easy to retrieve. It uses individual patient and clinician data. It focuses more on financial and administrative issues and less on clinical issues. It requires accurate underlying data because it is the foundation of critical operational decisions.[8] Overall, home care agencies tend to be relatively expert at gathering and using this type of information.

*Management Information.*Management information is used to evaluate agency progress toward meeting its mission and attaining its vision. It evaluates progress toward meeting performance indicators as well as planning, organizing, and evaluating agency operations. It answers such questions as:

- How effective is our referral process?
- What percentage of post–acute care wound patients develop infections within three weeks of hospital discharge?
- How much does it cost to provide care to a post–acute care hip fracture patient if there are no variances from the clinical path? If there are variances, what are the reasons and associated costs?
- Is the new pediatric asthma program cost-effective?
- Will this referral exceed the per-beneficiary cap?

Management information tends to combine data from different areas across the agency and may include external data to forecast trends and compare performance. It uses aggregate and statistical data rather than individual data and may tolerate limited margins of error within the data. It encompasses clinical, financial, and administrative data. Because it requires data from separate sources, it is more difficult to obtain than operational data, and home care agencies are still struggling with how to collect and retrieve these types of data. For example, only a few agencies have been able to determine cost of care for a defined group of patients and to link that cost with outcomes of care. Collecting clinical data alone has been challenging, with many agencies still struggling with the concept of clinical pathways and how to collect and monitor variances.

Outcome information has been defined as a subset of management information that focuses on meeting clinical outcomes.[9] It is a crucial part of managing data within the new paradigm and will be dealt with later in the book. Ultimately, outcomes information needs to address the following question:

- Given Mr. Jones' demographics (age, sex, caregiver status), health status, and environment, what is the most clinically effective and cost-effective course of treatment?

This type of information requires extensive clinical data collected over time, compared with external data and analyzed with cost and variance data. It is currently receiving much attention through the Outcome and Assessment Information Set (OASIS) and the Joint Commission's ORYX initiatives for home care, as well as from managed care organizations.

External Information Requirements

Internally, agencies have a need for aggregate information on cost, quality, and utilization in order to manage their organization. In addition, each year a greater percentage of a home care agency's information will be created for external use.[10] This is due to a need for standardized information that will allow agencies and others such as regulators, payers, and consumers to describe the scope of home care services, analyze utilization and costs of services, and evaluate the comparative effectiveness and quality of services.[11]

Standardized external information is dependent on overcoming three barriers to collecting reliable interagency data.

1. the varying capacity of more than 17,000 home care providers to compile, collect, and report data
2. the unwillingness to report data due to competitive concerns and the lack of confidentiality safeguards
3. data incompatibility due to differing definitions or reporting methods[12]

There are several initiatives underway that are addressing these barriers, including the Uniform Data Set for Home Care and Hospice, the proposed regulation requiring Medicare-certified agencies to collect the OASIS, and the nursing profession's work on a Unified Nursing Language System.

Uniform Data Set for Home Care and Hospice. The Uniform Data Set for Home Care and Hospice was begun in 1993 by the National Association for Home Care (NAHC) to advance the possibility of obtaining reliable interagency information. It is comprised of a minimum set of uniformly defined items for home care and hospice services that meet the essential information needs of multiple data users within the health care system. Data items are divided into two levels: (1) organizational and (2) patient/client. Under organizational data are the subcategories organization/services, utilization, financial, and personnel. Under the patient/client data are the subcategories demographics, clinical items, and service/utilization.[13]

Proposed Condition of Participation to Include OASIS. The March 10, 1997, *Federal Register* proposes the required use of OASIS as part of a comprehensive patient assessment. OASIS is a uniform data set comprised of 10 identifying information items and 79 patient assessment items of health and functional status that are patient oriented (i.e., discipline neutral) and when measured at two or more points in time serve as outcome measures. Development of OASIS began in 1988 as part of a contract by HCFA with the Center for Health Policy Research at the University of Colorado to develop, test, and improve a system of outcome measures.[14] The items in the data set are considered reliable and valid and provide for uniform data collection within an agency and across agencies for computing outcome measures. The current regulations call for the individual agency collection and use of these items only. With future regulations, however, HCFA hopes to establish a national database in the public domain to make data available, such as home health agency outcomes to consumers, purchasers, home health agencies, and HCFA.[15] OASIS will be discussed further in a later chapter.

Unified Nursing Language System (UNLS). Languages are made up of vocabularies (terms and definitions) and grammar (the rules for using the terms). There have been several recent efforts in nursing to identify nursing vocabularies in order to have a unified nursing practice language that fosters understanding and communication. Until nurses in various settings use the same terminology to document their assessments, diagnoses, interventions, and outcomes, nursing will not be included in the national databases used for health care policy decisions. Once nursing can name what it does, then nursing practice can be measured, evaluated, recognized, and reimbursed.[16] A UNLS would identify the semantic linkages among different nursing vocabularies and extend those linkages to other health care–related vocabularies such as the National Library of Medicine's Metathesaurus of the Unified Medical Language System. The UNLS is seen as essential for the establishment of national nursing practice databases that would make possible the study of variations in nursing practice and in patient outcomes across the country.[17] Four vocabularies are currently recognized by the American Nurses Association. They are

1. the North American Nursing Diagnosis Association (NANDA) list of nursing diagnoses: list of accepted diagnostic labels
2. the Nursing Interventions Classification (NIC): standardized nomenclature for nursing treatments
3. the Omaha System
4. the Home Health Care Classifications (HHCC)[18]

The last two vocabularies are home health care specific and include terms for problems (diagnoses) and interventions. The Omaha System also includes a series of rating scales (knowledge, behavior, and status) that can be used for measuring outcomes. The HHCC provides a method for coding the expected outcome. The challenge for home care is the multiple disciplines involved with no current linkages to terms the other disciplines use for problem identification or intervention.

DATA MANAGEMENT: THE OLD PARADIGM

Home health, as a highly regulated element of the health care delivery system, has significant data requirements. As has been mentioned, data creates information, information creates knowledge, and knowledge creates opportunity. In the old paradigm, data are made available only to a chosen few because information is viewed as the domain of senior management. This supports the hierarchical organizational structures and concepts of the paradigm. Data collection, tracking, and management rely heavily on paper forms and most of the data collected focus more on the management and financial issues rather than the clinical ones.

Clinical documentation is usually on a manual chart with little or no ability to longitudinally track the care provided. Patient data are entered in multiple places on the chart, by multiple disciplines. The purpose of documentation is to note patient events, to establish a need for services and a legal record, and to refresh clinicians' memories. It is in narrative format listing fragmented tasks. Not only does this make the data difficult to access or share, but it also increases staff time and agency resource consumption. The task of aggregating data across a large number of patients or across a specific patient population is almost impossible! Furthermore, definitions of terms and abbreviations are not standard and are left open for individual interpretation leading to data misinterpretations. Handwritten notes are often illegible, service provision is not completely documented, and the rationale behind the diagnosis and care choices is often ill-defined.[19] And then the chart is misplaced, misfiled, or filed with notes from contracting disciplines missing.

These data associated with providing patient services, however, are required from multiple layers of customers with a dependence upon a diverse workforce. Home health managers need to compile data to satisfy regulatory and business requirements. Unfortunately, the ability to develop comprehensive electronic information systems to meet many of these requirements has been thwarted for many reasons, including the fact that home care is not as big a business as acute care, and thus it does not get the same attention from outside vendors. This has led to the development of smaller, focused electronic data processing systems starting with billing requirements. What exists now is system fragmentation, where home care agencies purchased one system to meet billing requirements, one system to satisfy general ledger and business requirements, and possibly a system to meet clinical needs and then purchased an off-the-shelf software package to satisfy analytical and ad hoc reporting requirements.

The development of software solutions and the subsequent approach to data management has been consistent with the old paradigm. Management of data within the old paradigm deals with compliance. This approach satisfied the basic need for external reporting to payers and regulators, allowed agencies to bill and generate cash flow, and fulfilled basic management requirements; however, it created significant inefficiencies from an organizational perspective. Inefficiencies were created because of basic software design that did not share data among applications, forced data to be rekeyed when used for multiple purposes, and forced the use and development of applications that were flexible enough to capture and manipulate data outside of the limitations of hard-coded software programs.

In addition to the inefficiencies created by software, there is the tendency to approach data management in a haphazard fashion thus causing suboptimization, at best, and, at worst, an adversarial approach to the purpose of gathering data. Suboptimization is the underachieving of results and occurs when a segment or department of an agency begins to develop sophisticated reporting and analysis of data. The department uses the resulting information exclusively, viewing it as a source of power. The information is often used as a tool to say, "I gotcha." An example of suboptimization could be the use of financial and budget data to force accountability or the development of patient profiles to support the provision of care beyond clinical pathway resource requirements. Use of information as a club creates a climate of control and subsequent mistrust. Mistrust fosters a we-they division and more suboptimization occurs.

DATA MANAGEMENT: THE NEW PARADIGM

Data management in the new paradigm is facilitated by a new focus on software development. Software developers are already beginning to build information systems instead of data processing systems. Data processing systems were created to enter data such as patient demographics, visit information, accounts payable information, and journal entries for the purposes of producing canned reports, UB92s (Medicare billing forms), visit summaries, and trial balances. Developers in the new paradigm are creating information systems that allow for

- the manipulation of data to create information and knowledge
- relational databases that facilitate the retrieval and manipulation of data to look at the relationships between organizational approaches and results
- clinical repositories as a strategic resource for quality and practice and to gain a better understanding of predictors of care requirements
- electronic interfacing systems to facilitate the sharing of data

The outcome of this transition will be the creation of management information systems instead of data processing systems.

Furthermore, software developers have entered the world of clinical information systems, shifting their emphasis from task support for caregivers to providing clinical information as a strategic resource for practice. The goals of a computerized patient record (CPR) are to

- Increase the quality of information throughout the continuum of care

- Decrease the cost of care over time
- Improve the effectiveness of care by providing a longitudinal record, instant access to clinical data, on-screen alerts and reminders, and real-time data entry[20]

As the need increases for tracking relevant patient information to verify the effectiveness of service, the clinical record becomes more of a decision-making and informational tool and not just a diary for documenting patient events. Accurate clinical documentation becomes the basis for analyzing outcomes of care.

The new paradigm is about quality outcomes and performance excellence. Therefore, the management of data and the subsequent information that can be created provide an opportunity to create a source of competitive advantage for home health agencies. But to get there, data management cannot be random or haphazard: It must be focused and based on defined outcomes and the pursuit of a shared vision.

> A shared vision is not an idea. It is not even an important idea such as freedom. It is rather, a force in people's hearts, a force of impressive power. It may be inspired by an idea, but once it goes further—if it is compelling enough to acquire the support of more than one person— then it is no longer an abstraction. It is palpable. People begin to see it as if it exists. Few, if any, forces in human affairs are as powerful as shared vision.
>
> At its simplest level, a shared vision is the answer to the question, "What do we want to create?" Just as personal visions are pictures or images people carry in their heads and hearts, so too are shared visions pictures that people throughout an organization carry. They create a sense of commonality that permeates the organization and gives coherence to diverse activities.[21] (p.206)

The concepts of vision, mission, and values will be addressed later in Chapter 5. From the perspective of data management, however, shared vision facilitates the development of a strategically driven, customer-focused approach that emphasizes continuous improvement. Building upon the premise that shared vision requires the buy-in, commitment, and enrollment of all levels of staff, it is an easy transition to realize that all levels of staff must have access to data in order to pursue organizational strategies and achieve organizational goals. This transition will be consistent with organizational change as layers of management are flattened to reduce overhead costs and to allow an agency to be more responsive to changing requirements. It is also consistent with access to data extending beyond agency walls and being shared with suppliers, payers, physicians, and patients.

This concept can be illustrated by building upon the basic elements of a process. Figure 3–1 illustrates these three elements of a process: input, activities, and output. There are multiple processes within the agency, and when viewed as a whole, they represent a system. The system is made up of staff and activities associated with the processes. It produces outcomes that hopefully will exceed customer expectations. The system is designed by the organization's leaders and, if strategy driven, will focus the efforts of all resources toward the provision of value to multiple stakeholders. Therefore, the concept of shared vision becomes more important as leaders attempt to eliminate suboptimization and pursue something larger than the sum of the pieces, the organization's shared vision.

STRATEGY

The real question is What approach should agencies adopt toward data management in the new paradigm? This approach is one of alignment of organizational performance. Figure 3–2 illustrates the relationship among current reality, vision, and strategy. Current reality is where the organization is today. This may be its financial condition, its ability to satisfy customers, or any other measure that is meaningful. Organizational vision is a desired state in the future that is based upon a synthesis of the organization's values, strengths, weaknesses, potential to take advantage of opportunities, dreams, aspirations, and ability to avoid threats. The difference between current reality and a desired state is referred to as a gap. A vehicle to close the gap is strategy. Strategy requires the channeling of resources toward focused objectives.

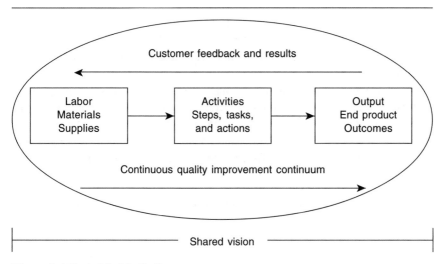

Figure 3–1 Basic Model of a System

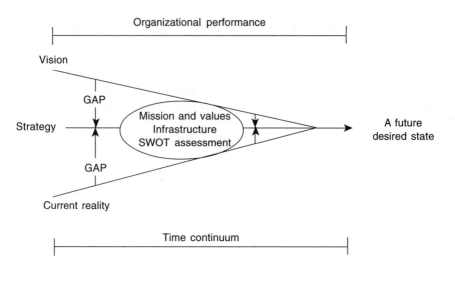

Figure 3–2 Alignment of Organizational Performance

A tool for identifying objectives is the SWOT analysis, formatted in four columns. The first two columns of a SWOT analysis identify organizational strengths (S) and organizational weaknesses (W); and the second two columns identify external opportunities (O) and external threats (T). Strengths and weaknesses primarily focus on the present while opportunities and threats have a future perspective.

- *Strengths* are the major advantages on which one should capitalize.
- *Weaknesses* are the major disadvantages that will impede performance and must be overcome.
- *Opportunities* are the external advantages that can be exploited in the agency's favor. The more opportunities identified, the more flexibility the agency will have for allocating resources to the areas of greatest return.
- *Threats* are the external major changes that may have a significant impact on the agency's performance. Every attempt should be made to minimize these threats, or at least to create a plan for dealing with them.[22]

Completion of a SWOT analysis provides a starting point for strategy identification and prioritization.

To be successful, strategies depend on the development of common values and purpose (mission), an infrastructure that will support the pursuit of objectives while being flexible enough to respond to opportunities and threats, and a performance measurement system that facilitates the assessment of organizational progress. If strategies are realized, then as time passes, the gap between vision and reality will close and the desired state will be realized.

Strategies are realized through the development of a strategic performance measurement system.

> A strategic performance measurement system can lead a company to make a quantum leap in performance. A strategic performance system achieves a balance of cost, quality, and time measures at the organization, process, and people levels. It is driven by market-differentiating strategies that are focused on customer needs yet are still tied to vision, mission, and values of the company. It is based on the organizational goals and the critical processes that must be managed to achieve these strategies.
>
> In addition, a strategic performance measurement system provides leadership with the necessary input to drive strategic thinking and identify changes. The right performance measures inherently communicate the strategy of the company, create buy-in, and promote a cross-functional perspective by guiding appropriate employee behavior.[23] (p.22)

Therefore, to support strategy, it is necessary to define what data are critical to assessing organizational performance with respect to the organization's vision. Defining data requirements helps to focus the agency's staff on common objectives by identifying what is important to the agency. Once objectives and performance measures are defined, then it is possible to define what data are necessary to collect in order to support organizational strategies and performance measures. Because collection of data is resource intensive, collection of data that does not support the achievement of organizational goals is superfluous and a non-value-adding activity.

The following illustration will demonstrate the concept. The local home health agency has decided that in order to be a player in the health care delivery system it has to pursue four major strategies. Its leaders believe that if they pursue four strategies they will obtain their vision. The four strategies are cost effectiveness, demonstrable quality, customer satisfaction, and employee satisfaction. Table 3–1 identifies several of the performance measures they utilize to monitor where they are in the pursuit of their goals.

Table 3-1 has identified four major strategies and four performance measures or indicators associated with each strategy, current results, and agency goals. (Obviously, the local agency will want to track additional performance metrics to gauge progress toward the achievement of organizational strategies.) Their strategy of pursuing cost effectiveness is identified in relationship to a one- and two-year goal. The development of strategies in relationship to goals identifies how

Table 3–1 Agency Strategy, Related Performance Measures, Current Reality, and Goals

Strategy and Related Performance Measure	Current	Goals 1 Year	2 Years
Cost effectiveness			
(cost per visit)	$75	$68	$61
Demonstrable quality			
(% patients with improved ADLs)	70%	80%	90%
Customer satisfaction			
(% patients satisfied with service)	80%	88%	95%
Employee satisfaction			
(% staff satisfied)	50%	65%	80%

much gap there is and focuses organizational efforts. Further information could be provided by including competitive data or benchmarks from within or outside of the home health care industry.

Figure 3–3 illustrates a basic premise related to data management and performance measurement. First, data needs to be aggregated. Table 3–1 is an example of aggregated results. Aggregated results have very little meaning to the majority of staff, however, because they do not know how their job relates to the aggregate performance measure.

As illustrated in Figure 3–3, the challenge in designing data management systems is to identify what data are necessary to collect to measure organizational strategies, identify how agencywide performance measures cascade down to the different process levels or owners, and discover how process-level metrics

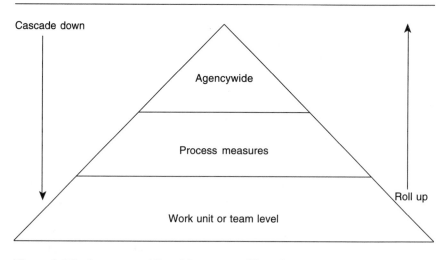

Figure 3–3 Performance and Data Management Hierarchy

cascade down to the work unit or team level. Conversely, work–unit or team-level indicators need to roll up to facilitate organizational review that is not mired in detail. Once there is agreement on the type and composition of performance measures, action plans can be developed that identify goals, intermediate milestones, and other indicators that will assist the periodic evaluation of progress toward organizational goals.

Data management in the new paradigm is multidimensional. Successful agencies will combine multiple performance measures into their data collection strategies and assessments. The new measures will include quantitative and qualitative indicators of clinical quality, customer perceptions regarding satisfaction with services and staff, staff satisfaction, cost, and time. The integration of performance measurements into the agency's data management strategy will assist in

- defining what data are critical to collect
- providing guidance in the identification of systematic approaches to collection
- developing sound approaches to analysis

Once collected, performance measures and the underlying detail will provide the basis to implement improvement initiatives and design experiments. Ultimately it will be the shift in focus from data management for compliance purposes to data management for continual improvement. This organizational growth will create viable, customer-focused home health agencies.

MANAGEMENT OF DATA: A SYSTEMS PERSPECTIVE EXAMPLE

How an agency chooses to manage its data is an individual decision, but an important one. Data become the basis for an agency's operation, improvement, and—ultimately—its survival. Analyzed data provide the information for strategic planning, process and outcome management, and more. An illustration of the pervasiveness and critical nature of data is offered by the framework for the Malcolm Baldrige National Quality Award as pictured in Figure 3-4.

The framework consists of seven categories: leadership, strategic planning, customer and market focus, information and analysis, human resource development and management, process management, and business results. Collectively, the first six categories represent an organization's system, and the seventh category, business results, represents the collective outcomes of all efforts within that organization. Of specific interest is the placement of information and analysis. Information and analysis (category 4) crosses the entire organization. It is a major process within the system. "Information and analysis are critical to the effective management of the company and to a fact-based system for improving company performance and competitiveness."[24]

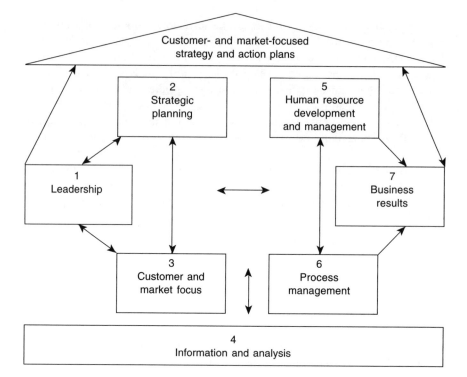

Figure 3–4 Baldrige Award Criteria Framework—A Systems Perspective. *Source:* Courtesy of Malcolm Baldrige National Quality Award, 1997.

Information and analysis come from data. The flow of data (the process of data management) that supports the information and analysis is depicted in Figure 3–5.

Understanding this flow of data provides the foundation for managing the process of data management. This process can then be used to support an organizational system such as the one depicted in the Malcolm Baldrige framework, or however defined by an agency. Managing and improving this process can be accomplished by using the steps for managing a process found in Chapter 11.

DATA MANAGEMENT PRINCIPLES

Agency data management strategies include a methodology for identifying required data, collecting or gathering the data for defined categories, and integrating and reporting the data. Once data are reported, strategies need to consider how

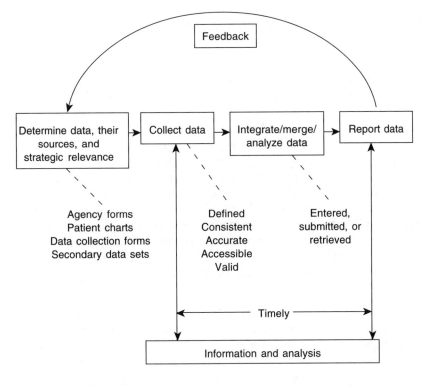

Figure 3–5 The Flow of Data

data can be used to focus improvement efforts; to develop, implement, and improve customer-oriented services, strategies, and business results; and to foster an environment of perpetual growth consistent with the organization's vision and values. Some key principles to follow in this process are discussed below.

Data Need To Be Relevant. Data collection efforts should focus on accumulating data that are consistent with the mission and objectives of the agency. Data used for measuring patient quality should be the same as that used for patient care—there should not be a separate data set. Data collection needs to be unobtrusive to clinical practice. Remember that data that are easy to collect may or may not be relevant. Relevant data are a beginning point for understanding the business, patient problems, demographic variables, perceptions, and trends. Nonrelevant data are expensive. It is better to collect too little data than too much. Collect only what is needed and use all the data collected. Always know how the data fit into the greater picture. Also be aware that relevancy changes over time.

What was relevant yesterday may not be relevant today and probably will not be relevant tomorrow.

Data Requirements Need To Be Continually Updated To Meet the Changing Information Needs of Patients, Stakeholders, and the Changing Health Environment. As consumers of health care (patients, payers, families) become more knowledgeable, they will require more information regarding the value of an agency's services. Updating data collection requirements forces providers to assess what information is critical to the achievement of strategic goals. It may be that a particular strategy is no longer relevant because of some internal or external factor. Therefore, to continue to collect data that are no longer being used, produce reports that have minimal meaning, and burden system resources by keeping outdated data represents an inefficient use of resources. A potential strategy to keep data relevant is to conduct an information needs analysis, which takes into consideration strategy, changing patient and stakeholder requirements, the needs of employees, and the marketplace. Once developed, a needs analysis can be used to fine tune source data for the purposes of creating meaning and clarity.

Relevant Data Need To Be Consistent, Accessible, Accurate, and Shared in a Timely Fashion. The purpose of providing data is to create information. Valid information relies on accurate, timely, and statistically stable data. If the data cannot be retrieved or merged into a single database over time, they are not available to create information. Without information, staff and managers cannot find new ways to improve their department operations or the care they provide to patients and families. Sharing the data is also important. Staff who are the "data providers" who never get to see the resultant information never see the benefit and rapidly become frustrated with increased documentation requirements.

DATA MANAGEMENT SHORTCOMINGS

The need for a well-organized information system has arisen quickly and is growing out of a quagmire of fragmented, inconsistent, obsolete, or missing data elements that are identifiable at best. Developing an integrated, organized information system requires defining, retrieving, classifying, integrating, and reporting the data successfully. This is a growth process with many shortcomings that need to be addressed. No one shortcoming is insurmountable, but taken together they may impede progress toward obtaining needed information. Some identifiable shortcomings to address include the following.

Collecting Data in a Massive and/or Haphazard Manner. This is the antithesis to collecting relevant data. Information gets lost in a massive data set or when there is no hypothesis. Many times data are collected because they are easiest and most available, or because they might be beneficial later on. Decide first what you want to address and collect only the data that support the problem/measurement that you are seeking to address. Whether they are collected manually or electronically, be sure that the data are collected in a manner that is retrievable.

Ineffective Analysis of Data. Most providers do not have specially trained data managers or data analysis staff. There are many reasons for this: It is hard to find experienced people and when they are found they are costly; data analysis professionals will not necessarily be familiar with the home care business so there will be a learning curve involved in teaching them; it is a non-revenue-generating function; and there is a nonlinear return on investment.[25] Working with aggregate data, however, requires different aptitudes than working with individual data. It requires the ability to abstract, categorize, summarize, and synthesize. It also requires a level of comfort with statistical tools and conclusions. It is important that the person responsible for data collection and analysis have these talents.

Using a Poorly Defined Clinical Data Set. A clinical data set includes demographics, patient/family assessment indicators, statements of patient needs or problems, expected outcomes or goals, and interventions, including physician orders. Aggregating clinical data sets of patients with like conditions provides the basis for standardizing and tracking processes and outcomes of care. Aggregating clinical data sets for all patients provides an overall case mix data set for the agency and provides the evidence the agency needs to show the results of various services in terms of value, quality, and cost-efficiency. Unfortunately, most clinical data sets are inconsistent, ill-defined, piecemeal, and nonreflective of the scope of agency services. To be effective, data set terms must be commonly defined (see section on UNLS) and detailed. The more detailed the elements in the data set, the more standardization there will be in the delivery of care. An example is the intervention *wound care*. Wound care itself can be performed many ways; therefore, including protocols to describe the exact care for different types of wounds such as a Type III decubiti, or a surgical incision, would improve the degree of standardization and subsequent understanding of the process of wound care that leads to the outcome of a healed wound. Adding defined steps for procedures, such as how to remove the sutures, would further assist with standardizing care. Without standardization of the care processes, it is difficult to determine what clinical processes need to be improved to enhance the effectiveness of obtaining healed wounds.

Neglecting To Measure All Dimensions Relevant to the Services Provided. With all the focus on outcomes, it is easy for quality improvement personnel to get caught up with outcomes (outputs) and forget about inputs and processes. When an outcome is not met, however, it is probably because of something in the process. When an outcome is met, there are still ways of improving the process that may yield efficiency and cost savings. Assessment of inputs could include considerations such as: Is equipment in good order (e.g., sphygmomanometers calibrated routinely)? Are the knowledge and skills of caregivers up to date? Are professional licenses current? Process quality can include systems beyond the care process; it can also include relationships with consumers (patients, payers, suppliers, physicians) and support processes such as the data management and information systems.

Neglecting the "Soft" or Human Elements. Data management as a system itself has inputs, processes, and outputs. Identifying these components helps to identify the weaknesses of the system. One part that is often neglected is the human element, the attitudes, feelings, resistance, and conflict that impact job performance and productivity. Some staff are data providers and others are information consumers. Each is dependent on the other. If the data providers do not see reason to be accurate, timely, and complete, then the information suffers and the information consumers become frustrated at not being able to get answers to their questions. The data provider sees data as more work; the information consumer sees it as essential. These conflicting attitudes create tension and negative attitudes overtake the functioning of the system.

Understanding attitudes of persons in the data-to-information continuum is actually a great way to uncover many of the shortcomings of data management. Staff cope with the shortcomings every day by inventing and using *workarounds*. A workaround is an improvisation to bypass the system and get the work done.[26] To find data management shortcomings, ask staff about the workarounds they have created and their causes. For example, if adding an intervention to a patient's clinical path requires extra documentation, including reasons and validations, staff may elect to do the intervention and just not document it. After all, documentation in home care has always been "creative." Unfortunately, the intervention and its impact on the clinical path and resulting outcomes are lost.

CONCLUSION

Data management is evolving from the data processing that agencies have always performed in order to comply with external requirements such as providing data to satisfy regulatory standards and providing numbers to support the billing and financial processes. It is evolving to information systems that allow for the manipulation of data to define cost-effective, quality practice. Today, all agency documents (clinical, administrative, and financial) are seen as a potential source of data to be used as the basis for information to improve decision-making abilities and patient services. Data demands are even extending beyond agency walls to allow for comparisons across sites. The goal is to understand the value of the services offered by home care from the global perspective to the smallest detail of what is done.

The challenge is overcoming the inconsistencies, voids, and other shortcomings of past data collection and use. With such rapid change, many internal shortcomings and external barriers still exist. Each of these must be addressed and corrected. Some are more difficult to see; others are more challenging to address. Some require a change in attitude; others require a change in behavior. Some require new expertise; others require new technology. Some can be simply corrected by better organization and understanding. It is these weaknesses that the authors seek to address.

NOTES

1. I.B. Cohen, Florence Nightingale, *Scientific American* 250, no. 3 (1984): 128–137.
2. J.R Pratt et al., A Study of Home Care Quality Management Data-Collection Systems, *Caring Magazine* 13, no. 11 (1994): 10–11.
3. R.W. Paul and P. Heaslip, Critical Thinking and Intuitive Nursing Practice, *Journal of Advanced Nursing* 22 (1995): 40–47.
4. Paul and Heaslip, Critical Thinking, 40–47.
5. N.C. Facione and P.A. Facione, Externalizing the Critical Thinking in Knowledge Development and Clinical Judgment, *Nursing Outlook* 44 (1996): 129–136.
6. Paul and Heaslip, Critical Thinking, 40–47.
7. C.W. Tidd, From Data to Information: Management Tools for Home Care Clinical Directors, *Home Health Care Management and Practice* 10, no. 2 (1998): 1–10.
8. Tidd, From Data to Information, 1–10.
9. Tidd, From Data to Information, 1–10.
10. Tidd, From Data to Information, 1–10.
11. K.B. Pace, The Information Challenge in Home Care. Unpublished manuscript.
12. Pace, The Information Challenge, 1–18.
13. Pace, The Information Challenge, 1–18.
14. National Association for Home Care, NAHC Outlines HCFA's Proposed Changes to Conditions of Participation, *Homecare News* 12 (April 1997): 4–6.
15. National Association for Home Care, NAHC Outlines HCFA's Proposed Changes, 4–6.
16. D.K. Milholland, Naming What We Do—Nursing Vocabularies and Databases, *Journal of AHIMA* 63, no. 10 (1992): 58–61.
17. D.K. Milholland, Naming What We Do, 58–61.
18. American Nurses Association, *Nursing Data Systems: The Emerging Framework* (Washington, DC: 1995).
19. A. Bender, Management Information Systems—A Required Tool for Survival, *Home Health Care Management and Practice* 10, no. 2 (1998): 42–47.

20. J.L. Usher, *Protecting the Home Care Patient: Electronic Patient Record Confidentiality* (Paper presented at Home Care Informatics, New Orleans, LA, March 13, 1997).

21. P.M. Senge, *The Fifth Discipline* (New York: Doubleday, 1990), 206.

22. D.D. McConkey, *How To Manage by Results*, 4th ed. (New York: AMACOM, 1983).

23. Compiled by L. Struebing, News: Strategic Plans Don't Produce Desired Results, *Quality Progress* 29, no. 6 (June 1996): 22.

24. 1997 Criteria for Performance Excellence, Malcolm Baldrige National Quality Award (Milwaukee, WI: American Society for Quality, 1997).

25. M.N. Warren, National Data Comparisons: Opportunities and Risks from the Provider's Perspective (Paper presented at the Disease Management Congress, Phoenix, AZ, April 1997).

26. Tidd, From Data to Information, 2.

PART II

The Necessary Components for Survival

CHAPTER 4

A Perspective on Environment: The Beginning

It has been said that there are only two events that are absolutely certain: death and taxes. Change, however, is an event that has been omitted from the preceding statement. We live in a world that is constantly changing. Change can be good or bad, depending upon one's perspective.

Perspective is how you choose to look at events, influences, and occurrences. For instance, the transition to a prospective payment environment is an event that is external to agency operations. Prospective payment can be viewed as a threat, a foreshadowing of a changing health care delivery system, or an opportunity. Therefore, perspective affects how one relates to events or relationships. Perspective will be shaped by whether agency management is greatly or minimally influenced by changing external circumstances. Ultimately, perspective is the result of an agency's relationship to its vision and the alignment of the agency's infrastructure toward the achievement of its vision. Otherwise, perspective will be akin to a vessel sailing on the open seas. Without a desired future state or outcome (vision) the sailing vessel will be bounced around the ocean by the changing winds. In this scenario, the vessel's infrastructure reacts to the changing environment and the vessel's management believe they are being proactive by steering into waves instead of being hit broadside. Regardless of belief, this vessel's infrastructure and management are in a reactive mode based upon changing external events. With a vision in mind, however, strategies can be developed to reach desired outcomes. The development of strategies considers the changing environment of transoceanic travel and creates a system to respond to those circumstances. Once the requirements of transoceanic travel have been addressed, it will then be possible to create a sailing vessel that will focus on performance excellence and meet and exceed the needs of its customers. In this scenario proactive management and infrastructure development are based upon interrelationships that include, but are not limited to, the needs of customers being served, staff, suppliers, and the resource requirements necessary to obtain future goals.

When these interrelationships focus on a common outcome, an inner harmony prevails even though the external environment is turbulent.

This chapter discusses perspective, clarity of purpose, and customer/community focus. Perspective addresses the external environment and requirements of operating a home health agency. Perspective, however, goes beyond regulatory requirements and accreditation standards. Perspective is really about answering a very basic question: What is it that we want to create? Do we want to create organizations to meet the needs of regulatory and accrediting bodies, or do we want to create organizations that are driven by the needs of our customers and honor our desire to go beyond mediocrity to performance excellence? The achievement of performance excellence requires a clear articulation of purpose and a focus on the actions and drivers that enable opportunity to be manifested and excellence to be exemplified. The key is to use the customer/community from the environment coupled with internal fiscal soundness to drive an agency's programming. It is defining the needs of the customer/community and using them to refine and clarify the agency's purpose that provides the beginning point for agencies under the new paradigm.

In looking at perspective, clarity of purpose, and customer focus, this chapter deals with

- the external agency environment and its regulatory systems
- the internal agency environment and structure
- extrinsic and intrinsic motivation
- customers—individual and community
- scorecards
- strategy and strategic planning

So, when environment is considered from the perspective of quality, cost, and data management, it is seen as the beginning. It is the environment, and the customers in it, that determine the purpose of the business and its programs and services. Once these strategies are determined, then daily operations can be defined, measures of quality determined, the required data to measure the quality collected, and the cost of the operations estimated.

EXTERNAL ENVIRONMENT

Many practitioners entered health care out of a belief that they could help others. They felt their efforts would somehow contribute to the betterment of society or at least contribute to helping another human being regain health or get to a point where his or her condition had stabilized. Many of these same practitioners are beginning to question their motivation for getting involved with health care given the turbulent environment of the health care delivery system and the impact this turbulence has upon agency operations.

In preceding chapters, references were made to changing paradigms or going from an old paradigm to a new one. Most of the references have dealt with external events such as a move away from a fragmented delivery system to an integrated one, a move by the federal government to adopt a prospective payment system for Medicare, and the entry of managed care.

We are in the middle of a changing paradigm with respect to the way health care services are provided in the United States. The old paradigm was characterized by "more is better." The new paradigm is "providing more with less." The old paradigm was comfortable; we had learned the rules and knew how to act accordingly. The new paradigm is not comfortable; it represents change, the rules are not clear, and similar to the aforementioned example of the ship, if an organization's strategy isn't firmly anchored to its vision, it will be at the mercy of external events.

What is the underlying cause of the changing paradigm? The root causes can be attributed to events that took place decades ago. Multiple, complex systems were developed to meet the needs and characteristics of a population that existed then. Furthermore, because the larger system was fragmented, system participants learned how to optimize their specific element of the larger system. Lack of alignment occurred by developing one payment system for hospitals, another for physicians, a third for home health agencies, and then other reimbursement formulas as well. Other factors influencing the changing paradigm include inflation, population growth, rising health care costs, and intensity of care.[1] Intensity of care is influenced by an aging population. "On average, the aged tend to be sicker and consume four times as much health care expenditures per capita as the under-65 population. Specifically, persons 85 years of age or over represent the highest-cost cohort in terms of the healthcare expenditures they incur." [2]

The need for change became obvious as symptoms of the dysfunctional health care system appeared. Symptoms have taken the form of personal health care expenditures increasing from $23.9 billion in 1960 to an estimated $832.5 billion in 1994. This represents an average annual rate of change of 11 percent. Spending is expected to reach $2.0 trillion by 2005.[3]

These symptoms became a catalyst to change the health care delivery system paradigm. Several of the changes include the introduction of health maintenance organizations (HMOs), a payment system for hospitals comprised of diagnosis-related groups (DRGs), changes in Medicare coverage provisions, and the foreshadowing of prospective payment for home health agencies.

All of these changes are influencing the external environment in which home health agencies operate, and are part of a larger evolutionary process. In order to identify strategic responses to a changing environment, however, it is first necessary to understand agency infrastructure and the driving forces in the design of that infrastructure before identifying a proactive or reactive action plan.

REGULATORY SYSTEMS

The federal government is the largest purchaser of health care services and, as such, needed to identify rules, regulations, and procedures for suppliers of health care services to follow. The rules, regulations, and procedures will differ depending upon whether a hospital, rehabilitation facility, or home health provider is the supplier. Collectively, these specifications provide a mechanism to identify minimum standards that providers of health care services must follow in order to receive payment for the provision of services to Medicare enrollees. The goal of the specifications is to develop a uniform approach to dealing with thousands of suppliers. The federal agency that administers the Medicare program is the Health Care Financing Administration (HCFA).

For home health providers, becoming a certified supplier of home health services entitles the certified agency to bill HCFA for services provided to Medicare enrollees. Certification represents a barrier to entry for agencies interested in providing care and billing for Medicare patients. Most industries have barriers to entry. Barriers to entry can include personal licensure for a certified public accountant (CPA), facility licensure for a restaurant or drinking establishment, or major capital investment for entry into the airline business. Other barriers to entry could include access to natural resources, human resources, or intellectual capital. Barriers to entry represent a minimum hurdle all potential business operators or owners must face before starting a business. Specific barriers will differ by industry. Some barriers are designed to protect society and purchasers of service, or are a result of the requirements of the industry.

Non-industry-specific barriers are regulatory requirements that all businesses encounter. These are laws and requirements that businesses must adhere to and satisfy. Requirements can range from filing quarterly and annual tax returns to having building inspections to ensure minimum code standards are being met for occupancy (e.g., proper fire exits and functioning fire alarms). All employers must adhere to specific laws regarding the payment of minimum wages and overtime and must contribute to the Social Security fund and to federal and state unemployment funds on behalf of their employees. In addition to specific payroll-related requirements, businesses must respect the rights of their employees. Employee rights include, but are not limited to, family and medical leave, proper notification before termination, the ability to purchase health care insurance under the Consolidated Omnibus Budget Reconciliation Act of 1985 (COBRA), and workers' compensation insurance that is paid by the employer. All laws and requirements related to employees are compliance oriented. Compliance means you follow the laws, regulations, or rules. Noncompliance means you do not follow the laws, regulations, or rules. There is no in-between. It is a binary equation where there are only two answers—yes or no, or true or false. This means that taxes were or were not paid on time, or policies and procedures do or do not exist. Compliance-driven systems represent minimum standards for maintaining certification or licensure.

The certification process enables HCFA to determine whether an applicant has the systems in place to provide appropriate patient care and a steady stream of information to HCFA. The certification process determines whether the applicant agency has sufficient human resources to provide care to Medicare enrollees, to maintain appropriate documentation and financial records, and to report on a timely basis. Once certified, all home health providers need to follow the rules and regulations associated with the Medicare program. Rules include but are not limited to ensuring that all patients are homebound and services rendered are reasonable and necessary as prescribed by a physician. Home health providers need to follow specific formats for billing and reporting and to satisfy state survey requirements or accreditation regulations by the Joint Commission on Accreditation of Healthcare Organizations (Joint Commission) or the Community Health Accreditation Program (CHAP).

HCFA has had the power to put "teeth" into its supplier agreements. Suppliers who do not follow the rules and requirements of the Medicare program may have committed fraud and abuse against the program and can be legally prosecuted. Prosecution could result in restitution, fines, imprisonment, and exclusion from further participation in the Medicare program. Prosecution for fraud/abuse can result from billing for services that were not provided, offering or paying cash or in-kind services for referrals, and misrepresenting the type of services provided. This has led to the development of federally mandated compliance programs such as Operation Restore Trust (ORT).

AGENCY INFRASTRUCTURE

An approach to dealing with the bureaucracy created by participating in the Medicare program has been to create compliance-driven organizations. HCFA expected information to be submitted in a specific format, on specific forms, and classified for its purposes. Therefore, to meet the needs of their largest customer (Medicare), agencies built their systems around meeting external regulatory and accreditation requirements. Perhaps the clearest example can be demonstrated by thinking about which customer an agency's financial systems may be serving.

Currently, agencies are required to file an annual cost report. The annual cost report requires the summarization of general ledger data into specific rows and columns in order to determine agency reimbursement for services provided to

Medicare beneficiaries. To facilitate accurate cost reporting, financial systems have been designed to capture data in a format that is easily transferable to the cost report. Financial systems also are set up to facilitate compliance with the federal Internal Revenue Service and state regulatory agencies.

Systems were also developed to gather all financial transactions into the general ledger. Many general ledger coding schemes were designed for ease of summarization and subsequent entry into the cost report. These coding schemes made meeting compliance-oriented requirements easier. Financial statements and management reports became byproducts of meeting third-party reporting requirements. This goal displacement occurred because management was more interested in meeting third-party reporting requirements than in addressing its own internal management requirements. Nowhere in the cost report or traditional financial statement can one learn how well agency services are satisfying customers or how effective operations are in assisting patients improve their ability to perform activities of daily living (ADLs).

This lack has led to the development of multiple tracking systems within an agency. In order to meet the diverse needs of clinical operations, human resource management, and fiscal management, organizations have had to purchase multiple off-the-shelf and industry-specific software packages to track data and support their evolving management requirements. These purchases have helped to meet short-term needs but have also created suboptimization at a systemic level. Suboptimization occurs through adding duplicative reporting and data entry requirements, creating inaccurate or conflicting reports, and causing difficulty in translating or transferring data between multiple software packages and platforms.

The emphasis on compliance is evident through the historic perspective of regulators and accrediting bodies whose primary concern is to verify that specific policies and procedures are in place. Policies and procedures provide a basis to evaluate agency structure and an agency's approach to dealing with areas critical to the delivery of home health services such as patient care and human resource administration. Policies and procedures, however, are often created in back rooms or purchased from consultants. The result usually represents a picture of the way things should run and does not always reflect current reality.

Compliance-driven systems tend to be costly to maintain because they are not closely linked to an agency's reason for being, or vision. Although the concept of vision will be addressed more fully in Chapter 5, it is logical that if you are a member of a compliance-driven organization, then all efforts expended toward the collection of data and subsequent reporting will be driven by the needs and requirements of a third party, such as a regulatory agency or accrediting body. In this scenario, organizational emphasis is placed on satisfying external requirements instead of pursuing the collective dream of the organization. The scenario can be easily illustrated. If an agency has developed a values-driven infrastructure that is linked to its vision, then it will collect data to measure whether it is on target in achieving its vision. Its entire infrastructure will have been developed based upon its values. The values will be evident in its policies and procedures, performance measurement systems, approaches to team development, and data gathering and reporting. On the other hand, a compliance-driven organization conducts business on an as-needed basis up until the impending visit from the accreditation body or state surveyors. Then there is a mad rush to make sure all the forms are in place and that all physician orders have been received and filed in the proper records. To reconcile the two approaches requires a shift in perspective.

A SHIFT IN PERSPECTIVE

A shift in perspective is evident by HCFA's proposal to change the conditions of participation (COPs) for home care agencies. HCFA's goal in updating the COPs is to move away from their historic perspective of regulatory compliance and instead to develop a partnership with all certified agencies. This shift is consistent with the statement by Bruce Vladeck, former head of HCFA, almost a decade ago, "External controls may focus on relatively secondary or tangential aspects of service quality not because anyone really believes they constitute high-quality service, but because that is what they are capable of focusing on."[4] HCFA's approach is to identify areas where minimum performance is required and to mandate that all agencies begin to focus on performance improvement, the actual care delivered to the patient, whether the provided care has improved the health status of its patients, and the performance of the home health agency as an organization. The primary focus will be on patients' rights, the provision of a comprehensive assessment, patient care planning and coordination, quality assessment, and performance improvement. HCFA's goal is to

- Improve outcomes of care and satisfaction for patients
- Reduce the burden on providers
- Increase flexibility and expectations for continuous improvement
- Increase the quantity and quality of information on which to base health care choices and efforts to improve quality
- Improve stakeholder relationships, specifically the supplier-customer relationship

It has been said that the proposed changes parallel the 1997–1998 Joint Commission standards for home care accreditation. Joint Commission standards typically have been compliance oriented except for the addition of a section on improvement of performance. This section, similar to HCFA's proposal, shifts responsibility to agency management for the continual improvement of performance and operational results. Both the Joint Commission and HCFA have identified the need to collect data in order to improve performance. The challenge will be to identify data that are critical to pursuing organizational strategy and performance excellence as opposed to those required for regulatory compliance.

Obviously, there is a cost associated with data collection. To collect data for the sake of collecting data and to do nothing with collected data are non-value-adding activities. Therefore, it is important to understand why data are being collected. For instance, are data going to be used for regulatory compliance or to improve the agency's approach to the delivery of care, to increase patients' satisfaction, to improve support processes, or to reduce cycle time associated with performing admission visits? If data are collected solely for regulatory compliance, then the agency should try to minimize the cost associated with the data collection activity. Ideally, all data collection costs should be minimized; automation provides a vehicle to accomplish this goal. It may not always be possible to automate data collection requirements, however, so a critical review may be necessary to answer the following questions:

- Why are we collecting the data?
- Who uses the data?
- How are the data used?
- Is there a better way to collect the data?
- Once collected, how often are the data used?
- Should data be collected on an occurrence or sample basis?
- Are these data used to enhance clinical operations?
- Are these data used to enhance administrative operations?
- Are they collected solely to meet external requirements?
- Is data collection related to organizational strategy?
- Have the data been collected consistently and are they reliable for forecasting?
- Are our results comparable to industry benchmarks?

The primary purpose of data collection beyond regulatory compliance is to improve operations and processes. Data provide the basis for making decisions and forecasts about the future. The overriding question with regard to data collection is, Will the collection of data enable us to monitor the pursuit of our strategies and the satisfaction of our customers? This basic concept is illustrated in Figure 4–1.

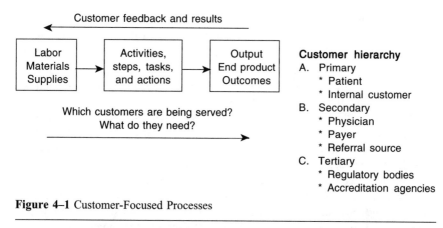

Figure 4–1 Customer-Focused Processes

Figure 4–1 builds upon the concept of processes initially identified in Chapter 1. An agency is made up of multiple processes. The questions are:

- Who are the customers of the processes?
- Are they being served?
- What do they need?

Once the initial questions have been answered, data need to be collected to determine whether process output is meeting customer needs and accomplishing agency goals. All processes can be broken down into three distinct elements: (1) input, (2) process or activities, and (3) output. Output is a result. It could be a finished report, a completed visit, a discharged patient, or the monthly financial statement. Historically, agencies have been designed to meet the needs of regulatory and accrediting bodies and, as illustrated in Figure 4–1, these customers represent the lowest level of the customer hierarchy.

The distinction between the historical design and the new customer-driven design is perspective and provision of value. Who is the agency serving? What is the primary purpose of the agency? Who pays the bills?

Therefore, the real question is, Does the agency want to make a difference? If the answer is yes, then the perspective needs to shift onto the primary and secondary customer groups and efforts to satisfy the needs of tertiary customers must be minimized. Yes, it is still necessary to meet the requirements of regulatory agencies and accrediting bodies. To make a difference, however, an organization's infrastructure needs to focus on meeting and exceeding the needs of the first two customer groups. This can be accomplished by transitioning away from meeting the minimum requirements established in the Joint Commission standards and HCFA regulations and instead asking your customers what they want. The shift in perspective is all-inclusive. It requires taking a step backward and asking, What are we really about? If answered honestly, the response will probably include serving customers instead of serving regulatory agencies. It will include critically looking at the processes that have been created within the agency and asking, "Who are we serving? Are we as effective and efficient as we can be? How can we improve?"

When this concept is followed through to the next step, management reporting contains multiple perspectives. Each perspective, if linked to agency strategy, will provide management with a gauge of where they are in relationship to their goals/vision. In the opening example, the gauge could be a compass, radar, sextant, or any other instrument that could keep the vessel pointed toward its ultimate destination regardless of the turbulence of its current environment. Therefore, agency management reporting could include results of customer satisfaction surveys, indicators reflecting percent of patients who met their expected outcomes on time, percent of patients achieving outcomes within anticipated pathway costs, financial results, and indicators of employee satisfaction. The shift in perspective channels all operational results into a common reporting tool that will inform everyone where the agency stands in relationship to its goals. Comparing actual results to goals provides an opportunity for corrective action, but more important, for continual improvement and pursuit of long-term goals. Ultimately, the aim is to track and trend improvements over time. Trending, or the graphing of data over time, enables the graphical illustration of an agency's progress toward its goals and will be key to satisfying the Joint Commission's improvement of performance standards.[5]

SCORECARDS

Management produces financial statements to convey results to board members, lenders, fiscal intermediaries, shareholders, and staff. Financial statements and ratios derived from the financial statements represent lagging indicators.[6] Stated differently, the results reflected in an agency's financial statements are the results of actions that were set in motion prior to the period recorded in the financial statement. These actions could have occurred a month, quarter, or year before a specific financial statement was produced. Actions taken by management today will not be reflected in the financial results until some specified period of time following their implementation. Reliance solely upon financial or lag indicators has the potential to jeopardize long-term viability.

This concept can be illustrated with a simple example. An agency begins negotiating with a managed care organization (MCO) to provide services. After a six-month negotiation the agency is awarded a two-year contract. During the two years, its financial statements reflect a significant profit margin due to this contract. The contract was not renewed or renegotiated at the end of the two-year period because of customer dissatisfaction with patient results and process reliability. This example illustrates two things. The first point is the concept of lagging indicators. The profits being reflected on the current financial statement (the last month of the two-year contract) were the results of actions taken two years and six months prior to the current financial statement (i.e., during the original negotiations). Financial indicators are usually lagging indicators. The second point is that the agency was not measuring or reflecting customer satisfaction, process improvements, and organizational growth. Customer satisfaction, process improvements, and organizational growth represent leading indicators.[7] They are leading indicators because they measure the current pulse of the operating environment. They are also an indicator of the effectiveness of the underlying processes that management has created. Leading indicators are rarely financial in nature. In the above example, if the agency had been paying attention to its leading indicators, it may have been able to salvage the contract. It would have known that the MCO was not pleased with the service it was providing because of the poor customer satisfaction results indicated on its surveys. Employees were not happy and this unhappiness translated to poor employee satisfaction. Agency processes were unreliable because of a lack of management and staff accountability. Had the agency paid attention to these leading indicators instead of the lagging financial indicators, it would not have been surprised that the contract was not renewed.

In the preceding example the agency had met all of the compliance-oriented requirements to get the initial contract. The agency, however, had not developed an internal assessment system to focus on the key elements of a successful organization: customer satisfaction, defined key processes, organizational learning, and continuous improvement. Its perspective was compliance-based instead of improvement-oriented.

A solution was developed by Robert Kaplan and David Norton from Harvard University. They developed an approach to measuring operations known as the Balanced Scorecard.[8] The Balanced Scorecard (BSC) provides a tool to assess an organization holistically. The BSC consists of four main categories: (1) financial, (2) customer, (3) organizational learning (and continuous improvement), and (4) internal processes. Within each category, performance measures are developed to assess agency operations from a strategic perspective. By combining leading and lagging indicators of agency performance, the BSC provides a tool to communicate agency vision and strategy, set goals, align processes, and align work groups or teams. The BSC provides the performance measurement system for setting agency strategy and providing a framework for the development of cascading objectives as illustrated previously in Figure 3–3. This approach facilitates the alignment of goals, clarifies objectives, and enables leadership to focus all resources toward strategic objectives. Moreover, by concentrating on lead and lag indicators there is an opportunity to create a balance between operational requirements and organizational results.

"Management reviews and updates the shift from reviewing the past to learning about the future. Managers discuss not only how past results have been achieved but also whether their expectations for the future remain on track."[9] This outlook is consistent with the direction that HCFA has decided to go in changing the COPs. HCFA is interested in having agencies track predictive measures that will be better indicators of factors that contribute to a patient's ability to achieve specific outcomes.

Exhibit 4–1 represents a list of possible performance measures that could be used in the development of a BSC using agency-specific metrics.

Scorecards can also be used as a marketing tool. For instance, if an agency is demonstrating significant results in customer satisfaction and clinical outcomes, it could use these results to approach potential referral sources and MCOs to generate additional business. Scorecards can also be used to compare results among different organizations. An example of this is the Health Plan Employer Data and Information Set, commonly referred to as HEDIS. HEDIS is sponsored by the National Committee for Quality Assurance (NCQA), and its goal is to provide purchasers and consumers with information in order to make educated choices among health plans.

The HEDIS scorecard measures results across eight dimensions. The goal of the scorecard is to provide consumers with information that goes beyond the cost of the health plan. The eight categories are listed below.

1. effectiveness of care
2. access/availability of care
3. satisfaction with the experience of care
4. health plan stability (disenrollment rate)
5. use of services
6. cost of care
7. informed health care choices
8. health plan descriptive information

Developing performance measures at an agency level that are consistent with the reporting requirements of MCOs provides a vehicle that can be used to meet the needs of the agency customers. For instance, developing indicators to demonstrate the effectiveness of care by patient problem or the satisfaction with the experience of care across service lines will be useful in meeting the needs of both the MCO and the agency. Moreover, using HEDIS can be a two-way street if an agency uses HEDIS to evaluate whether the MCO is a desirable customer. Stated differently, if the health plan is not stable the agency could be at risk for collecting receivables. The same is true for the BSC if creative leaders use results to share information with lenders, potential partners, and prospective staff. Such sharing

Exhibit 4–1 Possible Indicators To Use in Developing a Balanced Scorecard

Financial	Service line profitability Working capital turnover ratio (activity ratio) Return on equity (profitability ratio) Cash-flow-to-debt ratio (capital structure ratio) Economic value added Payer mix Risk mix Percent growth by service line
Customer	Market share Customer satisfaction: • by branch or location • by service line • by discipline • by program On-time delivery
Organizational learning and continuous improvement	Evaluation of staff competency by job category Continuous quality improvements Value-added vs. non-value-adding activities Percent of staff participating on teams Percent of employees vs. contract staff Staff satisfaction Access to information Staff productivity using an activity-based costing format
Internal processes	Clinical outcomes Medication management Cycle time reduction Measures of process efficiency: • submission of paperwork • initial assessment time frame • collection of accounts receivable Measures of effectiveness: • submission of claims (no re-billing or edit correction) • improvement in medical condition or ADL • payroll checks are correct Job-related injuries Internal customer surveys

enables outsiders to gain an understanding of the inner workings of the company that would not have been known solely from evaluating financial statements.[10] This information has the potential to create a competitive advantage for those providers who measure and manage both lead and lag indicators and demonstrate achievement of multiple goals.

The goal in using scorecards is to communicate information to internal and external customers. HEDIS primarily targets external customers. The BSC is used for aligning an agency's objectives so that all members of the agency can work toward a common goal. As depicted previously in Figure 3–3, once the performance measures are developed at the agency or strategic level, they must be cascaded down to the process and work unit or team level. This cascading provides an opportunity for the development of metrics that everyone can relate to their specific job, helping employees understand how their unique functions contribute to the accomplishment of strategic goals. Furthermore, by shifting away from a compliance-oriented perspective to one based upon continuous improvement and organizational growth, there is an opportunity to create a sense of shared vision and community. This "glue" creates a common platform for alignment of objectives and a focusing on vision-oriented goals and provides clarity when making value-based decisions.

EXTRINSIC VERSUS INTRINSIC MOTIVATION

Both HCFA and the Joint Commission are providing a source of extrinsic motivation to continually improve processes. There is an inherent problem with extrinsic motivation, however. Extrinsic motivation is doing something for someone else. Extrinsic motivation can be used to capture market share, have everything polished before the visiting dignitary arrives, or have all of the standards and guidelines updated and records in place before the surveyors arrive. Once the moment passes, however, staff fall back into habitual patterns.

Intrinsic motivation comes from within. It is done because of an individual or collective need to accomplish a goal, pursue a vision, or live by consistent values. The goal could be continuous improvement, the pursuit of higher learning and integration of one's learning into daily work life, or the intent to become "world class." The result is an organization that views customers and co-workers as dignitaries, satisfies operational requirements (regulatory and accreditation) as an inherent part of daily operations, and is concerned with exceeding goals more for the inherent challenge than to meet someone else's expectations. Intrinsic motivation is a long-term strategy. It is a way of life based upon heartfelt desires, not a head game. At its most basic level it is akin to doing what you do because you want to, not because someone (e.g., your mother, regulatory agencies) told you to.

Several environmental conditions or prerequisites must be present to build intrinsic motivation. They are

1. personal security
2. psychological safety, established by having an environment in which one's worth is accepted and one is treated with recognition and respect
3. psychological freedom; the freedom to think, feel, be whatever is most true for oneself. It is permission to be free, which includes permission to be responsible, to be afraid, to be wrong, and to be confused[11]
4. true participation, embracing the values of empowerment and trust

A culture that fosters these conditions will promote the benefits that come from the breakthroughs within it. Organizational culture and values will depend upon leadership's approach to its employees. For instance, if leadership is actively engaged in field visits with the professionals, has lunch with clerical staff, and is genuinely concerned about them, their issues, and work-related problems, it is creating a culture that says the customer and staff are important. A leadership team that views staff as a commodity, never leaving its ivory towers or visiting clients, is making an adversarial statement to its staff. It is extremely difficult to motivate staff if they feel that the words of leadership are not consistent with their actions.

This can be illustrated another way. Human beings need interaction. They need to be acknowledged for their efforts. Acknowledgment can be as simple as a genuine "Well done" or "Good job." Often it is the little things that make a difference and, if done sincerely and on a regular basis, will contribute more to the creation of intrinsic motivation than the more grandiose events such as a big summer picnic or holiday party. Think about your relationship with your spouse or significant other. Wouldn't you rather have an occasional flower bouquet handed to you, a special dinner prepared, a back rub, or any other act of kindness on a regular basis than nothing all year long except for a big birthday gift? It is the regular and unexpected acts of kindness that warm our hearts, create intrinsic motivation to work toward goals, and help us to believe in an organizational vision.

An underlying value here is commitment: commitment to agency mission, vision, and values, and to the customer at every level of the organization, from the chief executive officer to the maintenance worker who cleans up at night. Without commitment the best one can expect is compliance. Complying to someone else's mission or vision is boring at best, and may yield quality, but not performance excellence. An analogy is the patient who is asked to comply with a care plan, let's say a diet plan, that was devised by a well-meaning health care team to assist the patient in losing weight to alleviate hypertension. Some patients may do well with the diet plan, at least in the short run, depending on how "good" they are and how supportive the team is, and some patients will be "noncompliant." However, getting the patient involved in the development of his or her own diet plan that addresses the required changes (reduced sodium, reduced fat) and accommodates his or her "likes" gets the patient interested in his or her health state and *committed* to reducing the weight as a means to be healthier. It gives the patient his or her best chance to get the weight off and keep it off. So it is with getting employees committed to their work. It gives them their best chance to perform at their optimum level.

> Concerning all acts of initiative (and creation) there is one elementary truth, the ignorance of which kills countless ideas and splendid plans: that the moment one definitely commits oneself, then Providence moves too. All sorts of things occur to help one that would never otherwise have occurred. A whole stream of events issue from the decision, raising in one's favor all manner of unforeseen incidents and meetings, and material assistance, which no (human) could have dreamed would have come his or her way.
>
> —Goethe

Building commitment is based on alignment of staff and agency vision, mission, and values. This alignment is a result of a dynamic interaction between staff and administration. It means that administration includes staff in all aspects of agency strategy and operations in order to establish a milieu of ownership.

A CUSTOMER-ORIENTED PERSPECTIVE

To move beyond mediocrity and pursue performance excellence requires developing a customer-oriented perspective. A customer-oriented perspective deals with the external environment. It requires understanding what actions are necessary to satisfy patients and payers. It occurs through developing the systems to continually assess customers' requirements and measure changing perceptions of how well you are doing in meeting their requirements. This process could be as simple as meeting with payers on a monthly or quarterly basis to discuss results and to learn about their expansion plans or new offerings; or, if they are MCOs, to see how you could help them exceed their NCQA requirements.

Listening to the voice of the customer is an important strategy for long-term survival. Strategies can be as simple as having coffee on a regular basis with referring physicians, having a cookie break with nurses and aides who have returned from the field, or following up with patients and staff on written survey suggestions. More sophisticated methods include conducting focus groups, organizing telephone surveys, or hiring an external market research company. The goal is to learn what customers want and to develop programs or protocols to meet and anticipate their evolving needs.

Ways to listen can be formal or informal. Formal examples are the annual written surveys that are sent to referring physicians, referral sources, and MCOs. On a more frequent basis, patients and families receive surveys upon admission, while they are on service, and after they have been discharged. The survey questionnaire may be completed by the patient or family or conducted by an interviewer via telephone or in person. Data gathered during these formal processes are summarized, and the summaries provide the basis for process improvement plans.

Informal listening can include any patient feedback such as interaction with staff at a physician's office or at the local hospital, or even in the supermarket. Informal sources of information can lead to the identification of opportunities to correct problems, improve services, or meet an unexpressed customer need. Collection and usage of informal data to drive strategy and improvement efforts can be as valuable as formal methods. The challenge is to provide a format for the collection and evaluation of data to obtain meaningful information.

The internal customer includes all clinical and administrative staff members, suppliers, and the board. These people represent the agency's customer service agents or goodwill ambassadors. Collectively, these individuals are responsible for understanding customer needs and requirements and developing the processes to measure, evaluate, and improve the services that are being offered. It is through the continued efforts of all staff members that organizations can create an unique culture that differentiates them from competitors, and more important, will provide the intrinsic motivation to achieve performance excellence.

Performance excellence is holistic in nature. The human body is an example of performance excellence. There are major systems within the body that all work in unison, adjust to changing circumstances, and regenerate and repair themselves. Performance excellence is possible in organizations as well. It requires a shift in perspective from mere compliance to adhering to values. The challenge is to have a consistent understanding and application of values in order to succeed. In the preceding example of the body as a system of performance excellence, it is possible to demonstrate how dysfunction can occur. In the case of paralysis, nerve impulses do not connect with the muscles that they were intended for, so muscles do not function correctly. This is the same in organizations. When organizations are not aligned to common value and measurement systems, then dysfunction occurs. Using the preceding analogy, if an agency transitions to an environment utilizing teams and does not change its individual performance review processes to reflect this transition to teams, an inconsistency exists. This inconsistency will prevent team-level optimization because staff know they are not judged by their peers but instead by a supervisor, or manager, who may not have an understanding of their contributions and efforts on behalf of the team.

The above is one example of an impediment to performance excellence. Performance excellence is achievable by involving all agency staff, board members, and suppliers. It requires rethinking old strategies that may have served the agency well in the past but are outdated and prevent the organization from moving forward.

THE COMMUNITY AS A CUSTOMER

What is your agency's contribution to your community? Home health agencies have traditionally provided various gratuitous services during community fairs such as blood pressure screenings and flu shots. The real question is how community need is assessed. What role does agency administration play in assessing the needs of the community and working to develop a plan to meet those needs? Obviously, there is a resource limitation from an agency perspective. But if agencies work in conjunction with other providers such as physician groups, hospitals, outpatient clinics, and local businesses, there is no reason that the local community could not adopt specific strategies for community wellness. For instance, there may be a need for Meals on Wheels, volunteers to drive the elderly to their physician offices, or providers to educate new mothers. Everyone in the community can contribute to meet the needs of the community.

Hopefully, the movement to managed care will have a positive impact upon community health. For instance, as larger regional health care centers begin to move toward self-insurance, they will have a vested interest in the well-being of their community. This investment is especially true if community well-being translates into fewer emergency visits, fewer hospitalizations, and less need for services that are prevented through routine checkups, a balanced diet, or a community support system. In fact, this is the nucleus of public health. Wouldn't it be wonderful if the MCOs, the regional health systems, and the physicians realized that home health represents a mobile delivery arm of the health care system that could be an effective way of delivering curative, preventive, and educational services to the elderly, disabled, and poor? The reality is that where community members are under a managed care contract, they become the customers of the agency even when they are well. Using the public health model, agencies can conduct community assessments that focus on the prevalence of disease or risk factors and establish preventive programs accordingly.

Community assessment is, in fact, the keystone of public health practice. The appraisal of the community involves the collection and analysis of various kinds of data and the combined judgment of many disciplines. Some of the data will be precise while other data will be inferences. Ultimately, the level of community health is decided based on three interdependent, interactive, and constantly changing conditions.[12]

The Health Status of the Community. The health status of a population involves people and their environment.

* people factors:
    –the characteristics and growth trends of the population (e.g., changes in birth rates; age, sex, and racial characteristics; educational achievements)
    –trends in the death experiences, especially untimely deaths
    –prevalence of presymptomatic illness
    –number and location of vulnerable or special risk groups
    –number and characteristics of those functioning below their potential health level[13]
* environment factors:
    –physical environment (e.g., air and water quality, adequacy of housing)
    –social environment (e.g., use of drugs, prevalence of gangs, provision for recreation)[14]

The Health Capability of the Community, or the Ability of the Community To Deal with Its Health Problems. A powerful determinant of the ability of a community to address its health issues is the general economic situation and the distribution of wealth. Within this context it is important to know to what extent the available institutional and human resources (professional and volunteer) are able to address the well-being of the population.

The Health Action Potential of the Community, or the Ways in which the Community Is Likely To Work with Its Health Problems. Every community will differ in how it deals with its health problems based on the values and beliefs of the individual and corporate community members, the political system by which it is governed, and community response to health problems.[15]

Assessing need, providing necessary services, and meeting the needs of communities cannot be done single-handedly. It will require resources in multiple forms. Home health can be the leader in assessing community need, acquiring and channeling resources, and assessing community impact. Every cause needs a champion, and this may be a natural calling for home health leaders.

AN APPROACH TOWARD A CUSTOMER-FOCUSED SYSTEM

One approach toward developing a customer-focused system is to involve all staff, board members, and suppliers in an agency's goal setting process. If the goal is to develop a customer-focused system of performance excellence, then management will need to focus its resources toward common goals. Therefore, to achieve this result, everyone needs to know what goals are important to the agency. Once goals are understood, then it is possible to identify how each group will work toward the common goals.

Let's say an agency has determined that its strategy for growth will be to compete for managed care contracts. It has completed an assessment of what managed care companies are paying for services in its area, it has completed an analysis of its competitors' cost structure, and it knows how much its cost structure needs to be modified. This information can be used as part of a planning session to identify the agency's current cost structure, its goals, and potential interim milestones for cost reductions. By looking at this systematically, the agency could break down the composition of cost into primary and secondary processes. Once this has been accomplished, the agency could then begin to examine data within each of these subsets. The aim is to get all staff thinking and working toward the common goal of achieving an agreed-upon cost reduction. This may be accomplished through the elimination of activities (not necessarily personnel) that do not add value to the agency's customers, automating manual processes to reduce repetitive data entry, or eliminating reports that were asked for once and produced ever since.

Cost reduction is a concern to most employees because of the horror stories they have heard regarding downsizing, reengineering, delayering, and rightsizing. The missing element is values. If the organization values its staff, it will be up-front with them about strategies, the need for cost reduction, and the need to work toward collective goals. If everyone is in the same boat (working toward a common cause), the usual behavior is to rally toward the cause. If however, the staff sense an inconsistency between the speech and subsequent actions, then there is a values disalignment and a dysfunctional organization. To avoid this scenario is a leadership challenge. It is a leadership challenge to be honest and open and not misplace the trust that staff have placed in your words and actions.

The same can be said for any other strategy the agency may embark upon, whether it focuses on increasing customer satisfaction, improving medication management, improving staff satisfaction, improving staff competency, or reducing cycle time. The point is that leadership, values, and vision provide the foundation for systems thinking. It is the focus on staff development, process design, and improvement with respect to vision, values, leadership, and systems thinking that will ensure the achievement of organizational outcomes. This concept is illustrated in Figure 4–2.

Figure 4–2 illustrates the concept of a system alignment. At the pyramid's base, or foundation, are values, vision, mission, and culture. This foundation is created and influenced by the organization's leaders. This influence will be evidenced by what values they create. Values and vision will influence the selection, hiring, and training of management and staff. Management will create the processes to meet customer needs. It is the activities of staff within the processes designed by

Customer and market focus

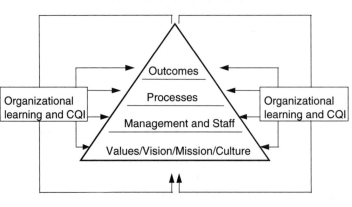

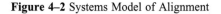

Leadership

Organizational Alignment

Figure 4–2 Systems Model of Alignment

---

management that produce results or outcomes. In this illustration, leaders, the culture they create, the staff that are hired, and the processes that are created represent the organization's infrastructure. It is the infrastructure that enables outcomes to be achieved. Outcomes should be designed to meet the evolving needs of the marketplace and the customer base that is served. Paying attention to the needs of customers, the external marketplace, and the larger health care delivery system will provide an opportunity for agency leadership to continually revise its infrastructure to deliver ever-improving outcomes. Therefore, outcomes can be influenced by changes made in any of the enabling elements of the infrastructure. One approach for changing the infrastructure is to create an environment that thrives on continuous quality improvement (CQI) and organizational learning. Once created, however, the environment needs to align reward systems to stimulate momentum, to encourage experimentation, and to share, encourage, and reward learning across all levels. The power of this approach is in involving all staff members, suppliers, and board members in achieving the larger goals of the agency. This is where the "rubber hits the road"; when the plan becomes part of the everyday perspective or an intrinsic drive to accomplish something bigger than the self . . . to be part of a winning team.

STRATEGY

The purpose of strategy is to gain a competitive advantage. This means that an agency needs to evaluate the external environment and determine what course of action would be most successful. The essence of a home health agency's strategy is to differentiate what it can do best from all its possible choices (services) and pursue the best choices. This concept is particularly important for home care agencies that attempt to be all things to all people (i.e., provide all services requested of them). This way of conducting business is contrary to strategic thinking.

Strategy answers the basic question, Where are we going? Strategic planning, then, is concerned with establishing the major directions for the agency: its mission, the customers it chooses to serve, the services it wants to offer, and the geographical region it wants to cover. It is this strategic planning that is used to cope with the changing external environment. Once the strategic planning has been done, then agency operations determine the best way to provide the services.

To meet the purpose and fulfill the essence of strategy, two major questions need to be answered:[16]

1. What major changes will take place in our industry in the next several years? The answers focus on the opportunities and threats that will be presented to the agency from the external environment in the coming years.
2. What role should the agency play in the changing industry? The answer focuses on the strengths and weaknesses of the agency and its internal capability.

THE LARGER PERSPECTIVE

The larger perspective is that the health care delivery system is changing. Being compliant with regulatory requirements will not ensure profitability or long-term viability. By understanding trends occurring within the community, region, state, and nation, the agency has an opportunity to increase the probability for long-term viability and improved quality. Focusing on internal infrastructure will provide a vehicle to strengthen the agency. By developing relationships with the payers, MCOs, physician groups, hospitals, long-term care facilities, and employer coalitions, an agency will enhance its opportunity for favorable positioning in the changing delivery system. Again, this is about perspective; clarity in goals, objectives, and strategies; and focusing on how the organization can serve the community or participate in the larger picture. It is through the expansion of customer focus and negotiation with payers that opportunities will arise. Opportunities could initially look like losses. For instance, perhaps a major referral source has been lost and it is questionable whether it makes sense to remain in business. If the larger perspective is shifted to recognize opportunities that may exist, based upon agency strength, values, and employee suggestions, a new service line might develop in response to lost business. Although this may be an extreme case, it underscores several key points. First, if survival is threatened by an external event, draw upon your internal resources for ideas and suggestions. Involve employees in the decision-making process and future directions. Second, opportunities are never pursued by maintaining the status quo. It may have been that if the managed care contract was won, it would have consumed more resources than anticipated, thereby weakening other programs. Agency personnel can now use this experience and rally to land a more reasonable contract. Finally, developing a strong relationship within and outside of your organization will provide a vehicle for self-renewal. It is no longer one person solving all of the world's problems, but the working of many people who have multiple talents and abilities. If these talents are harnessed properly, the ability to create results far exceeds the capabilities of any one individual, as in the old saying "many hands make light work"—and many hands make it better.

CONCLUSION

Laws and regulations are created to protect purchasers, citizens, and communities. Following laws and regulations is the first step in being a community player. Focusing on the requirements of regulatory and accreditation bodies will satisfy these tertiary customers, however are these regulatory bodies the customers upon whom you really want to focus your major efforts? This chapter has discussed perspective, clarity of purpose, and focusing on customer/community service. If your perspective is about getting by, then follow regulatory guidelines for data collection and improvement activities. But if you want to make a difference, then elevate your perspective to meet the evolving needs of a diverse customer base, by interacting with the community and aligning performance measurement systems with strategic objectives. Accomplish all of this by utilizing the unique talents of your staff.

Albert Einstein believed we use only a small portion of our brain matter. If we were able to tap into all the additional potential, imagine what amazing individuals we could be. The same is true for organizations, except when you apply the preceding concept to an organization its potential grows exponentially. The challenge begins with whether leadership is willing to be honest with itself and its staff—whether leadership is willing to stand up and say that it doesn't have all of the answers, is human, and is willing to walk its talk. Furthermore, if an organization decides to pursue performance excellence, it will not happen overnight; it will be an uphill learning process. But imagine, once you got up to the top of the hill and accomplished your dream, what a rush that would be. If people in all organizations invested their unique talents toward accomplishing this common goal, then there would be no need for organizations like the Joint Commission and CHAP.

NOTES

1. Health Care Financing Administration, *Health Care Financing Review*, 1996 Statistical Supplement, 10.

2. HCFA, *Health Care Financing Review*, 1996 Statistical Supplement, 20.

3. HCFA, *Health Care Financing Review*, 1996 Statistical Supplement, 10.

4. B.C. Vladeck, Quality Assurance through External Controls, *INQUIRY* 25 (Spring 1988): 103.

5. Facing a Survey? Watch for More "A" Standards, *Homecare Quality Management, American Health Consultants* 3, no. 3 (March 1997): 36.

6. R.S. Kaplan and D.P. Norton, *The Balanced Scorecard* (Cambridge, MA: Harvard Business School Press, 1996), 24.

7. Kaplan and Norton, *The Balanced Scorecard*, 73.

8. Kaplan and Norton, *The Balanced Scorecard*, 7.

9. Kaplan and Norton, *The Balanced Scorecard*, 15.

10. P. Bierbusse and T. Siesfeld, Measures That Matter, *Strategic Performance Measurement* 1, no. 2 (April/May 1997): 6–11.

11. W. Harmon and H. Rheingold, *Higher Creativity* (Los Angeles: Jeremy P. Tarcher, Inc., 1984).

12. S. Clemen-Stone et al., *Comprehensive Community Health Nursing* (Philadelphia: Mosby, 1995), 429–459.

13. R.B. Freeman, *Community Health Nursing Practice* (Philadelphia: W.B. Saunders Company, 1970), 254–256.

14. Freeman, *Community Health Nursing Practice*, 256–257.

15. Freeman, *Community Health Nursing Practice*, 259–260.

16. D.D. McConkey, *How To Manage by Results*, 4th ed. (New York: AMACOM, 1983).

CHAPTER 5

How Firm a Foundation?

The dictionary defines foundation as a basis upon which something stands or is supported. Foundation in the context of an organization addresses the guiding principles or tenets that were instrumental in creating the organization. Most important, it provides a framework for developing the ongoing organizational infrastructure and philosophy for dealing with internal and external customers. Many people instinctively think of foundations as made of bricks and mortar. Our prior experiences lead us to view an organizational foundation as solid, financially secure, privately held, public, or nonprofit. These descriptions tend to be impersonal and factual and do little to explain the inner workings of the organization, which are represented by the values and beliefs of the individuals that make up the organization. It is this inner foundation that inspires and sustains individuals to come together collectively as an organization with a specific mission or purpose and to take responsibility for their future.

This chapter discusses

- vision
- mission
- values

Vision, mission, and values are collectively referred to as an organization's governing ideas.[1] It is an agency's governing ideas that will dictate how it deals with patients, payers, partners, staff, the community, regulatory agencies, and accreditation bodies. It is the governing ideas that will provide a sense of meaning for staff, and a focus for short- and longer-term strategies, while providing a framework for the design of the organizational infrastructure. "Taken as a unit, all three governing ideas answer the question, 'What do we believe in?' "[2 (p.224)] Understanding an organization's governing ideas provides context for all operating decisions, such as how the agency defines and measures quality, what data it collects, and how it incurs costs for these operations. Of equal or greater importance is that the development and refinement of an organization's governing ideas provide a common platform for all staff to interact with one another, interact with the external community, and align their own personal vision, mission, and values with that of the organization. If there is no alignment, there is no match and no amount of time, training, or coaching will make a difference. If on the other hand there is alignment, then there is an opportunity for an individual to grow within the organization. This creates a value-adding process for both the individual and organization.

VISION

In the context of an organization's governing ideas or foundation, vision is an ideal or desired future state into which the organization will eventually evolve. In Proverbs 29:18 it states, "Where there is no vision the people perish." Vision often has been thought of as having a mystical connotation or dreamlike quality, perhaps because it implies something that has not happened or because visioning also had roots in many of the Native American cultures, where the act of visioning was left to tribal elders and shamans, and/or induced through ingesting a hallucinogen.[3] These individuals were responsible for forecasting the future and protecting their people. Regardless of whether vision and visioning has a mystical root, the ability to create a robust image for human beings to believe in and work toward serves an extremely powerful purpose in today's health care organizations. "A vision must give people the feeling that their lives and work are intertwined and moving toward recognizable, legitimate goals."[4] (p.85) Vision creates a "cause," something that is bigger than one individual, worth working or fighting for, and is intrinsically motivating.[5]

What is vision? Vision is a picture or image of something we want to create. It identifies how an individual or an organization will be of service to mankind. Vision provides context for the development of a mission statement, values, and identification of strategic direction. Vision also becomes a tool to motivate, focus, and align individuals within an organization. Alignment is an extremely important concept and is critical to organizational success. Vision provides a picture, an image, and a sense of urgency about a desired future state that all work units, teams, or departments can work toward. The challenge is to provide a unifying framework so that everyone works toward the achievement of a common vision and not individual interpretations of the organization's vision. If there is no framework a dysfunctional organization can result.

A dysfunctional organization can occur when the individual in charge of clinical services has one interpretation of the agency's vision, the financial manager has a different interpretation, and the chief executive officer (CEO) has yet another interpretation. Each individual shapes the elements of the organization they control based upon their interpretation of the strategies critical to achieve the organization's vision. In a cost-reimbursed world this approach would not have been detrimental to the agency's long-term viability. In a risk-based environment characterized by capitated managed care contracts, severely discounted per-visit payments, and shifting referral streams, however, multiple strategies are detrimental to long-term viability.

More than ever, agency vision must be clearly defined and quantifiable. Otherwise, there is no way to focus staff and align them toward common goals. In the preceding example, clinical operations and financial operations could have been at odds if the agency vision was *to provide and promote effective and efficient health care services in the home.* The clinical operations person could interpret that statement to mean that effectiveness requires many visits to achieve clinical outcomes, highly trained and competent staff, and the latest in medical equipment and supplies. The financial person could interpret the same statement to mean that efficient services require low utilization, higher staff productivity, and a smaller overhead structure. The result is a duality in perspectives that will probably be manifested by wasted time and activities spent defending opposing actions and perspectives.

If on the other hand the same vision statement was developed and supported by specific strategies such as providing cost-effective services, demonstrable quality, and stakeholder satisfaction, then it would be possible to develop performance metrics to evaluate what the desired future state will look like. Furthermore, when compared against current reality, the difference between the desired future state and current reality creates a gap. This is illustrated in Figure 5–1. Gap identification enables an agency to align human resources and devise a strategy for closing the gap. The strategy depends upon organizational mission, values, infrastructure, and the agency's assessment of internal strengths and weaknesses and external opportunities and threats (through a SWOT analysis). Pursuing vision-oriented performance metrics will enable the achievement of a future state. Attainment of future-oriented goals will take time. Performance measurement systems may also change during this time as organizational performance responds to the changing external environment. This is not problematic, however, if the revised performance measurement systems remain vision oriented.

It is interesting to note that a study of publicly traded companies that were driven by organizational vision yielded a return to their shareholders 15 times greater than the general market.[6] Moreover, "the use of vision as a management tool is the most significant determinant for easing from a bureaucratic to a flexible organization. When combined with top management commitment, vision accounts for the success of quality management programs." [7 (p.84)]

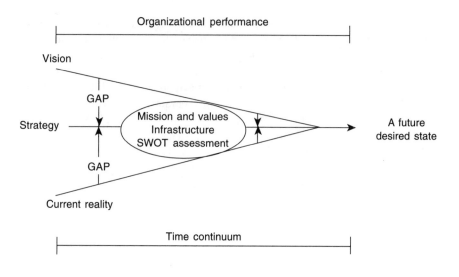

Figure 5–1 Alignment of Organizational Performance

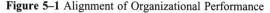

There is no magic template for vision statement development or style. Vision statements range from three lines to an entire page. The acid test, however, is whether the vision is meaningful to all staff. The objective is to organize the goals, dreams, ideas, and inspiration of the organization's staff and create a statement that provides meaning and inspiration to all members of the agency.

Peter Senge, in *The Fifth Discipline,* differentiates between positive and negative vision.

> "What do we want?" is different from "What do we want to avoid?" This seems obvious, but in fact negative visions are probably more common than positive visions. Many organizations truly pull together only when their survival is threatened. They focus on avoiding what people don't want: being taken over, going bankrupt, losing jobs, losing market share, having downturns in earnings, or "letting our competitors beat us to market with our next new product."
>
> Negative visions are limiting for three reasons. Firstly, energy that could build something new is diverted to "preventing" something we don't want to happen. Secondly, negative visions carry a subtle, yet unmistakable, message of powerlessness: our people really don't care. They can pull together only when there is sufficient threat. Lastly, negative visions are inevitably short term. The organization is motivated only as long as the threat persists. Once it leaves, so does the organization's vision and energy.

There are two fundamental sources of energy that can motivate organizations: fear and aspiration. The power of fear underlies negative visions. The power of aspiration drives positive visions. Fear can produce extraordinary changes in short periods, but aspiration endures as a continuing source of learning and growth.[8] (p.225)

It is however, the writing of the vision statement that gives form to the vision. This is similar to writing a book. It is one thing to have ideas, but it is putting them into the written word that provides form. Once form has been created, then it is possible to revise, expand, and to share with others. Form is, in a sense, commitment. Furthermore, once the vision has taken form, it helps to create alignment. Without alignment there is the potential for misinterpretation, loss of focus, and the wasting of resources.

The following are two examples of a vision statement for nursing:

Nursing is
  Helping
  Healing others and
    ourselves
  All in the same
    mind frame with
  Love,
  Understanding
  and Hope.

                     —Anonymous[9] (p.48)

. . . vision for nursing is a sisterhood/brotherhood of loving people who are fulfilled and dedicated through hard work, knowledge, caring and empathy to the calling toward helping those in pain and despair toward peace.

                     —Pat Simmons[10] (p.42)

Their form and content are very different. It can be seen that the first deals with the healing of all, including ourselves, while the second only addresses those in pain and despair. Neither is right or wrong. One's personal beliefs about nursing will determine which vision he or she will align with.

VISION STATEMENT DEVELOPMENT

The development of a vision statement is an evolutionary process. It is not something that can be performed in an ivory tower by senior management with the expectation that once it is written and distributed the vision statement will create instantaneous buy-in. A vision statement is an iterative or repetitive process. The iterative process begins with forming a vision statement creation team. The vision statement creation team should represent a cross-section of the agency, all disciplines, include different levels of staff, and be open to valuing all perspectives in the creation process. Team members may also include customers, suppliers, industry experts, and experts outside of the home health industry.

The actual process could begin by using a brainstorming exercise built around several core questions. The questions that form the basis for the brainstorming exercise could begin with, "What does the future of home health look like from the perspective of

- the customer?
- the staff?
- the community?
- the organization?
- offered services?"

Addressing strengths, weaknesses, opportunities, and threats as they are known today also provides the basis for projecting into the future.

The purpose of the brainstorming exercise is to collect everyone's thoughts in a free-form, nonlinear fashion. Expressed thoughts or ideas should be recorded for future reference. Once all thoughts have been expressed, the meeting can be adjourned and thoughts transcribed. Transcribed notes should be distributed to all team members for discussion at the next scheduled meeting. Team members have an opportunity to share results with their colleagues between meetings to see if there are any additional thoughts that could be added to the list at the next scheduled meeting.

Once the list is finalized the process of refinement begins. This could be accomplished by the team members choosing a fixed number of items that, from their perspective, would exemplify what the agency is all about. Further refinement could occur through a technique such as multivoting where items on the list are rank-ordered to eliminate those that do not fit with the majority of team members. Once the list has been further refined, it is time to write the vision statement.

All statements begin with a rough draft. The object is to capture the important points, meanings, and essence. The challenge is to have the words and sentences in the statement create a mental picture that will convey meaning to all who read the statement. This is an iterative process and requires a considerable amount of time and energy.[11]

Once the statement has been developed, a spot check is done. Does the statement address the criteria that are essential to the agency? Does it address the future needs of the patient, the organization, the staff, and the community? Will it provide motivation? Will it empower all staff to act? Does it provide a clear picture of the future and a sound base for strategy and goal formulation? The vision statement should conform to the following conditions:

- Be realistic, feasible, simple, and clear.
- Provide a challenge for the whole organization.
- Mirror the goals and aspirations of the constituents.
- Be far but close, in terms of time span and organizational commitment.
- Be able to focus the effort with respect to scope and time.
- Be translatable into goals and strategies.
- Be endorsed and frequently articulated by top management.
- Be derived from a sense of direction.[12]

If the vision statement has passed the first round of review, then expand the review process to include multiple levels of staff: clinical and administrative staff, inside staff, and field staff. Ask them to rate the vision statement on a scale of one to five using five as the most meaningful level. Find out whether the vision statement is clear or requires explanation. Determine whether or not the vision statement is meaningful for those who read it. Ask for feedback and be willing to revise the statement until it provides meaning to all.

Once a meaningful statement has been developed, ensure there is a strategy to support the pursuit of the vision. This will provide constancy of purpose or alignment toward common goals.[13]

CHALLENGES TO ORGANIZATIONAL VISION

How many people can relate to the following slogans: "The flavor of the month," "The walk doesn't match the talk," or "This is what the consultant said we must do"?

Why have so many of management's good intentions fallen by the wayside? Is it because we associate ourselves with those things that are perceived as being sexy, the latest trend, or buzzwords? Is it because there is a lack of commitment to follow intentions through to completion, to live them on a daily basis, and to be willing to hold oneself up to personal scrutiny?

Creating a vision statement is not a quick fix. It is not a magic bullet, the holy grail, or the winning lottery number. It is, however, a concept that is strategically driven, influenced by organizational culture and values, and mission dependent. If a vision statement is seen as something "hokey" or that provides no value or meaning to staff, then it will amount to nothing more than a string of words.

Vision statements must be consistent with organizational culture, leadership's behaviors, and customers' expectations. Many organizations have realized too late that their customers are interested in the truth, not optimistic forecasts and reassurances.[14] Poor management participation, complacency, and lack of a creative process have been reasons cited to explain why an organization's vision statement never enlisted the hearts and minds of staff.[15]

Perhaps the biggest challenge is the willingness to share, be open, treat everyone within the organization as equals, and commit to the future. Vision is a tool that, if shared, can inspire people to go beyond their self-imposed limits to participate in creating something that is beyond the scope of any one individual. Vision, if lived, can be future oriented and provide guidance for all daily activities. Vision, if merely espoused, can be perceived as another ploy by management. It is a leadership challenge to inspire, motivate, and create the environment that will foster the pursuit of vision. "Visions spread because of a reinforcing process of increasing clarity, enthusiasm, communication, and commitment. As people talk, the vision grows clearer. As it gets clearer, enthusiasm for its benefits builds."[16] (p.227)

SHARED VISION

Shared vision occurs when the entire organization owns a piece of the vision. It is when all members of the agency have an equal understanding of their unique contributions to the whole and how their efforts contribute to the realization of the agency's vision.

Figure 5–2 uses eight different groups to demonstrate the concept of shared vision. Actually, this illustration should indicate every staff member as a circle; however, the point remains the same. Shared vision occurs when all groups and individuals view each other as contributing members of an organizational team. This is where individual and professional diversity are checked at the door to work toward a common goal. Is it possible for clinical and financial operations to see "eye to eye" on every issue? Well, the answer is yes, no, and maybe. Through the use of metrics (agency measurement systems), however, it is possible to define goals that support both clinical and financial operations instead of "either/or" and work toward the larger goals of the agency.

The dotted line in Figure 5–2 indicates a sense of connectedness. Similar to Jung's theories on the collective unconsciousness, the dotted line illustrates an informal support system or a "sense" that occurs and helps to hold people/groups together in times of stress. It is this togetherness that helps to hold the group energy, to encourage, and to offer support when an individual or group begins to question whether it is contributing to the larger goal. It is the informal system that will either facilitate the growth of shared vision or block access to it. It is the

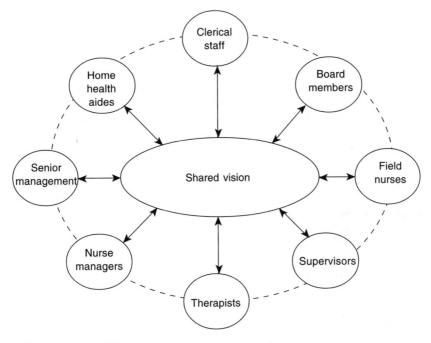

Figure 5–2 Shared Vision

---

willingness of every individual to move beyond the "What is in it for me?" syndrome toward a willingness to honor common values that ultimately will create shared vision. Without a willingness to move beyond "me" to "us," partnership and shared vision will never happen.

MISSION

An organization's mission defines its purpose, its reason for being, and its broad objectives, or how the organization will provide value to its customers. For instance, the following could be used as a mission statement: "We serve the elderly and homebound in the five-county region by providing nursing and related health care services in the home." The preceding statement identifies the agency's objective, how it will provide value, and the services it will provide. For example, the above agency would be providing nursing and other health care services to all homebound elderly in the five-county region. It will not take maternal and child health cases or provide clinic services. The preceding mission statement also provides a framework for developing strategic initiatives or directions, and resource allocation and action plans, and can be used to support behaviors and values.[17]

The concept of mission applies to an organization, departments within the organization, and even to teams and individuals. In fact, mission helps to clarify objectives and focuses all members on specific goals. Mission is instrumental in inspiring the emotional commitment of managers and staff who are responsible for implementing the mission.[18] Mission deals with the present. It is not future oriented like an organization's vision although, if constructed properly, it can be a timeless concept. Unlike vision, mission is never achieved. The mission does, however, address the specific services and customers that will be impacted by the organization's services, and the mission needs to support the achievement of an organization's vision. Vision and mission are interdependent, however. It is not enough solely to state an organization's purpose or mission; by including vision to provide future context, there is an opportunity to address today and tomorrow. Together the two statements inspire and create an image of where we will be going tomorrow given today's objectives.

PERSONAL MISSION

In addition to organizational mission, there is also personal mission. Every individual has a personal mission, whether they know it or not. Once this mission is put into an identified statement, it becomes the basis for making both major life decisions and for making daily decisions in the midst of the circumstances and emotions that affect our lives.[19] Since mission sets the direction in which one can be impassioned and committed, it is important as employees are brought into an organization with a well-defined strategic focus (vision, mission, values) that the aspects of their personal mission that deal with their work be complementary to the agency's mission. Otherwise, it is impossible for new employees to commit to a peak performance.

Personal mission has two elements: one aspect addresses self-development and the other, how the individual will be of service. These two aspects can be independent or interdependent. If they are interdependent, there will be a sense of self-fulfillment associated with personal development because one has an opportunity to apply personal growth through being of service. That is not to say that one cannot have self-fulfillment by being of service and not pursuing self-development. Nor is it to say that one cannot have self-fulfillment by pursuing self-development without being of service. It is the combination of the two, however, that lends itself to inspiring others. It is the combination of the two that fuels the concept of mentoring: to learn from another's experiences and to be able to apply that knowledge to a real-life situation. How many of us have been in a work situation, for instance, and a new associate impresses us because of his or her technical competence, education, or worldly experience. In that situation, the new associate is being of service to the organization and at the same time may be inspiring others to renew their self-development, pursue additional training, or further their education.

This is an extremely powerful concept and supports the idea of organizational learning, which begins at a personal level. If everyone in the organization is working toward a common cause (being of service), then the collective consciousness of the team, department, or organization is being raised. If on the other hand, there is not harmony of actions, then there is not a compatible match between staff, organizational values, and organizational mission. At that point, one may want to consider evaluating personal vision, mission, and values with respect to organizational vision, mission, and values using the common format illustrated in Table 5-1 later in this chapter. Then, if inconsistencies are discovered, revisions can be made to remove them, or action taken to find an organization compatible with one's personal service and development goals.

Garfield defines six guideposts to formulating a workable mission. They are:

Put Preference before Expertise. Mission starts with determining what one really cares about and wants to accomplish and then committing to it. One can always develop the expertise later. First, discover your preference.

Draw on the Past. Look at the times in the past when you felt truly committed and ask what was it about those situations that brought out the best in you.

Trust Intuition. An intuitive feel for the way something fits, its natural "rightness," accelerates the creation of a mission that is both powerful and workable.

Have No Preconceived Limitations. Mission is not bound by preconceived limitations. It inspires one to reach for what could be and to rise above the fears and preoccupations with what is.

Combine Profit with Contribution. One cannot separate the mission from the context in which it intends to succeed, whether it be social, financial, cultural, or corporate. Agencies that profess and operate under the belief that "people are our greatest resource" make it very easy to align individual and organizational missions.

Be Pulled by Values. The sustaining source of a mission is what one cares about most, or one's values.[20]

VALUES

Similar to *vision*, an organization's *mission* faces developmental and operational challenges. One of the ways to provide context for an organization's vision and mission is to identify organizational values and related behaviors. Identification of values not only provides a context for daily operations, but can also support the pursuit of organizational objectives and strategies.

Values are beliefs that are instilled in us at a very young age. Some values are instinctive, such as curiosity, while others are learned, such as honesty and integrity. Learned behaviors are the result of parental leadership, the environment in which we are raised, and parental and environmental reward systems. Everyone has values. Many have values that are different than ours, many have values that are similar, and sometimes we encounter individuals who seem to have "negative" values. It is these values and beliefs that guide us, shape our experiences, and influence our actions. It is the combination of inherent and learned values that we bring forward into adulthood.

The following is a short listing of personal values:

- humor
- integrity
- respect and goodwill for all
- self-fulfillment
- compassion
- honesty
- openness
- truth telling

An organization is a collection of individuals. Each individual brings to the organization his or her unique experiences, backgrounds, and values. Without management intervention to provide structure and leadership, however, there would be a free-for-all, with each staff member doing what she or he thought appropriate. One of leadership's many challenges is to create an organizational value system.

An organizational value or belief system provides a context for decision making. It provides context for strategic thinking, human resource management, service offerings, relationship management, and everyday operational decisions. A value system is not simply a listing of words that have a specific meaning to the organization. A value system provides context; it spells out exactly what type of behavior is expected when one exhibits a specific value. The preceding listing of personal values provides the basis for the following example. On a personal level we all have values. All of us may say that one of our values is honesty. If this is an organizational value, however, then it must be supported. This means that if an employee makes a mistake, such as charting that a Medicare patient (who by definition should be confined to the home) took a walk around the block and was therefore not homebound, and is honest about the mistake, he or she is not disciplined. Instead, the employee should be instructed in how to correct the charting error and be accurate next time. This is the proactive approach to mistakes: acknowledge them, correct them, and learn from them. It supports individual honesty because covering up a mistake involves rationalizations (rational lies) to self and others.[21] It also supports agency honesty because it does not discipline the honest behavior. Perhaps one of the best known examples of honesty is George Washington and the cherry tree. Like George, are we willing to tell the truth, regardless of the subsequent consequences? If we tell the truth, is this action rewarded with support rather than punishment? This is an example of illustrating values through actions.

Peters and Waterman, who wrote *In Search of Excellence,* noted that excellent companies had several beliefs that supported their individual value systems.

1. a belief in being the *best*
2. a belief in the importance of the details of execution, the nuts and bolts of doing the job well
3. a belief in the importance of people as individuals
4. a belief in superior quality and service
5. a belief that most members of the organization should be innovators and subsequently, the organization's willingness to support failure
6. a belief in the importance of informality to enhance communication
7. explicit belief in and recognition of the importance of economic growth and profits[22]

To merely list these seven points as organizational beliefs is meaningless. This is what Deming addresses as the need to eliminate slogans, exhortations, and targets for the workforce; they are simply the equivalent to lists.[23] So the question becomes, "How does the organization, its staff and management, exemplify these beliefs on a daily basis?" Words or beliefs that are not backed up by actions are meaningless. Similar to a mission or vision that is not lived on a daily basis, exemplified and rewarded by management, and an inherent part of daily operations, values and beliefs that do not provide context for subsequent actions amount to nothing more than meaningless rhetoric. The words are impressive, but when the going gets tough, reality becomes obvious. The reality is that the values exhibited are different from the ones professed, and mission divergence results.

Values provide staff and management with a framework for making daily decisions and realizing results. Therefore, management needs to identify organizational values and also provide a context for putting into operation the actions that support organizational values and produce desired results.

THE DEVELOPMENT OF ORGANIZATIONAL VALUES

A framework for values identification begins with the identification of characteristics, beliefs, and a cultural infrastructure that will enable the organization to differentiate itself from its competitors. What are the values that will provide a foundation for future growth, customer satisfaction, business excellence, and the achievement of organizational vision? What are the values that will honor your customers, your staff, and your partners?

These values can be extracted from the agency's vision, mission, standards, and guidelines. Once values are identified and agreed upon, agency standards and guidelines need to be reevaluated for consistency with the values. Processes and programs also need to be reviewed using the values as guides to determine the appropriate activities for the agency.

The Values of the Malcolm Baldrige Award

The Malcolm Baldrige National Quality Award was designed to help companies enhance their competitiveness through focusing on dual, results-oriented goals. They are: (1) the delivery of ever-improving value to customers that results in marketplace success, and (2) the improvement of overall company performance and capabilities.[24]

The Baldrige Award Program was developed to stimulate competitiveness among businesses within the United States. The Award represents the nation's highest honor and recognition for companies that are values driven, customer focused, and performance driven. The Award program currently does not have a specific award for health care and education; however, the concepts provide a model for organizational development, internal assessments, and analysis that is nonprescriptive and more robust than the Joint Commission's Improvement of Performance Standards. (See Exhibit 5–1.)

Exhibit 5–1 Core Values of the Malcolm Baldrige Award

1. Patient-focused quality and value
2. Leadership
3. Continuous improvement and organizational learning
4. Employee/health care staff participation and development
5. Management by fact
6. Results orientation
7. Community health and public responsibility
8. Partnership development
9. Design quality and prevention
10. Long-range view of the future
11. Fast response

Source: Courtesy of Malcolm Baldrige National Quality Award.

The 11 core values[25] presented in Exhibit 5–1 were determined as being an initial starting point for health care organizations that are interested in achieving performance excellence.

Management by fact is an organizational value that creates an operational paradigm that is data driven. The gathering of data provides factual results of operations. For instance, anyone can say that his or her organization has satisfied employees and customers. Organizations that truly manage by fact, however, will have the data to back up this claim. Management by fact, as an organizational value, is more than collecting data to demonstrate claims and results. Data are gathered to track continuous improvement, to assess pursuit of organizational strategy, and to dig below the surface of symptoms to resolve problems at the source.

The Quality Award Criteria go one step further to identify generic concepts that need to support each value. The following example will illustrate the concepts involved in management by fact.

An effective health care services and administrative management system needs to be built upon a framework of measurement, information, data, and analysis. Measurements must be derived from and support the organization's mission and strategy, and encompass all key processes and services, and their outputs and results. Facts and data needed for organizational improvement and assessment can be of many types, including: patient, employee, community health, epidemiological, critical pathways and practice guidelines, administrative and business, payer, competitive comparisons, and "customer" satisfaction.

Analysis refers to extracting the larger meaning from data to support evaluation and decision making at various levels within the organization. Such analysis may entail using data to reveal information—such as trends, projections, and cause and effect—that might not be evident without analysis. Facts, data, and analysis support a variety of purposes, such as planning, reviewing performance, improving operations, and comparing performance with competitors, similar health care organizations, or "best practices" benchmarks.

A major consideration in the use of data and analysis to improve performance involves the creation and use of performance measures or indicators. Performance measures or indicators are measurable characteristics of health care services, processes, and operations the organization uses to track and improve performance. The measures or indicators should be selected to best represent the factors that lead to improved health care, improved operational and financial performance, and healthier people. A system of measures or indicators tied to patient and stakeholder satisfaction and/or organizational performance requirements represents a clear and objective basis for aligning all activities with the organization's goals. Through the analysis of data from the tracking processes, the measures or indicators themselves may be evaluated and changed. For example, measures selected to track health care service quality may be judged by how well improvement in these measures correlates with improvement in patient satisfaction and health care outcomes.[26 (p.4)]

Presuming that an organization believed in management by fact as a core value, it would be necessary to understand its approach to demonstrating that value, its approach to putting the value into operation, how actions or operations would translate into results, and finally, how the value is linked to continuous improvement efforts.

Demonstrating Value

What is the organization's approach to demonstrating a value? Using the preceding example of management by fact it would be necessary to identify how data are collected, measured, analyzed, and turned into information. Merely collecting data for the sake of collecting data, however, is similar to meaningless rhetoric associated with slogans. Data collection needs to have a purpose, be linked to strategic objectives, and provide a baseline for continuous improvement activities.

Figure 3–3 illustrates the flow of data. Data collected at the work unit or team level roll up into processes, and then process indicators can be aggregated to support strategic or agency indicators. Stated differently, agencywide performance measures are supported by strategically oriented data collected at the work unit or team level. These measures cascade downward to the process and work unit or team level. Figure 3–3 illustrated a framework for identifying data collection activities. Analysis of these data provides management, staff, and teams with feedback on how their efforts are contributing toward strategic goals.

Figure 5–3 illustrates a slightly different perspective to demonstrating the value management by fact by looking at an organization systemically. Figure 5–3 illustrates seven elements of a system where data collection is required. Each category—leadership, strategic planning, customer and market focus, information and analysis, human resource development and management, business results, and process management—will require that specific metrics be developed to assess the effectiveness of the efforts. Analyzing business results over time will indicate whether there has been improvement in organizational efforts.

An organization's approach also addresses how data will be collected. Is there one integrated information system that is the repository of all organizational data, or is there an in-house database system that collects application-specific data,

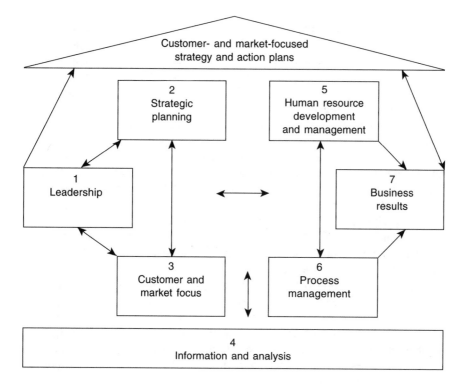

Figure 5–3 Baldrige Award Criteria Framework—A Systems Perspective. *Source:* Courtesy of Malcolm Baldrige National Quality Award, 1997.

survey results, and data that is outside the realm of application-specific programs to measure organizational progress? The key is not just to gather data; data are easy to collect. The key is to collect data that will enable the agency to accomplish its vision.

Putting a Value into Operation

Once an approach to demonstrating a value has been identified, it needs to be put into operation or deployed. Using the example of management by fact, deployment would involve sharing information with all staff, an action that moves beyond the old paradigm where knowledge and information were the domain of senior management only. It is the sharing of results with all members of the agency, regardless of discipline or position; it is the involvement of suppliers, customers, and multiple staff levels in the review of results and the subsequent efforts for continuous improvement. Sharing information with all staff on the surface sounds simple, and indeed it is. Its ramifications are far reaching, however, and it is easy for administration to come up with reasons not to do it. For example, handing staff financial information that shows a poor management performance can be threatening to managers. A good excuse is that management doesn't want it to fall into the hands of competitors. The real reason is fear that staff will denegrate them. Thus, the situation comes back to one of trust and willingness to work together as a team.

Management by fact is different from a management system based upon whim, or anecdotal information—it is management based upon data. It is the development of quantitative measures to guide the organization, assess customer and staff satisfaction, and utilize the unique strengths and abilities of all stakeholders. If done in a supportive, creative environment, the result will be an organization that will succeed in achieving its objectives.

From the perspective of the performance and data hierarchy (Figure 3–3), management by fact would require that all work units and teams understand how their data measures contribute to process and agency efforts, and are knowledgeable about performance results, and about how these results provide a baseline for agency operational improvements. From the system perspective, as demonstrated in Figure 5–3, management by fact would identify critical data to collect in order to monitor human resource alignment with organizational strategies, customers, and processes. Supporting the value and philosophy of management by fact requires the collection of data to evaluate how leadership creates and sustains organizational vision and creates an environment that enthusiastically pursues operational and business excellence.

How Operations Translate into Results

Results are dependent upon what is being measured. Results can include financial indicators, measures of customer and staff satisfaction, process improvement indicators, client retention figures, and clinical outcomes. Results provide a feedback mechanism. Results that are trended over time, compared to internal and external benchmarks or goals, will provide an agency with an understanding of where they have been, where they are now, and where they need to be. These results reviewed within the context of management by fact provide a systematic format for involving all facets of the organization in achieving results instead of one person, the leader, being accountable for everything.

Results are also necessary as a basis for taking action. Reviewing results without taking action equates to "paralysis by analysis." There is the need for a balance between the two. It is important to have reliable and relevant data so results are reflective, but spending all one's time on "knowing" and none on acting creates a culture of risk adversity (e.g., not taking any action or risk to move the agency to its next level of service, whatever that may be). If an organization welcomes risk, it must balance acting with understanding results so that the risks it takes are calculated and programmed for success.

Continuous Improvement

It is not enough just to provide context for a value, such as management by fact. Certainly identifying how the organization's values are developed, supported, and put into daily operations, as well as how results are used to shape the organization's future, is critical to value-driven organizations. Value-driven organizations also need to examine how they improve their values' infrastructure. Using the example of management by fact, an organization would determine how it can improve data collection, measurement, analysis, and information sharing. An agency could also consider how better external data collection could improve internal operations.

Similar to personal values, the only way organizational values become stronger is to practice them on a daily basis. One must continually look inward and ask, Do I follow my beliefs in all of my daily encounters or do I merely revert back to following the crowd, doing what is expected? Reverting back is easy, even insidious, because old ways are known, safe, and more comfortable in times of crisis. Sometimes reverting back occurs because one is more at ease with the "Do as I say, not as I do" approach. Values, at a personal or organizational level, require personal honesty and a willingness to be self-critical.

CORPORATE CULTURE

Another influence in an agency's foundation is corporate culture. The bedrock of any corporate culture is values. Organizational culture dictates the political climate, how staff approach problems, and how staff respond to each other. The strength of the prevailing corporate culture is established by leadership. It is up to leadership to foster the subtle cues of a culture. These cues include the establishment of values and the inclusion of rites and rituals in the day-to-day life of the company. Rites and rituals are little ceremonies that portray and exemplify cultural values.

In organizations with strong cultures, leaders and managers discuss corporate values and beliefs openly and without embarrassment. There has already been much discussion on corporate values, but be aware that leadership values often dictate corporate culture. For example, look at the professional bias of the CEO. Professional bias is the result of previous training, prior experiences, and professional or group norms that one practices. An agency whose CEO is an RN will have a different culture than one whose CEO is a CPA. This does not imply that one is better than the other but does recognize that the top manager will influence organizational vision, mission, and values based upon his or her own value system. In this example, the value systems of the RN and CPA would have been influenced by their mentors, teachers, peers, and work experiences prior to becoming the agency's CEO.

Organizations with strong cultures also recognize the importance of play, ritual, and ceremony. Play is the creative side of corporate life that releases tension and encourages innovation. It has no real purpose or rules, but it bonds people together, reduces conflict, and creates new visions and cultural values. Rituals are actually dramatizations of an agency's basic cultural values. These can be

1. communication rituals (e.g., how formally or informally individuals are addressed, or who speaks first in meetings)
2. work rituals (charting in the office at the end of the day)
3. hazing rituals (new nurse always gets the difficult patients)
4. management rituals (how meetings are held)
5. recognition rituals (a chocolate bar is given to staff who have no deficiencies on their chart reviews)

Recognition rituals can be elevated into agencywide ceremonies. For example, there are retirement parties that can be particularly useful for recognizing the accomplishments of "old timers" and for reinforcing the importance of corporate values by telling stories, making speeches, and presenting appropriate gifts.[27]

A strong culture offers a system of informal rules that let employees know how to behave most of the time. By knowing what is expected of them, employees don't need to waste any time deciding how to behave. A strong culture also enables people to feel better about what they do so they are more likely to work harder. Signs to watch for to determine if an agency's culture is weak include

- the absence of clear values
- the presence of values and beliefs but no agreement on which are the most important
- various parts of the agency with fundamentally different values
- day-to-day rituals that are either disorganized, with everyone doing their own thing, or downright contradictory, with the left hand and right hand working at cross purposes[28]

The strength of an agency's culture can also influence its willingness to try new approaches. Strong cultures are able to respond to changing environments and circumstances by reaching into their shared values and beliefs for the truth and courage to see them through. An organization whose leadership has fostered a strong culture will find staff more willing to try new ideas and more receptive to risk, innovation, and flexibility. If an agency has a couple of successes under its belt in continuous improvement activities, winning contracts, or acquiring new referral sources, it can build upon the organizational momentum to continue to grow and attempt new projects. Conversely, if an organization's culture is weak, it will tend to wait until approaches are tried and true before changing existing programs. This symptom can be seen today in home care with some agencies experimenting already with the use of the Outcome and Assessment Information Set (OASIS) before it is mandated while others, with weaker cultures, are waiting to see exactly what the mandate is before they are willing to move forward. Their mantra is, "If it ain't broke, don't fix it." Their *esprit de corps* is weak or nonexistent.[29]

A strong organizational culture will facilitate the pursuit of vision, the obtainment of ever-higher standards and outcomes, and the achievement of performance excellence. Organizational culture begins with leadership and heroes. Leadership has the ability to develop and foster culture; heroes have the power to inspire and turn around any environment. Heroes are the motivators, the magicians, the ones whom everyone else counts on when things get tough. They are intuitive, have vision, and provide a lasting influence within the organization.[30] They are the ones within the organization that can replace the "if it ain't broke" philosophy with a "can-do" one. As agencies move toward the concept of shared vision, the opportunity expands for more people—including facilitators—to become heros.

COMMON PLATFORM

Throughout this chapter the concepts of vision, mission, and values have been addressed at a personal and an organizational level. At an organizational level, however, vision, mission, and values become blended in a multidimensional framework. They are specific to each employee (personal values), they are specific to the way staff members deal with each other within the organization (inner organizational values), and they are specific to the way the organization deals with its external environment and is viewed by people outside of the organization (external organizational values).

Figure 5–4 illustrates the interdependence between organizational values, vision, mission, the organizational structure, and the individual. In Figure 5–4, the individual is represented as the core of the system, which is comprised of all agency staff. This includes the CEO, managers, supervisors, clerks, and field staff. Everyone contributes to the larger whole. Each individual brings values and his or her personal mission to the organization on a daily basis. A zone of peak performance is created when (1) personal values and missions are consistent with

Job

* Positive descriptions
* Action plans
* Evaluation objectives
* Career development

Individual

* Personal mission
* Personal values

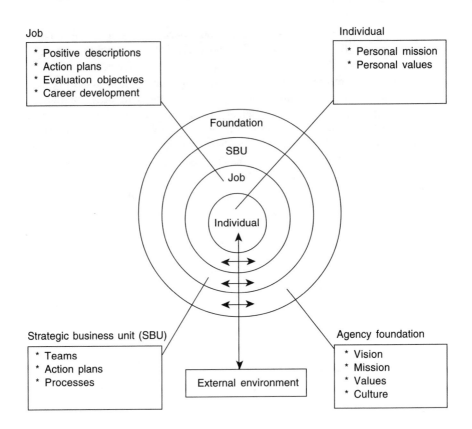

Foundation

SBU

Job

Individual

Strategic business unit (SBU)

* Teams
* Action plans
* Processes

External environment

Agency foundation

* Vision
* Mission
* Values
* Culture

Figure 5–4 Dynamic Interdependence between Alignment of Staff and Organizational Goals

organizational values and mission, and (2) individual missions are aligned with the specific demands of a job and the overall environment and goals of a strategic business unit and agency.[31]

This zone fosters a willingness to go beyond the mandated and accomplish the optimal. There is a shift in perspective from the daily activities being "work" or something unpleasant, to an adventure. A feeling of service grows; one is contributing to the agency, to society, and to a larger purpose than just one's self. The individual's placement at the core illustrates his or her central role in creating agency change in a flexible environment that is conducive to meeting the needs of the customers being served.

The next two circles represent layers of structure for the individual: job and strategic business unit. Each of these structures defines the activities and responsibilities that circumscribe the individual's area of contribution.

The outer circle depicts the foundation of the organization. It embraces the vision, mission, values, and culture of the agency. These pervade through the organization giving purpose, direction, and guidance to all that is done. This foundation is strategically drawn from the external environment, and reflects the needs and wants of the community/customer, as discussed in Chapter 4.

The cross-arrows represent the dynamic relationship of alignment. There is a give and take, a setting of priorities, and perpetual evolution of participation and ownership. Alignment from the greater whole through the agency structures to the individual and back out again offers the greatest opportunity for employee satisfaction and growth, and for providing services at a level of performance excellence.

A framework for aligning the multidimensional requirements of vision, mission, and values was developed by Richard Barrett. The format identified in Table 5–1 can be used for the alignment of personal and organizational values.[32]

At a personal level, Table 5–1 identifies the individual's vision, mission, and values. From a vision perspective, what will bring individual self-fulfillment? Being of service to others? Monetary reward? The pursuit of a dream? From the perspective of mission, Table 5–1 addresses the actions that will create personal self-development. Is it mastering a foreign language, obtaining a college degree, or becoming technically proficient? What are the values that individuals bring to the table to support their vision and mission? Being honest, trustworthy, and dependable?

Inner organizational motivation addresses how departments, teams, and process owners interact with one another. It addresses the "internal community" of the organization by addressing its vision, mission, and values. What is the vision for the internal community? Is it to be the best, to be recognized as a leader or innovator, or to be known for superior service? What mission will support the achievement of this vision? This is addressed in the organization's commitment to organizational development reflected through training efforts, continuous im-

---

Table 5–1 Development of a Common Platform

	Personal Motivation	Inner Organizational Motivation	External Organizational Motivation
Vision	Self-fulfillment	Organizational fulfillment	Societal contribution
Mission	Self-development	Organizational development	Service to customers
Values	Personal values	Community values	Organizational values

Source: Reprinted with permission of R. Barrett, *Liberating the Corporate Soul: A Value-Driven Approach to Building a Visionary Organization,* © 1998, Butterworth Heinemann.

provement objectives, and employee satisfaction. The values that support the vision and mission in this section are referred to as community values. These values are shared by all members of the organization and identify the beliefs that guide all interactions and relationships. Values could be a combination of personal values and core values from Exhibit 5–1.

The external organization motivation addresses how the organization interacts with its external environment: the community as a whole, referral sources, payers, physicians, and so on. In this context, vision speaks to what the organization is here to create; the "why" behind its mission. It identifies its societal contribution or how it will provide value to the community. Mission clarifies how the agency is of service to its customers while on the way to attaining its vision. Values support both mission and vision.

The common platform provides a framework for aligning personal and organizational values, mission, and vision. The common platform becomes a tool to assess whether there is a "fit" when hiring or recruiting new staff or even in helping existing staff members understand whether their values, mission, and vision are consistent with the agency's values, vision, and mission. In the case of new hires, early identification of a "bad fit" will help to reduce the amount of wasted resources for training, orienting, and investing in potential employees who would not be happy because of inconsistencies between personal and organizational perspectives. Comparing personal and organizational vision, mission, and values will help existing staff determine whether they need to move on or whether they have found a home consistent with their values.

The development of the tool is as follows. Begin with the center frame—organizational development in Table 5–1. Ask, "How is the organization (agency) going to develop?" Insert the answer. Then move above to organizational fulfillment, which is determined by asking "why" to the first answer. Then move to service to customers and again ask "why" to the first answer. Then move to societal contribution; the answer is in response to "why" from the organizational fulfillment box. Once these four boxes are complete, then community and organizational values can be completed. Finally, individuals can then add their personal mission, vision, and values that align with the other two columns.

Table 5–2 is an example of what the common platform might look like when it is completed for an agency. This table depicts one person's unique vision, mission, and values in the personal section but the inner and external organization vision, mission, and values would be the same for every staff member in the agency.

CONCLUSION

Vision, mission, and values together represent the organization's foundation. Once a sound foundation has been developed, it is possible to enlist the support of all staff and management to make long-term, strategically oriented decisions. This

Table 5–2 Example of a Completed Common Platform

	Personal Motivation	*Inner Organizational Motivation*	*External Organizational Motivation*
Vision	To participate in an organization that promotes the health and well-being of the elderly and disabled	To be the best at providing services within and outside the organizaiton	To provide and promote efficient and effective home health services
Mission	To advance my clinical, administative, and interpersonal skills	To foster staff development, continuous improvement, and personal creativity	To honor our obligations to our customers, their families, and the community
Values	Integrity Trustworthiness Honesty Humor	Openness Compassion Continuous improvement Results orientation	Management by fact Patient-focused quality Partnership development Leadership

chapter has addressed the development of vision as a tool to focus staff and align resources. Vision is future oriented, mission deals with today, and values provide context or a framework for decision making. These three themes represent an organization's governing ideas. These governing ideas help to create unique organizations that can differentiate themselves from their competitors. Moreover, these governing ideas provide a foundation for making the difficult decisions that will guide the agency through the turbulent waters created by managed care and the changing health care delivery system and reimbursement system. Beyond the difficult decision making, however, is the requirement that governing ideas enlist the support, participation, and interest of staff to contribute to working toward a common goal. Without their support and willingness to go beyond historical patterns, change will never occur. Change will be possible if people believe they can make a difference and are acknowledged and rewarded for their contributions. If the governing ideas are viewed as a tool to get us to work harder or if leadership does not exemplify the vision, mission, and values on a daily basis, then conditions will revert back to the status quo. In the long run, it really becomes a leadership challenge to not only walk the talk, but to be self-critical and extremely honest with themselves and their staff.

NOTES

1. P. Senge, *The Fifth Discipline* (New York: Doubleday, 1990), 223.
2. P. Senge, *The Fifth Discipline*, 224.

3. C. Castaneda, *The Teachings of Don Juan: A Yaqui Way of Knowledge* (New York: Simon & Schuster, 1968).

4. M. Lipton, Demystifying the Development of an Organizational Vision, *Sloan Management Review* 37, no.4 (Summer 1996): 85.

5. S.R. Covey, *First Things First* (New York: Simon & Schuster, 1995), 103.

6. Lipton, Demystifying the Development of an Organizational Vision, 83–92.

7. Lipton, Demystifying the Development of an Organizational Vision, 84.

8. Senge, *The Fifth Discipline*, 225.

9. C. McGuire, ed., *Visions of Nursing* (Sedona, AZ: Light Technology Publishing, 1989), 48.

10. McGuire, *Visions of Nursing*, 42.

11. J.R. Latham, Visioning: The Concept, Trilogy, and Process, *Quality Progress* 28, no. 4 (April 1995): 65–68.

12. M.S.S. El-Namaki, Creating a Corporate Vision, *Long Range Planning* 25, no. 6. (1992): 25–29.

13. W.E. Deming, *Out of the Crisis* (Cambridge, MA: MIT Press, 1982), 25.

14. Lipton, Demystifying the Development of an Organizational Vision, 83–92.

15. Lipton, Demystifying the Development of an Organizational Vision, 83–92.

16. Senge, *The Fifth Discipline*, 227.

17. A. Campbell and S. Yeung, Brief Case: Mission, Vision and Strategic Intent, *Long Range Planning* 24, no. 4 (1991): 145–147.

18. Campbell and Yeung, Brief Case, 145–147.

19. S.R. Covey, *The Seven Habits of Highly Effective People* (New York: Simon & Schuster, 1989).

20. C.A. Garfield, *Peak Performers* (New York: Avon Books, 1987), 93–106.

21. Covey, *The Seven Habits of Highly Effective People.*

22. T.J. Peters and R.H. Waterman Jr., *In Search of Excellence—Lessons from America's Best-Run Companies* (New York: Harper & Row, 1982), 285.

23. Deming, *Out of the Crisis*, 65.

24. 1997 Criteria for Performance Excellence, Malcolm Baldrige National Quality Award, (Milwaukee, WI: American Society for Quality, 1997), 39.

25. Malcolm Baldrige National Quality Award, 1995 Health Care Pilot Criteria, 3–6.

26. Malcolm Baldrige National Quality Award, 1995 Health Care Pilot Criteria, 4.

27. T.E. Deal and A.A. Kennedy, *Corporate Cultures,* 2d ed. (Reading, MA: Addison-Wesley Publishing Co., 1984), 59–84.

28. Deal and Kennedy, *Corporate Cultures,* 135–136.

29. Walt Disney, *Walt Disney's Treasury of Children's Classics* (New York: Disney Press, 1978), 195–205.

30. Deal and Kennedy, *Corporate Cultures.*

31. Garfield, *Peak Performers*, 276–282.

32. Richard Barrett, *A Guide to Liberating Your Soul* (Alexandria, VA: Fulfilling Books, 1995).

CHAPTER 6

The Art and Science
of Outcomes

One of the earmarks of the new paradigm is systems and results-oriented thinking. It is not enough just *to do* to follow the rules. Now, one needs to prove that what is done is effective. The winners in the new paradigm are those home health agencies that demonstrate they provide high-quality care at the lowest cost. In other words, to survive in the managed care environment, an agency must prove that the care given had a positive impact on the health status of the patient and that it saved money. The way to prove this is by focusing on outcomes, which are tools used to determine, monitor, and document the effectiveness of financial, clinical, and operational processes given certain inputs. They are used to

- improve processes
- improve subsequent outcomes
- create partnerships with managed care providers and other consumers
- create partnerships with staff

The tendency is to focus on clinical outcomes because so little is known about the care process (e.g., what interventions lead to what outcomes or what care improves health status) and because care is seen as the end point of the agency's service mission. As previously discussed, however, it is important to measure all aspects of an agency's operations, particularly financial and operational outcomes.

The concept of outcomes is not a new one for health care. Once again we can look back to Florence Nightingale for the origins of the concept. Nightingale compared the mortality statistics of the British armed forces during the Crimean War with civilian mortality in order to bring to attention the atrocious standards of care for military personnel.[1] What *is* new is the proliferation of the use of outcomes. This proliferation results from demands by payers, purchasers, physicians, providers, and consumers to determine and measure the value of care. Will Rogers' comment on nuclear power comes to mind: "It ain't new and there's nothing clear about it!" Some are able to picture outcomes and their subsequent process as a gestalt, others envision them as a linear process, and others see outcomes as a trip through a pinball machine.[2] There is much confusion and little clarity. Some confuse outcomes with assessments, care plans, critical pathways, utilization data, or even with home care services themselves. None of these are outcomes. It is true, that outcomes can be and are used in many ways and from different perspectives. This chapter will outline some of those differences. It will

- offer definitions for outcomes
- discuss various levels of outcomes
- provide insight into different perspectives on the use of outcomes
- outline challenges in implementing outcomes

DEFINITIONS

It was Avedis Donabedian who originally presented the notion of quality that incorporated the concept of outcomes with the concept of structure (replaced by the notion of inputs in system thinking) and process. (See Figures 2–2 and 2–3.) According to Donabedian, the concept of outcomes addresses the change in an individual's or population's current and future health and welfare status that can be attributed to the effects of the care provided.[3] The flow of the care process can be subdivided into minute parts each with its own outcome. For example, a completed referral form is an outcome (end result or output) of the intake process. Thus, there can be an infinite number of outcomes to be encountered on the way to achieving an ultimate change in knowledge, behavior, and general well-being.[4] Those processes that occur before the care process are upstream, and those that occur afterward are downstream. The intake process is upstream. Looking at outcomes from this perspective accommodates the financial and operational outcomes inherent in monitoring an agency's quality. There can also be parallel care processes, however. For example, there may be a separate but similar process for different groups of patients based on similar conditions or medical diagnoses. These are often put into care plans, critical paths, or clinical pathways, which will be discussed in a later chapter.

Outcomes are often confused with objectives. An objective or goal connotes the direction in which one wants to go. For example, an objective may be to improve toileting. An outcome signifies what it looks like once one gets to the destination. An outcome for the above objective could be to independently get into the tub and wash oneself, within two weeks.

Expected Outcomes

One way to define outcomes is simply as the picture on the puzzle box.[5] The picture on the box of the jigsaw puzzle depicts what the end point of the process will look like when the puzzle (process) is complete, or from a patient's perspective, what the patient will look like when care is complete. This type of outcome is also known as an *expected outcome*. Having an expected outcome is important for several reasons.

1. If you don't have a picture of what the patient will look like at discharge, it is hard to assemble the required care interventions to get there. This is like putting together a 2,000-piece jigsaw puzzle without the picture on the box as a guide.
2. Expected outcomes provide feedback on how care is affecting the patient: whether interventions are effective and whether changes need to be made in the patient's care.

The concept of feedback can be illustrated by using the example of a guided Tomahawk missile. These missiles are programmed with their destination and then given constant feedback to track whether or not they are on course. If they are on course, fine; if they are off course, they receive course corrections in order to reach their destination. If the destination is unknown or not programmed into the missile, however, there is no way to know if it is on or off course or to make course corrections. So it is with outcomes. Outcomes are a picture of the destination of the patient so that the effectiveness of the interventions can be monitored. If the care being rendered is not bringing patients closer to their destinations, then changes in care need to be made.[6]

Choosing expected outcomes not only focuses on where patients want to go; it also mandates that people know what people want, where they want to go, and when they want to get there. Many patients haven't really thought about where they want to be at the end of agency services, or that what they want may be beyond their own ability to commit resources or energy to achieve. By defining the end point, three very important contingencies occur.

1. Knowing what is wanted increases the chance of getting it. Denis Waitley has stated it this way: "Since the mind is a specific biocomputer, it needs specific instructions and directions. The reason most people never reach their goals is that they don't define them, learn about them, or ever consider them as believable or achievable."[7]
2. Knowing the end point makes the process clearer. If the outcome is negotiated with clients at the start of care, both client and caregiver are clear about the purpose and process of the services. Thus, it is easier to evaluate the success of the service, and clients are more satisfied because they are getting what they defined they wanted.

3. Knowing the end point defines for everyone, including the caregiver, the patient/family, and the payer, when the end has been reached. This makes it easier to discharge the patient in a timely fashion and rules out JIC ("just in case") visits.

Expected outcomes provide a dynamic interface with quality management. Outcomes provide the basis for determining which interventions are successful in reaching a certain destination and which are not. (More about quality management will be discussed later.)

There are three components of an expected outcome: (1) a measurable expected behavior, (2) a defined entity, and (3) a time frame.

Measurable Expected Behavior

Measurable expected behavior is the activity being sought. An example is to walk six feet with a walker. To improve walking is not measurable; it is the goal that you are moving toward, but it may mean different things to different people. For example, the therapist may think that getting the patient to walk five feet is an improvement because he or she was walking only two feet when they started. But what the patient had in mind was walking to the refrigerator, which was eight feet away. The patient did not accept anything less than that as an improvement.

Sometimes it can be difficult to define a single, or even a simple, expected behavior as an outcome. In these instances, performance indicators or measures can be used to make the outcome measurable. For example, a patient may want to be "happy" as an outcome. How do you measure "happy"? Well, there certainly are indicators of happiness such as: The patient has a smile on her face; and/or the patient has $100 in her pocket. These could be performance indicators for the outcome of "the patient is happy."

Defined Entity

A defined entity is the person or organization for whom the outcome is created. It may be a patient, the patient's family, a caregiver, the agency itself, an agency department, or an agency program.

Time Frame

Time frame is the expected amount of time required to reach the outcome. It can be expressed in actual length of time such as days, weeks, number of visits, or by a certain date. It is analogous in many ways to a deadline. We all live with deadlines. If something doesn't have a deadline it usually goes to the bottom of the pile and has the least chance of getting done. So it is with expected outcomes. Missing a deadline (or time frame) is usually not life threatening. We have all missed deadlines; we have all renegotiated deadlines. Missing and/or renegotiating time is also allowed with time frames. Missing a deadline does not mean that we self-destruct or are immediately deemed a poor performer. What it means is any or a combination of the following:

- The time frame was unrealistic.
- The interventions were not effective and should be changed.
- The outcomes were not negotiated with the client and thus she or he was not committed to achieving them.
- There were unexpected events that extended the time frame.
- New information became available after the time frame was established that altered the original plan.

What is important is that the outcome is evaluated at a predetermined time. If it is not met at that time, the appropriate corrections or adjustments are made to the outcome or interventions, or both, and a new time frame is established.

End-Result Outcomes

A second way to define outcomes is: a change in a patient's health status (physiologic, functional, cognitive, emotional, and behavioral) between two or more points of time.[8] These changes can be positive, negative, or neutral and are a result of the care provided, the natural progression of disease and disability, or both. These changes are intrinsic to the patient. This definition of an outcome is also known as an end-result outcome, and is identified by some[9] as a pure outcome. This type of outcome is currently exemplified in the Outcome and Assessment Information Set (OASIS).

These end-result outcomes are measured by quantifying the change in the patient's health status. It is important, however, to understand that this type of outcome is data driven rather than patient driven. This means that measuring the health status in a reliable way (e.g., measured the same way by everyone doing the measurement) is more important than whether the outcome is significant to the patient. For example, the functional status of a patient may deteriorate due to increasing arthritis. The choice of the patient, however, is to live with decreased functionality because it is too painful to do the exercises required to maintain the function. Thus, the negative outcome is due to patient choice, not agency performance. This type of outcome, however, is required for comparisons across agencies and over time and is important for the following reasons:

1. Outcomes can demonstrate the value of care to managed care organizations (MCOs) and other payers. Major payers of home care want answers to

questions regarding how or how much patients are benefitting from home care and whether the quality of care reflects the cost. Outcomes help to answer these questions. This provides agencies the opportunity to prove to payers that new diabetics, for example, learn to manage the disease better and faster at home than in an acute care setting, and that they experience fewer hospitalizations later in the course of the disease.

2. Outcome comparisons can respond to similar questions from consumers and consumer groups. One of the benefits of the health care reform movement has been more consumer empowerment and choice. As consumer groups such as the American Association of Retired Persons (AARP) and the National Citizens' Coalition for Nursing Home Reform (NCCNHR) advocate for more precise information on the quality of health care, providers will be expected to offer more information on outcomes.[10]

3. Accreditation/certification programs are emphasizing outcomes. These bodies have each become progressively more outcomes oriented. The Joint Commission has its new ORYX initiative; HCFA has its new conditions of participation; and the Community Health Accreditation Program (CHAP) has its benchmarking program built on outcomes.

4. Comparing outcomes provides a dynamic interface with quality improvement. Agencies have their own interest in self-analysis. Included in this analysis is how their agency is performing relative to other providers or standards. Outcomes are the primary reason for health care; focusing on what happens to outcomes provides the basis for strengthening and improving what we do in home care.

Outcomes and Assessment Information Set (OASIS)

As previously mentioned, the most predominant example of a quantification tool for end-result outcomes is the OASIS, developed by the Center for Health Services and Policy Research in Denver and funded by HCFA and the Robert Wood Johnson Foundation. The current version (OASIS-B) is a 79-item data set comprising clinical items that are usually assessed for adult patients. These items are more clinically precise than most existing agency assessment questions. This precision maximizes consistency of ratings among different caregivers collecting the same information. The items are also as discipline-neutral as possible. Table 6–1 shows a sample measurement scale from the OASIS-B instrument.

There are also 10 routine identifiers in OASIS-B (called clinical record items) that are used in tracking, managing, and organizing data collection and processing. These identifiers are: (1) agency ID, (2) patient ID number, (3) start of care date, (4) patient's last name, (5) patient's state of residence, (6) patient's ZIP code, (7) Medicare number, (8) birth date, (9) discipline of person completing the assessment, and (10) date assessment information recorded.

OASIS is used by collecting most of the data items at the start of care and then every 60 days until and including the time of discharge. Only collecting the data

Table 6–1 OASIS-B Rating Scale for M0700

Ambulation/Locomotion: Ability to *safely* walk, once in a standing position, or use a wheelchair, once in a seated position, on a variety of surfaces.

Score	Description
0	Able to independently walk on even and uneven surfaces and climb stairs with or without railings (i.e., needs no human assistance or assistive device).
1	Requires use of a device (e.g., cane, walker) to walk alone *or* requires human supervision or assistance to negotiate stairs or steps or uneven surfaces.
2	Able to walk only with the supervision or assistance of another person at all times.
3	Chairfast; *unable* to ambulate but is able to wheel self independently.
4	Chairfast; unable to ambulate and is *unable* to wheel self.
5	Bedfast; unable to ambulate or be up in a chair.
UK	Unknown.

Source: Courtesy of Center for Health Services and Policy Research, 1997, Denver, Colorado.

is mandated at this time. From these data, however, Shaughnessy and Crisler recommend the production of three basic types of reports: (1) an outcome report, (2) a case mix report, and (3) a patient tally report.[11]

Outcome Report. An outcome report provides a comparison of an agency's patient outcomes aggregated to the agency level for a given period of time. This comparison can be made with analogous agency-level outcomes for the preceding period, outcomes for a reference sample of patients from other agencies, or both. The outcome report usually contains statistics reflecting the percentage of patients improved or stabilized in certain health status indicators. Although submission of data to a national clearinghouse for comparisons or benchmarking has not yet been federally mandated, several states have begun their own projects for collecting and comparing data. Exhibit 6–1 is an example of such a report from the Indiana State "Outcomes USA" project, covering the period April 1, 1997, to June 30, 1997.

The purpose of this report is to compare agencies; therefore, the percent figures are more important than the actual number of cases. This fact is important to remember when reviewing this chart. The percent for each of the categories (improvement in ambulation, stabilization in ambulation, and so on) is calculated using the number of cases in that category divided by the number of cases that could improve or stabilize at the start of care. However, the former number (the number that improved or stabilized) is not shown in the chart except as a percentage (since that is what is important for comparisons) and varies by both category and time period. Therefore, even though the number of cases that could improve or stabilize shown for a category may be the same for both periods (e.g., improvement in ambulation), the percentage changed because the number of cases that did improve is greater in the prior period. Thus, this agency actually did slightly worse in the current period for improving ambulation than it did in the prior period.

Case Mix Report. A case mix report provides average values at the start of care for patient attributes on which data were collected that may impact resource consumption. Examples of OASIS data that appear on this report are: activities of daily living (ADLs) and instrumental activities of daily living (IADLs) disability scales; number of ADL and IADL disabilities; physiologic conditions; chronic conditions; prognosis; sensory impairments; pressure ulcers; mental/behavioral items; demographics; items regarding current residence, living situation, and sources of assistance; and presence of risk factors. Differences in case mix can be considered when interpreting the outcome report and are also important to monitor from the viewpoint of expected resource consumption and staff mix. Exhibit 6–2 is a sample report from the Indiana State project, using only a starter set of the health indicators.

Patient Tally Report. A patient tally report provides a listing of patient-specific outcome and case mix data. It provides an agency with the raw data for each patient, including the start of care value of the case mix items and the scores for the health status indicators. This report assists agency staff in choosing certain clinical records to investigate further if warranted in their quality improvement process. See Table 6–2 for an example.

Fifty agencies across the United States have been participating in a HCFA demonstration project on outcome-based quality improvement (OBQI) using

---

Exhibit 6–1 A Patient Outcome Report

OUTCOMES USA: All Patients Outcome Report						
Agency: 56789						
Current period: 1-Apr-97 30-Jun-97						
Prior period: 1-Jan-97 31-Mar-97						
	State		*Current Period*		*Prior Period*	
	Cases	*Percent*	*Cases*	*Percent*	*Cases*	*Percent*
Improvement in ambulation	2,775	23.53%	153	21.57%	153	28.76%
Stabilization in ambulation	3,825	85.36%	205	90.73%	214	93.93%
Improvement in bathing	2,814	39.20%	156	44.23%	145	55.86%
Stabilization in bathing	3,907	86.20%	206	83.98%	213	87.32%
Improvement in oral meds	2,128	28.38%	104	28.85%	105	39.05%

continues

Exhibit 6–1 continued

	State		Current Period		Prior Period	
	Cases	*Percent*	*Cases*	*Percent*	*Cases*	*Percent*
Stabilization in oral meds	3,910	89.36%	206	91.26%	213	93.90%
Improvement in pain interference	2,877	35.77%	162	45.06%	161	41.61%
Stabilization in pain interference	3,879	81.52%	205	83.90%	206	84.95%
Improvement in dyspnea	2,848	35.08%	174	43.68%	159	43.40%
Stabilization in dyspnea	3,915	78.11%	206	78.64%	216	83.80%

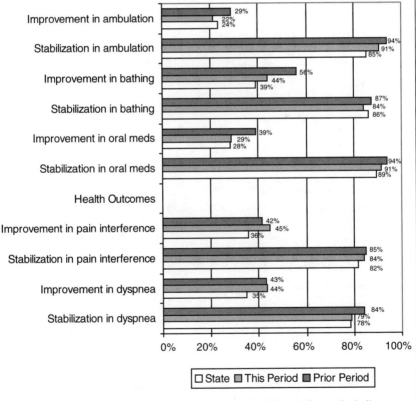

Source: Courtesy of Indiana Association for Home Care, Inc., Indianapolis, Indiana.

Exhibit 6–2 A Case Mix Report

OUTCOMES USA: Case Mix Report

Start-of-Care Patients   ABC Company (56789)

Aggregate Number of Admits in Current Period: 5,790
Agency's Number of Cards in Current Period: 604
Agency's Number of Admits in Current Period: 230

Report Period: 4/1/97–6/30/97
Report Date: September 9, 1997

Demographic	Agency Average	Aggregate Average
Age (Years)	74.25	74.05
% Male	30.26%	34.35%
% Female	69.74%	65.65%
Inpatient Discharge Point		
Hospital	63.06%	61.79%
Rehabilitation	3.15%	5.57%
Nursing Home	9.46%	6.46%
Other	5.86%	6.18%
Not Applicable	18.47%	20.01%
Prognosis		
Good Overall Prognosis	51.74%	72.11%
Good Rehab. Prognosis	35.53%	52.96%
ADL Disability Scales		
Ambulation (Note 1)	1.21	1.22
Bathing (Note 2)	1.88	1.76
Prevalence of Moderate ADL Disabilities		
Ambulation (Note 3)	20.87%	21.52%
Bathing (Note 4)	12.61%	11.40%
IADL Disability Scale		
Management of Oral Medications (Note 5)	0.62	0.68
Prevalence of Severe IADL Disability		
Management of Oral Medications (Note 6)	8.26%	14.87%
Health Status		
Pain Interfering with Activity (Note 7)	1.14	1.08
Dyspnea (Note 8)	1.99	1.52

Note 1: Ambulation: the agency and aggregate averages for this area represent the total patient average on a scale from 0–5 (0=independent, 5=bedfast).

continues

Exhibit 6–2 continued

Note 2: Bathing: the agency and aggregate averages for this area represent the total patient average on a scale from 0–5 (0=able, 5=unable/total).

Note 3: Prevalence of Ambulation: represents the percent of patients on the scale that are at or above 2 (i.e., patients that are coded as supervised or above).

Note 4: Prevalence of Bathing: represents the percent of patients on the scale that are at or above 4 (i.e., unable).

Note 5: Management of Oral Medications: the agency and aggregate averages for this area represent the total patient average on a scale of 0–2 (0=able, 2=unable).

Note 6: Prevalence of Oral Medications: represents the percent of patients on a scale that are at or above 2 (i.e., unable).

Note 7: Pain Interfering with Activity: the average profile of the total number of patients on a scale of 0–3 (0=none, 3=all).

Note 8: Dyspnea: the average profile of the total number of patients on a scale of 0–4 (0=never, 4=at rest).

Source: Courtesy of Indiana Association for Home Care, Inc., Indianapolis, Indiana.

OASIS. Having used OASIS for more than a year, 22 of these agencies responded to a survey, offering these advantages to using OASIS/OBQI:[12]

- Provided consistency in assessment that flows from start of care through discharge
- Provided focus on clinical quality improvement efforts as opposed to agency processes and procedures
- Afforded the opportunity to use outcome reports for managed care contracts, benchmarking, and marketing services
- Provided outcome measures that demonstrate the value and effectiveness of home care, showing that we can make a difference
- Identified patient problems more rapidly
- Demonstrated the importance of clear charting
- Provided data-driven direction rather than basing quality improvement on hunches, feelings, or reactions
- Brought quality improvement to the clinicians, rather than quality improvement just being the "QI nurse's job"

These comments reflect the points made throughout this book, demonstrating that OASIS can be a valuable tool in moving forward with quality and data management.

Utilization Outcomes

Utilization and costs of home care services are often regarded as outcomes. Shaughnessy and Crisler[13] define a utilization outcome as a proxy outcome. A proxy outcome is defined as a type of health care utilization, other than home care

Table 6–2 Outcomes USA, Patient Data Sampling

Date	Participant ID	Primary Dx	Secondary Dx	Birth Year	Sex	Inpt Disch	Amb Loc	Bathing	Meds	Pain	Dyspnea
3/11/1997	147018	296.30	724.3	1924	2	0	0	2	0	1	0
3/10/1990	147019	715.18	No ICD-9 Code	1926	2	1	1	2	0	1	3
3/14/1997	147020	996.59	No ICD-9 Code	1924	1	1	1	2	0	1	0
3/17/1997	147021	715.98	459.81	1916	1	0		2	0		3
3/22/1997	147022	414.9	250.00	1928	2	4	1	2	0	2	2
3/22/1997	147023	251.8	714.0	1948	2	1	1	2	1	1	3
3/29/1997	147024	458.9	429.2	1908	2	5	0	0	1	2	0
1/30/1997	153004	780.9	436	1902	2	1	1	5	1	0	1
1/5/1997	154013	333.7	465.9	1982	1	0	4	5	2	1	0
2/5/1997	157001	376.03	365.90	1934	2	4	0	0	2	0	0
2/7/1997	157003	673.61	No ICD-9 Code	1966	2	1	0	0	0	0	0
1/24/1997	157005	436	286.9	1932	2	1	1	0	1	0	1
3/24/1997	157005	436.00	286.90	1932	2	5	1	0	0	0	0
3/18/1997	157008	774.6	No ICD-9 Code	1997	2	1		5	2	4	0
3/23/1997	157008	774.60	No ICD-9 Code	1997	2	5	5	5	3		0
12/11/1996	2046003	496	196	1913	1	1	1	2	2	2	3
1/3/1997	204805	063.29	No ICD-9 Code	1920	2	0	0	0	1	1	2
12/30/1996	2046052	702.0	No ICD-9 Code	1902	2	5	1	2	0	1	1
12/21/1996	2046053	410.90	250.00	1920	2	1	1	2	0	2	4
12/21/1996	2046058	053.29	No ICD-9 Code	1920	2	0	0	0	1	3	2
2/24/1997	242024	493.90	496	1911	2	1	1	2	0	1	4
2/4/1997	242035	427.31	435.9	1911	2	5	0	2	1	1	3
3/7/1997	242035	428.0	427.31	1911	2	3	1	2	1	1	1
10/4/1996	242054	286.9	495	1905	1	5	1	2	0	0	3
2/10/1997	242967	533.40	436.00	1912	2	1	4	5	2	1	4

continues

Table 6–2 continued

Date	Participant ID	Primary Dx	Secondary Dx	Birth Year	Sex	Inpt Disch	Amb Loc	Bathing	Meds	Pain	Dyspnea
10/22/1996	243011	260.9	424.1	1921	2	5	0	2	0	1	1
12/23/1996	243037	486	428.0	1902	1	0	3	3	1	1	4
1/23/1997	2430372	486	428.0	1902	1	1	1	5	1	1	4
12/31/1996	2430372	486	428.0	1910	1	1	3	3	1	1	4
1/31/1997	2430373	486	428.0	1902	1	1	3	5	1	1	4
12/20/1996	243078	250.01	401.9	1915	2	0	1	2	1	0	0
12/28/1996	244002	250.01	414.9	1931	1	1	3	3	1	1	2
3/3/1997	244013	714.0	No ICD-9 Code	1918	2	5	1	2	0	2	2
2/8/1997	244032	722.6	203.0	1910	2	3	1	0	1	1	3
10/24/1996	244035	682.9	276.0	1934	2	0	0	0	1	1	3
3/7/1997	244050	715.93	250.01	1938	2	5	1	0	0	1	1

Source: Courtesy of Indiana Association for Home Care, Inc., Indianapolis, Indiana.

(such as a hospital admission, nursing home admission, or emergent care use during the home care episode of care) that infers a substantial change in patient health status. Thus, it can be regarded as a surrogate for a pure outcome.

Other service utilization and cost statistics, however (such as total number of home care visits, number of visits by discipline, number of visits by medical diagnosis, total costs per case, or total costs per medical diagnosis), are neither outcomes nor surrogate outcomes. In fact, viewing them as such can be precarious because it can lead to goal displacement and a subsequent potential for diminished quality. In other words, if an agency's expected outcome were to discharge all postacute, myocardial infarction (MI) patients in three visits, clinicians would focus on squeezing their care into three visits rather than assessing what patient outcomes were needed and whether or not they were accomplished. The number of visits, not the quality of care, would become the focus. Quality (and quality improvement) cannot be measured by utilization and cost figures. For quality care, the focus is on what patient outcomes were met or not met. The utilization and cost data are only significant once these measurements are made. Unfortunately, this is not always how these data are used.

Administrative Outcomes

A final type of outcome is an administrative or support outcome. It is a result of day-to-day agency operations that support the clinical processes. These are usually found at the agency level in the outcome hierarchy. An example is: All patient verbal orders will be signed by the physician and returned to the agency within 24 hours.

LEVELS OF OUTCOMES

One of the primary purposes for utilizing outcomes is for evaluation—How well are we doing? How well is the process going? What is our progress? What we want to evaluate will determine the level of outcomes to be used. For example, if we want to evaluate results of the specific care and treatment of individual patients and families, clinical outcomes are used; if we want to evaluate the effectiveness of agency systems or processes, agency outcomes are used; and we are evaluating the quality of services in regard to the health of a community (or region, state, nation), community outcomes are used. The following text further describes each level of outcomes.

Clinical Outcomes

Clinical outcomes take a microscopic view of the care being provided at the level of the individual patients, families, and their practitioners. They can also be called individual outcomes, although they may include the family and significant others. They are used to determine how much progress is being made toward individual patient goals and whether changes need to be made to the plan of care. Examples of health indicators or measures that have been used for measuring patient clinical outcomes include functional status, comfort level, response to treatment, and psychosocial status. An example of a family-sensitive indicator is caregiver burden.

An important health-related indicator that is beginning to generate interest is quality of life. Underlying this interest is the fundamental question about what difference health care really makes in a client's life. Health-related quality of life can include the client's perceptions of physical, social, cognitive, and role functioning; mental and general health; and pain and energy levels. Quality of life surveys allow clients to report the extent to which changes in functioning, or well-being, met their needs or expectations. The most popular of these surveys is the SF-12 or SF-36 by the Medical Outcomes Trust.[14]

To facilitate the organization of outcomes for analysis, clinical outcomes can be subdivided. For example, clinical outcomes can be broken down into subclassifications such as those dealing with health status, knowledge, behaviors, and/or general. Gingerich and Ondeck even divide this level into four levels (or sublevels):

1. Immediate: Outcomes that can be attained during the first encounter with the patient/family, such as during an emergency room visit.
2. Intermediate: Outcomes that can be attained during an episode of illness, such as returning a patient's blood sugar to within normal limits.
3. Long term: Outcomes that can be attained over multiple encounters within various health care settings, such as returning a patient to independent ambulation. Such an outcome would be addressed through repeated encounters in acute care, inpatient rehabilitation, home care, and perhaps an outpatient ambulatory care facility.
4. Lifelong: Long-term outcomes that are sustained throughout life.[15]

Agency Outcomes

Agency, or organizational, outcomes measure critical agency operations (processes or systems) and may form the basis of an agency's quality improvement plan, or scorecard. Many of these outcomes are the aggregate of individual patient outcomes; however, others may measure nonclinical functions such as accounts receivable. For example, an appropriate expected outcome for a billing department would be to reduce accounts receivable days for Medicare patients from 69 to 40 days within six months.

Customer satisfaction is an agency indicator that belongs in this level. Satisfaction outcomes can be measured by satisfaction performance indicators on surveys developed for patients, families, physicians, suppliers, payers, or agency staff. This area becomes more important as we take on the role of "consultant" or partner to our clients (patients, families, physicians, suppliers, payers, staff), rather than as "expert" as in the past. As consultants, it is important that we continually verify that our clients know what they can expect from our services and what effort they must extend in order to see results. If a client's expectations exceed our and/or the client's ability, dissatisfaction looms. Thus satisfaction surveys can provide one source of how well the agency defines mutual expectations.

Community Outcomes

Essentially the community is the external environment that influences or impacts agency operations or vice versa. One way to examine community outcomes is to consider the competition (e.g., the other agencies that provide similar services) and how well your agency performs compared to them. Regulators and accreditors are interested in community outcomes for just this reason. We have already mentioned the OASIS outcomes and the intent of the HCFA to mandate the collection of these outcomes so comparisons can be made. There is also the CHAP initiative, the Benchmarks for Excellence in Home Care. This initiative is collecting and tabulating outcome data from participating agencies and providing participants with all the information so that they can compare themselves with each other.

Another way of looking at community outcomes is to determine what impact, if any, your agency is having on the health of the community. Community can be defined as the geographical area serviced by the agency, or the persons covered by a managed care plan. These outcomes will probably not be available from aggregating patient outcomes, but will be separately determined. There are at least two communities across the nation that are beginning to look at health indicators themselves. One is Seattle, Washington, which is measuring 40 indicators of *sustainability*. The volunteer organization called Sustainable Seattle has defined sustainability as long-term cultural, economic, and environmental health.[16] Some of their outcomes are as follows:

- In 1981 there were 29 unhealthful air days; in the last five years there has been only 1.
- Percentage of low birthweight infants is steady.
- Emergency room visits at the public hospital went up 50 percent in the past five years, not for emergencies but for treatment of persons without insurance and no place else to go.[17]

The second city is Celebration, Florida. Celebration is a new town that incorporates into its plan a mix of ideas from some of America's best-loved small towns and from modern technology. Homes in Celebration are connected through fiber optics to the health campus. Residents are true partners in their health care. The focus is on lifestyles rather than the medical model. The Health Enhancement Program is based on eight universal principles of health: nutrition, movement, rest, choice, attitude, relationships, environment, and spirituality. The effectiveness of the program will be measured by five different health outcomes within the community.[18]

Outcomes across Organizational Levels

The definitions of expected outcomes and pure outcomes can be applied to each level. Expected outcomes, however, are more relevant at the clinical level. Because expected outcomes tend to be subjective and individualized, they are not as useful when aggregating data at the agency and community levels. Pure outcomes, or end-result outcomes, on the other hand, are more applicable at the community level because of their objectivity. They become less appropriate at the clinical level because they do not reflect an individual's needs. See Figure 6-1.

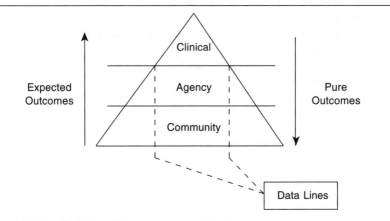

Figure 6–1 Applicability of Outcomes across Levels

Clinical outcome data are usually collected at the individual patient and family level and then aggregated to characterize the other units of analysis, such as the agency or community. These data are depicted within the dotted lines in Figure 6–1. Some outcomes, however (such as agency operational outcomes), may require the data to be collected at the agency or community level. These data are represented outside the dotted line at the agency and community level in the figure.

A MODEL FOR THE RELATIONSHIP OF MULTIAGENCY, CLINICAL, AND COMMUNITY OUTCOMES

A means for exploring the relationship of agency (provider), clinical, and community outcomes within a community can be seen in Figure 6–2. Clinical outcomes are codeveloped between the consumer and the practitioner. In this example, there are four types of organizations: physician group, hospital, home health, and ambulatory care. The consumer would negotiate with the clinicians affiliated with these organizations regarding the type of outcomes they want to achieve. The clinicians will be influenced by their responsibility to the community health initiatives for outcomes and as such will attempt to persuade individuals to adopt lifestyles that contribute to common community goals.

Similarly, agency (or in this case provider) outcomes will be influenced by community goals and objectives and the type of problems found in the community case mix. If community goals and objectives are clearly stated and each provider organization is aligned with these objectives, then all the clinical activities that each provider organization performs should be focused on achieving outcomes associated with community objectives. Their mission statement determines that area in which they have the most interest.

The mission statement will focus on and define various inputs necessary to compile their processes. Inputs represent staff, benefits, technology, and capital and are resources that are required to fuel a process. This is represented by the (I) in Figure 6–2. Individuals within an organization perform various activities (A) utilizing technology and capital investments. These activities (A) may be independent of the agency itself or a shared activity among other organizations that make up a provider alliance to accomplish community goals. Each activity has an output (O) that is measurable and should be focused toward the accomplishment of specific outcomes (organizational and/or community). When organizational outcomes are aligned toward community goals, there is an opportunity to have each element of the community care process (physician, hospital, home health, and ambulatory care) play a role in contributing value to the community as a whole. In doing so, however, organizations should assume the responsibility for their piece of the picture, not ownership of it. Once an organization moves toward

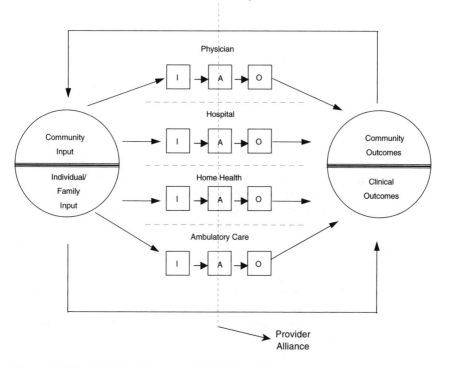

Clinical and Community Outcomes

Figure 6–2 The Relationship among Multiple Providers

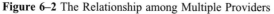

"owning," then turf issues arise similar to what is now going on between disciplines in determining who contributes what to each patient outcome. Owning contributes to the fragmentation that exists in the current system. Assuming responsibility for one's contribution to the whole as one views the whole picture is more congruent with systems thinking and a process orientation.

Not all activities performed within an organization will contribute directly to the community outcomes. This is the importance of differentiating between patient-focused care processes and secondary processes. The patient-focused care processes contribute to the community outcomes. Support processes contribute to the operation of the organization (operational outcomes). The more aligned the support processes are to the organizational goals, the more impact they have on the community outcomes.

In addition, the activities of the organization may not be the only reason, or sole cause, for the attainment of good health outcomes. The relationship between clinical or community health outcomes and the performance of a health care organization or clinician is complex. Other factors both known and unknown will affect the clinical or community health outcomes. For example, community-related factors that affect outcomes include

- the structure of the community's health care system
- the amount and allocation of health care resources in the community
- other factors that affect the population's health such as environmental pollution, workplace safety, and educational levels

There are also patient-related factors such as individual preferences; clinical-related factors such as level of knowledge; and provider organization factors such as the number and qualifications of staff.[19] It is important to consider these influences when defining outcomes. In the Joint Commission's ORYX initiative for example, it is a requirement when selecting the outcomes that the organization can directly attribute a change in health status to the care it provided.

One of the ways to define community is by the persons covered by a similar managed care payment system. So, if everyone in Figure 6–2 is part of the same capitated system, where a capitated system receives one monthly payment from an MCO for a given population, then everyone within the system will have a similar set of incentives and resource constraints. Financial viability will occur when all the providers work together to take care of the members and community outcomes. When this occurs, the concept of managed care transitions to managed health. Managed health will require all elements of the community to assess how the patient-focused care processes contribute to the good of the community. In doing so, all resources (I) become focused toward the accomplishment of community-oriented outcomes.

Capitation will also create opportunities for the development of economies of scale for support services. There will still need to be specific expertise related to each specialty, but there will also be an opportunity to consolidate those processes and activities that could be used by all. For instance, the management of data is a function that crosses all elements of the care delivery process and when integrated and stored in a common repository, will provide opportunities for the creation of value along the entire patient-focused care process.

How well the community services the needs of its members would be determined by how well community outcomes were met. It also would be evaluated by examining the efficiency and effectiveness of the processes (see Chapter 11 on process management). How efficient is it to have multiple services and duplicate processes? How effective are the different processes? Where is the most appropriate care provided and by whom?

The key to measuring these processes and outcomes is data. The data from the pure or end-result outcome measurement system would allow for comparisons across providers. Data from the expected outcome measurement system would provide input into how well the individual needs were being met and also give clues regarding the needs of the community. Both are necessary to complete the picture of what is happening.

VALUES

If an agency is transitioning into the new paradigm, and its methods of doing business are changing accordingly, the values associated with outcomes within the agency must reflect the new paradigm since it is values that provide guidance on how to act. Values are different from principles, however, because values reflect actions based on beliefs, not just what one applies regardless of what is believed. How a person acts needs to be consistent with anticipated results or outcomes of those actions. Following are some of the values for outcomes in the new paradigm. Listing them here, however, is like listing the ingredients for a recipe: Not until the ingredients are combined and eaten can one fully appreciate them.

Outcomes Are Consumer Determined, Not Provider Determined. Outcomes are actually most realistic when they are developed through an interactive negotiatory process. There is more to developing outcomes that just deciding what one wants. Also to be considered is what one is willing to do about it. For example, an agency may want to establish a preventive asthma program for school-aged children. There is no reimbursement available for such activities, however, so money would have to be raised through other means, and the agency and/or the local schools are unwilling/unable to devote the resources to raise the required money.

Outcomes Are Everyone's Job, Not Just Management's or That of the Quality Improvement Committee. This point seems relatively clear for clinicians at the clinical level, but often gets lost with other employees and/or at the agency and community levels. In the old paradigm, anything related to quality belonged to the quality committee or peer review committee, which spent its time looking for poor quality or poor performers. Everyone else's job was to keep from "getting caught." With outcomes as the basis for quality improvement, everyone is involved in developing, measuring, and managing outcomes. Ways to involve staff with outcomes include

1. Involving staff with decision making, such as having staff assist with determining which agency outcomes will be measured and how.
2. Supporting/encouraging/fostering creativity. Hold contests to come up with new outcomes or ways to meet or measure outcomes.

3. Letting staff know it is OK to make mistakes or to not meet outcomes. Staff should not feel like their jobs are on the line if they miss an outcome. If this is their perception, they will never try new things for fear of failure.
4. Providing opportunities for informal communication with and among employees. It is important for staff to have an opportunity to share experiences and ideas with their peers.

Outcomes Have a Positive Focus. This is important because experience shows us that we go where we place our attention. For example, if we look off into a field of flowers while driving a car, we will find the car heading in that direction if we don't return our gaze to the road ahead. So it is with outcomes. We get what we picture. If we want positive results we need to develop positive outcomes. The five Ds that have comprised the classic list of outcomes (death, disease, disability, discomfort, and dissatisfaction) are being replaced with more positive connotations of health—survival rates; states of physiologic, physical and emotional health; and satisfaction.[20]

Unfortunately, this value has not been embraced in many of our risk management programs or, for that matter, in many quality assurance programs. Typical programs still include outcomes relating to infection rates, medication errors, and falls. Besides fostering a negative outlook, using negative types of outcomes creates other problems. First of all, it is difficult to determine definitions that can be uniformly applied across clinicians and/or agencies. For example, what is a medication error? Is it wrong dose, wrong time, or wrong route? What is the wrong time? More than one half-hour from when it was scheduled to be given? If so, there certainly can be many medication errors! Or is a medication error only significant, and therefore counted, when there is an untoward patient reaction? And how do you define an untoward patient reaction? You begin to see the problem. Groups have been known to discuss these definitions for days and still not come to consensus. Furthermore, whatever is decided then has to be shared with all clinicians involved so that everyone is using the same definition in order to obtain accurate numbers.

Another problem with using negative outcomes in a quality assurance program is that people develop solutions that lower the scores for the negative outcome but don't necessarily solve the problem. In fact, the solution may create another problem. For example, nursing homes reduced the number of patient falls by restraining their patients. As a result of their overuse, regulations were revised to mandate that other less restrictive interventions be tried first, that restraints be removed when the nurse assesses that the patient is no longer in imminent danger to self or others, and that those patients in restraints be checked regularly. Why? Patients were developing skin irritation and breakdown that resulted from pulling against the restraint or from being bed- or chair-bound. Ambulation is more healthful but may contribute to falls. Another example is the commonly aspired-to outcome of reduced infection rates. One way to accomplish this rate reduction is to give prophylactic antibiotics. This is what has been done so extensively that now new drug-resistant organisms are appearing on the scene, giving rise to higher incidence of diseases such as pneumonia and tuberculosis.

Outcomes Are Holistic. Outcomes are greater than the sum of their parts and must be viewed in relationship with other situational, environmental, and personal values. For example, psychosocial factors can influence physical outcomes as much as clinical interventions. Take Mr. X. He lives alone, has no family, and cannot see well enough to drive by himself. Thus he must rely on others to either take him grocery shopping or do the shopping for him. Mr. X sees this as a weakness and therefore does not make the required arrangements to purchase items he needs for proper nutrition. As a result, his diet is poor, resulting in constipation and malnourishment. Attempts to improve his dietary outcome are futile without dealing with his perceived "weakness."

THE RIGHT OUTCOME

As has been discussed, there are many definitions of outcomes, levels of outcomes, and values for outcomes. In addition, there is much discussion about who owns outcomes. Most clinical outcomes are defined from the patient/family perspective. These outcomes are more than likely the result of interventions from multiple health care disciplines. Even so, outcomes are being developed that are discipline sensitive. For example, in nursing, it is felt that classification of nursing-sensitive patient outcomes is needed to complete the nursing process elements of the Nursing Minimum Data Set (NMDS) defined by Werley and Lang.[21] Such a project is underway at the University of Iowa, entitled the Nursing-Sensitive Outcomes Classification (NOC).[22] For this research, a nursing-sensitive patient outcome has been defined as "a variable patient or family caregiver state, behavior, or perception responsive to nursing intervention. . ."[23] It is also perceived that there are payer outcomes, although these are usually more along the lines of utilization requirements or limitations. So, the question is, What is the right outcome?

The answer can be all or none of the above. The right outcome is the one that best serves what is trying to be accomplished. For example, are outcomes being captured to document the effect of interventions on the patient's/family's health, or to allow an agency to justify both clinically and administratively the care it provides, or to allow a discipline to assess its practice? The secret to outcomes is not how well they are written, or by whom, but how thoroughly and thoughtfully they are integrated into an agency's way of doing business at every level. Thus, outcomes should reflect the values and mission of the agency and its providers.

The value of outcomes, therefore, is how well they are used. Outcomes provide the opportunity for an agency and its employees to shift their perspective from the number of tasks performed and/or how well those tasks were performed to the effectiveness of the outcome and the processes that contributed to it. There are two basic approaches to utilizing outcomes: (1) measurement and (2) management. Both are critical and each will be examined in more detail.

OUTCOME MEASUREMENT

Outcome measurement is a process-driven approach that utilizes outcome measures to determine the effectiveness of the process (i.e., measure the outcome and then find out how you got there). For example, outcome measurement can be used to determine what has actually happened to a patient(s) as a result of the care provided. An outcome measure is simply the subjective or objective quantification of an outcome. Measurement can be the response to met/unmet outcomes or can involve the use of scales. Each measure requires the collection of data (at the patient and/or aggregate level) and the calculation of a numeric result. Results can be trended, compared, evaluated, and incorporated into an agency's quality improvement program.

Outcome measurement is valuable because it

- Provides the foundation for sound decision making about patient care practice
- Directs an agency's attention to the performance effectiveness of a process(es)
- Establishes priorities for improvement of processes
- Allows an agency to determine the effect of implementing one or more changes to a process
- Provides a tool for agencies to expand their relationships with other payers and providers across the continuum of care

Essentials for outcome measurement include

- the use of a common set of well-defined outcome measures
- the uniform collection of outcome data
- quantification and tallying of the data
- periodic data analysis and distribution of the outcome information

These data are integrated into the quality management process by

- analyzing the process that led to the outcome
- determining changes to be made to improve the process

- developing a plan and timeline to implement the changes
- implementing the changes
- monitoring and evaluating the results (outcomes) of the change

If outcome measurement were applied in the model depicted in Figure 6–2, it would simply measure the outcomes that currently exist at the various levels (community, agency, and clinical) and jointly (physician, hospital, home care, ambulatory care) to determine the processes that led to those outcomes in order to combine processes and eliminate steps. This can be done by determining in advance which outcomes to measure concurrently across the community. The need exists for an effective data tracking system that collects, stores, and aggregates the required measures (disease related, health related, or functional). Some of this across-provider measurement is currently being done by hospitals and home care agencies as they combine clinical pathways for certain medical conditions, such as fractured hips. In some cases, old processes might even be discarded and creative new ways to meet the outcome may be developed. If no outcomes existed at the community level, aggregates of the clinical outcomes could be used as a starting point and as the driver of the process.

OUTCOME MANAGEMENT

Outcome management is an outcome-driven approach to ensure the delivery of effective interventions/services and to eliminate ineffective ones—determine what practices produce the desired expected outcome, follow that pattern, and measure the variance. It is both a strategy and operational approach for achieving targeted outcomes of patient care. Outcome management is especially useful in the management of diseases or in services to a homogeneous group. Too much care is micromanaged with the belief that if costs are watched closely they can be reduced, and magically the patient's health will improve. A more logical approach is to focus on the desired health status (outcome) of a patient or group of similar patients and attempt to improve that health status. If health is improved, the potential exists to reduce costs. The components of outcome management are

1. Strategic planning for health outcomes. This includes both a determination of what outcomes should be selected for management and a plan to prevent disease. These can be accomplished by considering the relevant mission and strategic plan, knowing the at-risk population in the community, and determining the high-cost, high-risk, high-volume, or known problematic cases.
2. Operational planning. Once the strategy is determined, it needs to be integrated into the community system, not just implemented within the agency. The plan also needs to include how data will be organized and collected. Data items and time points need to be determined and integrated

into current processes and procedures. Using tools such as case management and care guidelines, including clinical pathways is helpful. Having these "maps" of best practice processes for achieving the outcome(s) makes it easier to determine if a variation from that best practice is appropriate.

3. Communicating results. Outcome reports need to be produced with comments for further study and recommendations for change. These reports need to be shared with all involved in order to continue to evolve a best practice profile.

Using this systems approach at the community- or population-based level of outcomes can become the basis for transitioning the entire health care system. Bright and Beyt[24] cite the example of asthma treatment. Current treatment is fragmented and focuses on an asthma attack. Once an attack occurs, the patient experiences wheezing, coughing, and shortness of breath. Episodic treatment occurs in a physician's office or, more likely, an emergency room and results in frequent costly hospitalizations and absence from school and/or work. Over time, the dependence on the acute care system increases, the burden of responsibility for "health" is shifted from the patient to the health system, and the patient loses control over his or her own health. On the other hand, if the desired outcome for asthmatic patients is an improved quality of life, a best practice treatment of asthma can be established. In this case, asthmatic patients are actually members of the team. They measure their respiratory function at home and use preventive medications. They can intervene as soon as they notice changes in their respiratory function and, thus, reduce the need for emergency treatment. They are less dependent on the health care system and have greater control over their own health. Further, illness-related costs are contained.

Applying outcome management in the model depicted in Figure 6–2 would determine and adopt community outcomes which would then be used as the basis for provider (agency) focus and organizational outcomes and as the basis for clinical outcomes. This application provides a realignment of responsibilities from the beginning, with resultant new processes. The community outcomes become the driver of the care processes and priorities rather than the individual clinical outcomes. How this relates to outcome measurement can be seen in Figure 6–3.

The goal of outcome management is to maximize the health status and satisfaction of a patient or group of patients and minimize the costs of care by systematically

- defining effective interventions and planning for their efficient delivery
- noting ineffective interventions and reducing or eliminating their use
- ensuring the efficient use of effective interventions (by monitoring interventions and outcomes)
- changing practices if outcomes are suboptimal

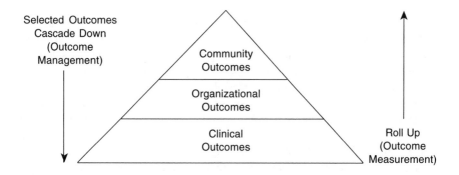

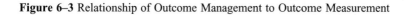

Figure 6–3 Relationship of Outcome Management to Outcome Measurement

The method for outcome management is to

- Review the agency's mission to keep focused and prevent overmeasurement
- Define measurable expected outcomes for a patient or homogeneous group of patients (a well-defined subpopulation of a disease group)
- Review the literature, research, established guidelines, and practices to determine the most effective interventions, and to eliminate questionable and ineffective interventions
- Establish best practice guidelines for care and who is responsible for implementing each activity
- Identify the gap (variances) between the best practices and existing performance in the agency (see Figure 3–2)
- Identify, develop, and implement strategies to reduce the gap (variances)
- Measure process and outcomes

OUTCOME MEASUREMENT VERSUS OUTCOME MANAGEMENT

There are several similarities between these two approaches to outcome utilization.

- similar basic tools
- sound data collection requirements
- usefulness in quality management

Despite the similarities, there are a few key differences that have a huge impact. Outcome measurement is process driven and outcome management is outcome driven. This means that with outcome measures, the process is already established and then the outcomes of the process are measured. With outcomes management, expected outcomes are determined and then the "best practice" process is defined. The impact of this difference is that outcome management is much more focused, with a well-defined goal and plan to meet that goal. A simple analogy involves an airplane pilot with a flight plan. All pilots flying similar courses (a homogeneous group, such as all pilots going nonstop from Philadelphia to Los Angeles) are then monitored for variances from that flight plan and for outcomes such as on-time arrival, smoothness of flight, and passenger satisfaction. Quality management focuses on maintaining best practice. In this example, it would be keeping to the flight plan and constantly improving the best practice. Using this same example, practices could be improved by utilizing the most modern weather prediction technology to determine where storms are located so flight plans can be filed prior to takeoff that avoid turbulence, rather than having to make those adjustments (variances) in the air at the last minute and possibly delaying arrival time.

Outcome measurement, on the other hand, is less focused on a specific group and needs to develop the means to address group differences (e.g., case mix adjustments). Outcome measurement would look at on-time arrival, smoothness of flight, and passenger satisfaction for all flights and then adjust for long flights, short flights, flights that were nonstop, and flights that had one or more stops. These outcomes could then be compared over time or among airlines. The focus of quality improvement is to change the practices for those outcome measures that are subpar. For example, if airline A had fewer on-time arrivals, this problem could be investigated for long flights, nonstop flights, and flights between certain destinations. Once the area of the problem is delineated, changes to the process can be made. If, for example, it was found that flights departing from major cities were always late taking off due to heavy air traffic and, therefore, always late arriving, changes could be made in their departure and/or arrival times.

Both outcome measurement and outcome management are useful and necessary. The challenge for outcome measurement is determining case mix (i.e., a method of risk adjustment to account for the differences in mix of patients served by different organizations); the challenge for outcome management is determining a homogeneous group (i.e., patients with similar needs). The opportunity with outcome measurement is to improve health service delivery practices; the opportunity with outcome management is to improve the health care system.

DOCUMENTATION

The primary purpose of home care documentation has been to show need. Most staff view documentation as burdensome paperwork, a necessary evil to substantiate the need for home care and receive reimbursement. Outcome measurement and outcome management require more. They require documentation that reflects the effectiveness of care as evidenced by changes in the patient's/family's health status. Data needs for outcome measurement and management require the documentation of outcomes, health problems, plans, changes to plans, interventions, and variances. They require the documentation of comprehensive assessments at the start of care and at selected follow-up points. This additional documentation, if continued to be viewed as a burden or threat, will never be done. The data to support these opportunities will continue to be incomplete, unreliable, and inaccurate. Using such data to determine process improvements may mean making decisions based on incorrect information. Therefore, in order for any outcome program to succeed staff must not only understand how to write and use outcomes for various purposes, they must also view documentation as an asset used to measure the value and contribution of their services to patient/family/community well-being.

DRAWBACKS OF OUTCOMES

Most home care agencies will have little choice but to involve themselves in outcomes, if they haven't already. If there is no internal impetus or commitment, the external demands of the Joint Commission, HCFA, and OASIS will force compliance to using outcomes. Payers and MCOs are already showing a growing sophistication in the area of clinical outcomes, rather than just hospital readmissions, infection rates, adverse drug reactions, or patient satisfaction.

The outcome movement is not without its drawbacks, however. In addition to the documentation challenges mentioned above, some of the other hazards facing outcomes programs are as follows:

Lack of Standardization of Definitions, Terms, and Measures. There is still much confusion over what an outcome is and how it is measured. Different measures abound, each with different definitions, so comparisons are difficult and the value of the data is limited. Furthermore, there is no standardized language so the same, or similar, outcomes are called different things depending on the whim of the provider. OASIS will assist with some of these difficulties, but OASIS alone is not a sufficient outcome program for an agency.

Outcomes Programs Are Resource Intense and Expensive. Data collection is always an expensive proposition, and the need for data must always be balanced with the burden of collecting it. Outcomes programs often are unfocused, implemented only to satisfy an external need, and lacking in expertise. This increases expense and diminishes the value of the return on investment. Voluminous and/or irrelevant data end up being collected, most of which are never used to improve patient care or agency operations. It has been shown that the ability to collect and analyze outcome data does not necessarily translate into the ability to utilize this information for improving performance.[25] The very first step to using outcomes needs to be answering the question, How will using outcomes enhance your knowledge and ability to improve patient care, knowledge, or attitudes, or a system? The second step is having the expertise available to operationalize and maintain the outcomes program.

Cost and time-consuming paperwork were also seen as drawbacks in the OASIS project. Pilot agencies reported that

- The amount of time that monitoring the program requires exceeded expectations
- They experienced additional costs—staff education, follow-up on required documentation, printing, and computer systems
- They experienced an increased workload for the primary care nurses and data entry staff[26]

Outcome Programs That Are Compliance Driven Rather Than   Patient Care Driven Often Collect Data Based on Ease of Collection Rather Than Relevancy. The result can be a lot of good data that does not mean anything or is not helpful in improving patient care. For example, one agency collected information about how many of its patients met their therapeutic goals at time of discharge because the data was readily available on its management information system. According to the results, 51 percent had their goals met, 6 percent had died, 4 percent had transferred to a different location, 4 percent were hospitalized, and the remainder were "other." Did those that died have their therapeutic goals met? Although these data might appear to be a good start, they really don't provide a good launching pad for improving care. At best, extensive investigation would have to occur before any changes could be made to practice patterns.

GETTING STARTED

The most important step in beginning the use of outcomes is creating the climate. Using outcomes is a different way of thinking and a different way of doing business. Staff need to feel safe in documenting care that reflects effectiveness or ineffectiveness. Sometimes they are going to make mistakes, as we all do, and they need to know they won't be punished for it. The changing need/value of documentation should be discussed so that additional paperwork can be incorporated into work routines without it being seen as more burden. The shift from evaluating tasks to evaluating systems needs to be started. Other suggestions for getting started include the following:

- Start slow—choose only one or two areas to start so that new ideas and processes can be piloted.
- Choose areas that are easy and manageable—don't use this opportunity as the chance to resolve a problem that you have never been able to resolve before. Instead, choose an area that is well-defined and manageable. Program the project for success. Remember that barriers are going to have to be removed. Expect mistakes, and offer rewards.
- Involve all levels of personnel—outcomes affect everyone since they affect how the agency operates. Involve support personnel, ancillary personnel, supervisors, caregivers, and clients.
- Be creative—remember, outcomes are something new. Everyone is learning. If it hasn't been done before it can't be done wrong, and once it has been done there is always another opportunity to do it better. Using outcomes is a process in itself that can be continually improved.

CONCLUSION

This chapter has described the concept of outcomes, their utilization, the need for the complete and accurate documentation of outcomes, and drawbacks to their use. The key to their successful use lies in understanding and defining why they are being used by an agency, department, or caregiver. Therefore, the best means to recapture all the ingredients is to examine the process of outcomes itself.

As we saw earlier in this book, in Figure 2–2, a process's components include input, activities, and output. Figure 6–4 depicts the process of outcomes. This is

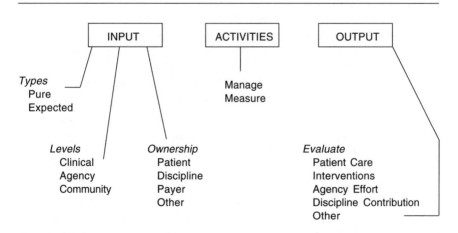

Figure 6–4 The Process of Outcomes

a conceptual-level depiction of the process of using outcomes that contains all the ingredients. Any of these ingredients can be appropriately selected for application at an operational level. The operational outcome process can then be managed using the steps found in Chapter 11.

Once the output is determined, selecting the inputs (type, level, and ownership) and the activities, either measuring or managing, is easy. The next challenge is to have the resources and expertise to implement and evaluate the program on an ongoing basis.

NOTES

1. N.M. Lang and J.F. Clinton, Assessment of Quality of Nursing Care, in *Annual Review of Nursing Research,* eds. H.H. Werley and J.J. Fitzpatrick (New York: Springer Publishing Co., 1984), 135–163.

2. N. Bauman, T. Mazich, and T. Reiff, Outcomes Analysis: How Substantial? *Homecare Providers Buyers Guide*, no. 2 (1994): 45.

3. A. Donabedian, Quality Assessment and Assurance: Unity of Purpose, Diversity of Means, *Inquiry* 25, no. 1 (1988): 173–192.

4. Donabedian, Quality Assessment and Assurance, 173–192.

5. D. Peters, Strategic Directions for Using Outcomes, *The Remington Report* 11 (June/July 1994): 9–11.

6. Peters, Strategic Directions, 9–11.

7. John Roger and P. McWilliams, *Life 101* (Los Angeles: Prelude Press, 1990), 234.

8. P.W. Shaughnessy and K.S. Crisler, *Outcome-Based Quality Improvement* (Denver, CO: Colorado Center for Health Policy and Services Research, 1995).

9. Shaughnessy and Crisler, *Outcome-Based Quality Improvement.*

10. Shaughnessy and Crisler, *Outcome-Based Quality Improvement.*

11. Shaughnessy and Crisler, *Outcome-Based Quality Improvement.*

12. L. Long, ed., Lessons from the OBQI Demonstrations Sites, *Caring* 16, no. 9 (1997): 46–50.

13. Shaughnessy and Crisler, *Outcome-Based Quality Improvement.*

14. C. Schaffer and F. Srp, Outcome Driven Home Care: Quality, Savings, and Results, *Caring* 15, no. 6 (1996): 8–12.

15. B.S. Gingerich and D.A. Ondeck, *Clinical Pathways for the Multidisciplinary Home Care Team* (Gaithersburg, MD: Aspen Publishers, 1997), 9:2–9:4.

16. D. Meadows, Measuring a City's Health, *The Systems Thinker* 7, no. 1(1996): 10–11.

17. Meadows, Measuring a City's Health, 10–11.

18. D. Tibitts, *Disney's Celebration Health* (Paper presented at the American Academy of Nursing Annual Meeting and Conference, Orlando, FL, November 1996).

19. Agency for Health Care Policy and Research, *Using Clinical Practice Guidelines To Evaluate Quality of Care,* Vol. 1, AHCPR Publication 95–0045 (Rockville, MD: 1995).

20. K.N. Lohr, Outcome Measurement: Concept and Questions, *Inquiry* 25 (Spring 1988): 37–50.

21. H.H. Werley and N.M. Lang, eds., *Identification of the Nursing Minimum Data Set* (New York: Springer Publishing Co., 1988).

22. M.L. Maas et al. Classifying Nursing-Sensitive Patient Outcomes, *Image* 28, no. 4 (1996): 295–301.

23. Maas et al., Classifying Nursing-Sensitive Patient Outcomes, 296.

24. S. Bright and G. Beyt, Lessons in Systems Thinking: A Tale from the Land of Middle Health, *The Systems Thinker* 6, no. 6 (1995): 1–5.

25. B.I. Braun and F.S. Zibrat, Developing an Outcomes Measurement System: The Value of Testing, *American Journal of Medical Quality* 11, no. 2 (1996): 57–67.

26. Long, Lessons from the OBQI Demonstration Sites, 46–50.

CHAPTER 7

How High Are Your Standards?

Standards are a carry-over from the old paradigm. The term *standards* is used more than it is defined, is used in many contexts, and is often misunderstood. There has been a prolific development of standards over the past several decades. Everyone got into the business of writing them because standards were perceived as having a direct connection to quality and, of course, everybody wants to be connected with quality. The number of standards has become so great it is difficult for any practitioner to know all of the standards to which he or she is accountable. The 1998 Health Standards Directory offered by ECRI indexes 32,000 health care standards, guidelines, laws, and regulations from more than 900 organizations. It is extremely important for clinicians to recognize these standards because, as a practitioner, one is legally accountable for practicing at the level defined by standards. The old paradigm viewed standards as mandated constraints and controls. In the new paradigm, the authority of standards comes from those who use them and, therefore, standards can become a foundation for improvement and trust. This chapter deals with

- defining standards
- identifying industrial (home care), professional, and institutional standards
- describing the relationship of standards to cost and quality
- implementing standards

DEFINITION

Standards are authoritative, descriptive statements of a level of performance against which quality or cost can be evaluated. They are a measurement of performance and are important elements to consider in measuring quality and/or

144

cost. At one time it was felt that standards represented excellence and the level of performance to which all should aspire. It soon became evident, however, that standards defined as excellence could actually constrain the industry, profession, or agency, because there was no incentive to do better than the standard that already defined excellence. Once someone met the standard there was no reason to try harder. Furthermore, it was difficult to be held accountable for excellence in every situation.[1] Therefore, the representation of standards was reevaluated, and organizations such as the American Nurses Association (ANA) are now defining standards as standards of competency.[2]

Standards can also be seen as a description of the responsibilities for which one is accountable. It is generally acknowledged and interpreted by the judicial system that standards are seen to be rigidly followed with few, if any, exceptions. This can be problematic, as it has been in nursing, where standards were either so general that they could not be easily applied to individual client situations, or so narrow that they were inappropriate in many situations. Thus they were largely ignored by practicing nurses.[3]

An argument also can be made that standards should focus on quality and not cost; if activities are carried out in an efficient manner, costs will be acceptable. In other words, costs are a byproduct (or lagging indicator of care) rather than the driver of care. Because of the many cost concerns regarding health care, and the unknowns facing the home care industry (e.g., managed care and prospective payment), however, finances are a priority. Financial standards, then, are often developed before quality standards and clinical guidelines and in these instances may become a driver of care. Financial standards reflect a uniform approach for the presentation of financial statements. They can include length of stay, resource utilization, and costs associated with the patient's care. They provide another view of agency operations that may offer clues to areas needing improvement. Financial standards also provide the perfect opportunity to build trust between payers and providers. Table 7–1 compares the focus, scope, intent, and application of quality and financial standards.

Table 7–1 Standards for Quality and Cost

	Quality Standards	Financial Standards
Focus	Agent responsibilities	Utilization (units and dollars)
Scope	Care provided to all consumers	Cost of care provided to all consumers
Intent	Efficiency—doing things well	Affordability—doing things well within cost constraints
Application	Rigid	Rigid

Standards are significant for many reasons. First, standards reflect the values, beliefs, and priorities of the industry, the profession, and/or the agency for which they were developed and provide direction for the provision and evaluation of services. They are designed to endure over time, compared to clinical guidelines, which are continually changing as care changes. Standards require modification only when changes occur in the values or priorities upon which they are based.

Second, standards provide a means for an industry or profession to exercise self-regulation. They focus on the agent (e.g., industry standards focus on providers, professional standards focus on the practitioner, and agency standards focus on agency employees). Nursing standards, for example, focus on nurses. If all nurses adhere to their professional standards, then the profession is ensured a competent level of performance because the nursing profession has promulgated the standards. Nurses have determined their own level of competency. This circumstance contrasts with situations where there are no standards and therefore standards are applied from the outside, mandating compliance by the profession. Types of external standards include governmental regulations, such as Medicare Conditions of Participation (COPs) and state licensing laws, which have been discussed in Chapter 4.

Third, standards provide a basis for trust. For example, in health care there are performance standards that payers use to determine the adequacy of service delivery. Because there are no reasonable performance standards in home care, payers have no way to measure the provider's performance. This absence of standards leaves the door open for concerns and worry about low performance. Thus the home care industry is placed in a position of having to respond to the overreaction of payer organizations to this concern or distrust in the form of unrealistic performance expectations.[4]

Next, standards provide a basis for determining negligence. For example, the procedure for establishing negligence in nursing performance consists of the following:

- determining the standard that governs the situation
- establishing that harm could be foreseen as a result of not meeting the standard
- proving that the nurse failed to meet the relevant standard
- determining that the nurse's failure to meet the standard caused harm to the client[5]

Finally, standards can be used as teaching aids for inexperienced staff and serve as the basis for performance evaluations because they provide a descriptive framework of the expected performance. Professional standards define the competencies expected of the professional. Agency standards define indisputable expected behaviors. Together they establish a foundation for employees to understand what is expected from them. Using those expectations as the basis for performance evaluations provides the practitioner with a framework for continually monitoring and demonstrating the employee's proficiency.

CATEGORIES OF STANDARDS

As mentioned previously, standards can be either external or internal. External standards are those to which one must comply and are imposed from outside, or the environment. Their intent is to control the level of performance, which is accomplished through a three-step process.[6]

Step 1. Develop and adopt standards. These standards focus on adequacy, or a minimum level of performance.

Step 2. Survey providers to assess the degree of compliance with the standards. There are many issues around the surveillance process itself, including the fact that not all surveillance activities are equally effective in promoting compliance with standards or in identifying noncompliers. Furthermore, there is little standardization in the surveillance process. For example, agencies without deemed status report passing their Medicare survey with no deficiencies one week and the next week having their Joint Commission survey and receiving deficiencies on numerous items that were supposedly surveyed by Medicare, or vice versa.

Step 3. Impose sanctions in response to reported deviations from standards. Noncompliance with Joint Commission standards can mean loss of accreditation. Noncompliance with Medicare COPs can mean even further loss. For example, there is Operation Restore Trust (ORT), an intensified effort to combat fraud and abuse in the Medicare and Medicaid programs. In its first two years, ORT has collected almost $188 million in restitution, fines, settlements, and other identified overpayments to patients from providers who did not meet the standards for providing services in the Medicare program. ORT has excluded 218 health care providers from the Medicare and Medicaid programs.[7]

One of the most challenging problems with external standards is writing them in a way that describes the level of performance such that control processes can be employed. In other words, the standard must be written so that it can be universally understood by the external surveyors and applied uniformly to all situations or providers to control the level of performance. External control processes work best in measuring structural aspects of quality. With more movement toward outcome measurement and management, however, it may be wiser to have external controls that intervene at a higher level by creating expectations for the process of quality assurance.[8] Interestingly enough, both accreditation standards and the new COPs are moving in this direction. The proposed COPs are changing the focus from the review of structure and procedural requirements to quality and the review of individual and aggregate outcomes. The core of these COPs is the presence of a self-sustaining system for performance improvement within an agency. The goal is to be able to demonstrate improved outcomes of care and patient satisfaction. To assist in this process, collection of the Outcome and Assessment Information Set (OASIS) questions is expected to be mandated. The role of the surveyor will be to confirm the agency's assessment of its performance. Ultimately, although not yet proposed, there will be a regulation to report outcomes to HCFA so that the surveyors can direct their review toward the poorest outcomes.

All that being said, it is internal standards to which an industry, professional, or agency commits that are the main focus of this chapter. Three categories of internal standards will be addressed: (1) industry, (2) professional, and (3) institutional.

Industry Standards

Industry standards focus on the performance of home care providers. No internal standards currently exist for home care and, until recently, no process existed to define appropriate performance standards. Providers have been fearful of standards because of the wide variation among patients, providers, and circumstances. The increase in home care providers contracting with MCOs, however, has promulgated the need and interest of the providers to establish fair and consistent standards for travel, distance, and service times.

This process has been assumed by the Institute for Ancillary Network Standards (IANS), a group of more than 20 home care professionals with extensive experience in managed care contracting and home care operations.[9] The goal of IANS is to develop reasonable standards for agency performance that would assist in establishing equitable payer expectations. IANS has developed standards for services to patients located in urban, suburban, and rural areas for

- travel time—the time it takes a professional to reach the patient
- geographic distance—the miles to the patient's home
- service time—the time between when a referral is received and when home care is rendered

These standards are represented in Table 7–2.

Table 7–2 Standards for Home Care Provider Performance

Provider Type		Urban	Suburban	Rural
RN	Travel time	Within 1 hour	1 hour	1.5 hours
LPN				
Infusion RN	Distance	2 providers with-in 35 miles	2 providers with-in 45 miles	1 provider with-in 60 miles
HHA				
MSW				
	Service time	24 hours	24 hours	24 hours
Hospice	Service time	24 hours	24 hours	48 hours
Therapies (PT, OT, ST)	Service time	48 hours	48 hours	48 hours
Others:				
Psych nurse Enterostomal T	Travel time	1 hour	1 hour	1.5 hours
MCH Peds nurse	Distance	1 provider with-in 35 miles	1 provider with-in 45 miles	1 provider with-in 60 miles
Cert diab. ed.	Service time	24 hours	24 hours	24 hours

Source: Reproduced by permission of the National Association for Home Care, from *Caring Magazine*, vol. XVI, no. 6 (June 1997). Not for further reproduction.

Standards for travel time, distance, and service time are shown for urban, suburban, and rural agencies. Travel time and distance standards listed above the bold line apply to all provider types (RN, LPN, infusion RN, HHA, MSW, hospice, and therapies) above the line. Service time standards differ for the hospice and therapies so they are listed separately. Different standards for travel time, distance, and service time apply for the psychiatric nurse, enterostomal therapist, MCH, pediatric nurse, and certified diabetic educator and they are listed below the bold line by the urban, suburban, and rural provider designations.

This group of home care experts felt that meeting these standards would require operational efficiency and strong management leadership, and that over time more detailed standards would evolve. These more detailed standards would be directly linked to financial, operational, and clinical performance indicators and integrated with broader, more comprehensive systems of provider evaluation. This implies a sense of excellence to accomplishing these standards rather than either competency or minimal performance. Thus IANS was challenged by the aforementioned issue of how to be held accountable for excellence in every situation. They agreed that meeting all of the standards all of the time was not realistic due to conditions beyond their control, such as bad weather. Their solution was to establish core rules of performance to determine aggregate thresholds of overall performance. These rules are

- 90 percent of the network providers will meet the standards
- 90 percent of the time, selected providers will comply with the standards
- 90 percent of the patients will be served within the standards[10]

Establishing these rules may appear contradictory to the definition of standards, but standard setting is an evolving concept from the old to the new paradigm. These standards represent a beginning approach for the home care industry to self-regulate, rather than having to respond to the demands of managed care, and that is significant. Moving from one paradigm to the next is not a simple event. It is a slow evolution, similar to peeling the leaves from an artichoke until one gets to the heart. During the entire process, old thinking is likely to slip in unnoticed, and one must always be alert for this.

The group acknowledges that there is much work and cultivating to be done. The immediate plans of the IANS are to

- Develop a plan for acceptance of these standards by other provider organizations
- Approach professional trade associations, such as the National Association for Home Care (NAHC) and the National Association of Medical Equipment Suppliers (NAMES), for support
- Approach payer organizations that are interested in using these standards in their managed care contracts
- Begin developing more specific clinical and financial standards

Development of more specific clinical and financial standards is a natural evolution. It would also be natural to base them on data that are beginning to become available. For example, the following (Table 7–3) appears in the *Home Health Data Quarterly*[11] published by Aspen Publishers. Data such as these collected over time could result in regional or national standards for how many days it should take to transmit bills to payers. The sooner bills go out, the sooner agencies can receive the reimbursement and have that money working for them. Table 7–3 illustrates current variability in the average number of days to bill Medicare, ranging from 9.6 days in the Southeast to 18.5 days in the Southwest. For all other payers, the range is from 8.8 days in the Northwest to 29.2 days in the Southwest. Based on these data, for whatever reason, it seems to take agencies in the Southwest longer to transmit a bill to their payers than it takes agencies in other regions of the country.

Table 7–3 Agency Billing Summary

	All Agencies	Northwest	Southwest	Midwest	Northeast	Southeast
Average number of total bills per month	1,003.1	381.2	767.9	647.4	2,123.8	530.5
Average number of days to bill Medicare	14.6	10.2	18.5	17.2	12.7	9.6
Average number of days to bill all others	21.8	8.8	29.2	25.5	20.1	14.6

Source: Adapted from S. Davis, *Home Health Data Quarterly*, Vol. 1, no. 1, p. 25, © 1997, Aspen Publishers, Inc.

On the surface, developing more specific standards for home care sounds like an ideal way for home care to continue to regulate itself. Caution is the word, however. Too many standards become constraining. For example, using the data in Table 7–3, say a standard was developed that said all bills had to be submitted to payers within 21 days (the current national average). A standard delineating the number of days an agency has to bill a payer may seem strange, but it could be offered as a means to regulate an agency's efficiency in order to keep the agency viable. It may be a real challenge for the Southwest, however, to take a week off their billing cycle. Also, it may constrain agencies from accepting contracts from payers that may have unusual billing requirements for fear they couldn't meet the standard. Thus, creative payment systems to support home care could be lost. A better approach may be for individual agencies to use these data as benchmarks in their quality improvement programs. In the industry's enthusiasm to self-regulate, it is important not to lose sight of the purpose of standards as well as their shortcomings.

Professional Standards

Professional standards focus on the professional care provider, such as the nurse, and articulate the scope of nursing practice. They focus the effort and interest of professional practice and provide a framework for the evaluation of that practice. Professional standards assist the profession in articulating what it encompasses (e.g., its scope of practice) and the activities for which it can be held accountable. In addition, they define the profession's accountability to the public.

The ANA has been involved in standard development for professional nurses since the late 1960s. ANA published its first standards of practice for the nursing profession in 1973. These standards were updated, and the revised standards were published in 1991 in a document entitled the *Standards of Clinical Nursing Practice*.[12] This revision included participation by state nurses associations and more than 30 specialty nursing groups from the National Organization Liaison Forum (NOLF). This collaborative approach yielded a framework developed by nurses that is applicable to all nursing practice. In 1995, the ANA charged its Committee on Nursing Practice Standards and Guidelines with reviewing the standards every five years and revising if necessary. This committee is currently undertaking such a process, and updated standards will be released shortly. Based on current feedback, revisions to the standards are expected to be minimal. In addition, specialty standards continue to be developed by specialty nursing organizations to reflect their unique areas of practice. The shared framework and standards from the *Standards of Clinical Nursing Practice,* however, are supported by these groups and unify this multifaceted profession.

The *Standards of Clinical Nursing Practice* apply to all professional nurses engaged in clinical practice regardless of specialty, practice setting, or educational preparation. They are generic in nature and address the care that is provided to all clients (individual, family, group, or community). The *Standards of Clinical Nursing Practice* include both standards of care and standards of professional performance. Exhibit 7–1 identifies the areas addressed by both the standards of care and standards of professional performance. The standards of care reflect a competent level of nursing provided to all clients as embodied in the activities and behaviors of the nursing process. The standards of professional performance address other professional role activities and behaviors appropriate to one's education, position, and practice environment.

The standards of care are enumerated in Exhibit 7–2 and use the nursing process as the framework to describe nursing practice. They address the activities of assessment, diagnosis, outcome identification, planning, implementation, and evaluation. The inclusion of a separate standard focusing on outcome identification reflects the importance of this activity in providing nursing care. The results of a recent survey conducted through *The American Nurse* revealed this standard and its associated criteria to be highly utilized by nurses in their practice, but to be generally the least used standard of the six.[13]

Also included in the standards of care are relevant measurable criteria that further define and demonstrate commitment to each standard. For example, the criteria for the standard on Outcome Identification is found in Exhibit 7–3. There are some common threads found in the criteria that weave throughout all the standards of care. These common threads define the following responsibilities for nursing practice:[14]

Exhibit 7–1 Areas Addressed by the Standards of Clinical Nursing Practice

Standards of Care
I. Assessment
II. Diagnosis
III. Outcome Identification
IV. Planning
V. Implementation
VI. Evaluation

Standards of Professional Performance
I. Quality of Care
II. Performance Appraisal
III. Education
IV. Collegiality
V. Ethics
VI. Collaboration
VII. Research
VIII. Resource Utilization

Source: Courtesy of American Nurses Association, Washington, D.C.

- A practice that sets priorities, is realistic, and is relevant to the client's immediate condition or needs
- A practice that is documented in a retrievable format
- A practice that includes the client, significant others, and other health care providers, as appropriate.

Exhibit 7–2 Standards of Care

I. Assessment
The nurse collects client health data.
II. Diagnosis
The nurse analyzes the assessment data in determining diagnoses.
III. Outcome Identification
The nurse identifies expected outcomes individualized to the client.
IV. Planning
The nurse develops a plan of care that prescribes interventions to attain expected outcomes.
V. Implementation
The nurse implements the interventions identified in the plan of care.
VI. Evaluation
The nurse evaluates the client's progress toward attainment of outcomes.

Source: Courtesy of American Nurses Association, Washington, D.C.

Exhibit 7–3 Criteria for the Standard on Outcome Identification

---

Standard III. Outcome Identification
THE NURSE IDENTIFIES EXPECTED OUTCOMES
INDIVIDUALIZED TO THE CLIENT.

Measurement Criteria:

1. Outcomes are derived from the diagnoses.
2. Outcomes are documented as measurable goals.
3. Outcomes are mutually formulated with the client and health care providers, when possible.
4. Outcomes are realistic in relation to the client's present and potential capabilities.
5. Outcomes are attainable in relation to resources available to the client.
6. Outcomes include a time estimate for attainment.
7. Outcomes provide a direction for continuity of care.

Source: Courtesy of American Nurses Association, Washington, D.C.

The standards of professional performance include activities that may not be directly evident in providing care to clients but are an integral part of the professional nurse's role. These activities include quality of care, performance appraisal, education, collegiality, ethics, collaboration, research, and resource utilization. Exhibit 7–4 enumerates the standard for each of these areas. All nurses are expected to engage in these activities appropriate to their education, position, and practice environment. Because of the wide diversity in these areas, the measurement criteria in these standards identify a broad range of activities that can demonstrate commitment to the standard. For example, the quality of care standard includes criteria that range from identifying aspects of care that are important for monitoring its quality to developing policies and procedures to improve care. Similarly, the research standard has diverse criteria that range from identifying clinical problems suitable for nursing research to conducting research projects.

These *Standards of Clinical Nursing Practice* are used as discrete entities to shape, define, and measure nursing practice. They can also be used as the foundation for other activities such as quality assurance, database development, documentation system development, and educational and certification activities. They also can be used to develop institutional standards such as policies, position descriptions, and performance appraisals.

Exhibit 7–4 Standards of Professional Performance

I.   Quality of Care The nurse systematically evaluates the quality and effectiveness of nursing practice. II.   Performance Appraisal The nurse evaluates his or her own nursing practice in relation to professional practice standards and relevant statutes and regulations. III. Education The nurse acquires and maintains current knowledge in nursing practice. IV. Collegiality The nurse contributes to the professional development of peers, colleagues, and others. V.   Ethics The nurse's decisions and actions on behalf of clients are determined in an ethical manner. VI. Collaboration The nurse collaborates with the client, significant others, and health care providers in providing client care. VII. Research The nurse uses research findings in practice. VIII. Resource Utilization The nurse considers factors related to safety, effectiveness, and cost in planning and delivering client care. *Source:* Courtesy of American Nurses Association, Washington, D.C.

Institutional Standards

The third category of standards is institutional standards. Institutional standards focus on the personnel and their care delivery systems within a given agency. They include policies, flowcharts, and position descriptions. Often these items are overlooked as standards, but do in fact serve as authoritative statements by which agency personnel are held accountable.

Policies

Policies are inflexible declarations that establish the foundation for the provision of care. They allow for no professional judgment or interpretation. They do not focus on clinical practice itself, but rather on the resources and conditions under which care is provided (e.g., who is to do what under what circumstances). These resources and conditions can be divided into three general categories:

1. Conditions that require delineation of responsibility. Specifically considered are those areas in which confusion about the focus of responsibility might result in malperformance of an act necessary to a patient's well-being. An example is a policy that defines admission and discharge criteria.
2. Conditions surrounding the protection of patients' and families' rights. An example is a policy on informing patients (and their families) of their rights.
3. Conditions surrounding personnel management and welfare. An example is a policy on staffing levels.[15]

The tendency is to write too many policies, or to categorize statements as policies that are really some other standard or guideline. Because policies are ironclad statements, there should and need to be only a few policies within a given agency. Because staff are held legally accountable for policy standards, it is important that they are reviewed periodically to be certain that they are relevant. Policies by definition are considered relatively stable, but with the rapidly evolving system of health care, they may become outdated.

Flowcharts

A flowchart is the depiction of all the predetermined sequential steps of a process. It is used as part of quality improvement to ensure that everyone knows the required steps in a given process. A flowchart provides easy identification of deviations from the process, sources of problems, and inefficiencies. Philosophically, both quality improvement and reengineering concepts assert that there are a limited number of key processes that are crucial to the organization of an agency. Once these processes are identified, the ideal steps to the processes are diagrammed using the shapes found in Figure 7–1. For example, a box symbolizes steps/activities and a diamond symbolizes a decision point. Processes that have been defined earlier in this book that would benefit from flowcharts include the support processes and the processes upstream and downstream from the patient-focused care process.

The resulting flowchart (once tested, revised, and retested until it is deemed the most efficient and effective means of performing a process) becomes the standard to which agency employees are held accountable when enacting that process. Figure 7–2 is an example of a flowchart for the referral process, one of the upstream processes of patient-focused care.

Position Descriptions

Position descriptions establish the standard qualifications and responsibilities for all persons within a position or job category. They reflect the competence, education, and experience required for all persons in a category and describe the

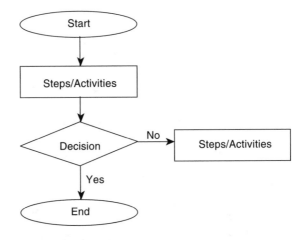

Figure 7–1 Shapes Used in the Flowchart Process

set role for which they are compensated.[16] Position descriptions are important because they present the responsibilities of the position and the qualifications of those who carry them out. As such, they define the role of each position of the "team" that is carrying out the mission of the agency. Charles Garfield reminds us of a simple fact of teamwork: "If my end of the boat sinks, so does yours."[17 (p.192)] Position descriptions help keep the boat afloat by defining who maintains the hull, who keeps the pump running, and who starts bailing when the water starts coming in. In this manner, team members can support each other's goals and apply peer pressure to other team members to maintain the position standards. One way this is accomplished is through performance evaluations.

Performance evaluations measure the degree to which a team member is meeting the competencies in the position description for his or her job. As mentioned earlier, professional standards define competencies for a profession. Where appropriate these can be used in a professional's position description and performance evaluation. For example, one position description in an agency may be for a clinical nurse or home care staff nurse. The position description would be the same regardless of individual professional differences or differences in geographical setting or caseload. It would be appropriate to use the ANA standards of care and standards of professional performance as the basis for competencies required for that position. Whatever competencies are identified, an agency must establish a system for measuring these competencies on a regular basis.

The evolving nature of the health care system, however, may require health professionals who possess different competencies and attitudes, and some of these differences may be in conflict with the traditional professional boundaries. For

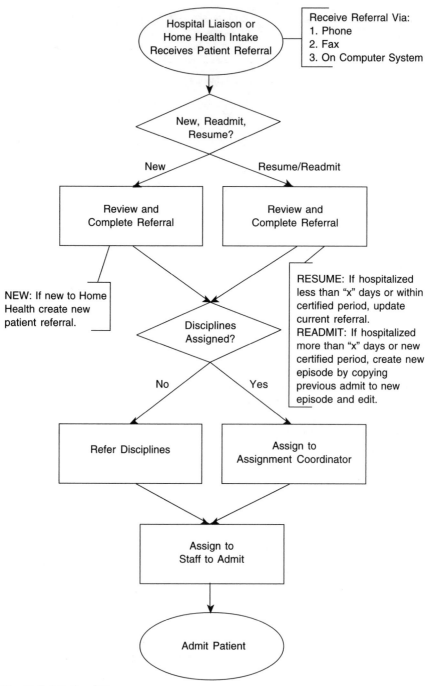

Figure 7–2 Referral Process

example, the emerging health care system has already allowed for a broader range of providers to have more responsibilities for the delivery of many aspects of patient care, as evidenced by the growing use of advanced nurse clinicians as primary care providers. This will require greater skill at collaboration, communication, and teamwork. Some of the required competencies that the Pew Health Professions Commission has identified for health care workers in the year 2005 include[18]

- Work to improve the health of the community
- Understand health care needs within a cultural context
- Provide contemporary clinical care
- Function in new health care settings
- Respond to increasing levels of public, governmental, and third-party participation in the health care system
- Ensure cost-effective care
- Use technology appropriately
- Emphasize primary and secondary preventive strategies for all
- Assist individuals, families, and communities to maintain and promote healthy lifestyles
- Involve patients and families in the decision-making process
- Manage and use scientific, technological, and patient information to maintain professional competence
- Continue to grow throughout practice life

Furthermore, as the relationship between the patient and clinician becomes more of a partnership, and patients assume more responsibility for their care, treatment will be more educational than therapeutic. The role of the clinician, therefore, will be more of an educator and coach.

It may be that these competencies could become the basis for all professional job descriptions including those of nurses, social workers, and the rehabilitation therapies. Another important competency that is already being added to position descriptions is computer literacy.

Position descriptions do not, however, define the unique skills, qualities, and values that the individual brings to the position. These attributes are the capabilities and characteristics of employees that set each person apart from others. Each person has something to contribute to the organizational team. The challenge and opportunity is to define those skills and qualities and then maximize the employee's use of those skills. Employees are an agency's most important asset and its greatest expense. Therefore, maximizing performance is a way to minimize cost and improve quality. It is also a way to increase job satisfaction.

Performance skills can include any type of special certification, such as venipuncture, or special knowledge, such as a second language. Performance qualities can include abilities and qualities that affect the relationship with the client. For example, one ability may be the capacity to relate to difficult patients. A characteristic to consider in placing home health aides may be whether or not they are smokers. Other considerations to make when assigning patients are personal growth experiences. For example, whether a care provider has experienced the death of someone close may be a factor in assigning that caregiver to a dying client.[19]

Considering these unique individual attributes, two approaches can be used to maximize performance. The first is to match talents and qualities with patient needs. Two examples were cited above. Agencies do reasonably well in matching performance skills with patient needs, but fall considerably short when attempting to match other qualities and characteristics. With better means of tracking these attributes, such as through electronic computer scheduling systems, it should be easier to identify such matches. Electronic scheduling systems can track these attributes and then match "qualified" staff to patient needs. The savings from the improved pairing of patient to caregiver may in itself pay for the electronic system. This can be illustrated using the home health aide example above. It is quite expensive to remove a home health aide from a case and assign another one. This is a common occurrence, however, when an aide who smokes is placed in a nonsmoking residence. To replace the aide, the agency must once again go through the difficult process of finding an aide who is available. This time the selection is narrowed to only those aides who are nonsmokers. Next, the nurse must make another supervisory visit, which in all likelihood is not billable. And of course, the agency has to deal with the unsatisfied patient, a potentially time-consuming undertaking.

The second approach to maximizing performance is to establish work teams. Instead of relying on autocratic, controlling systems to make decisions, there is the opportunity to develop empowered work teams to take on the responsibility for the assignment and distribution of work. In this approach, team members self-select their varying levels of skills to meet the group goals. For example, if a nurse has a talent for assessing clients' needs, but falls short when it comes to defining a plan of action, the team has the freedom and creativity to mix and match that nurse with someone with complementary talents or to use peer pressure to obtain improvement. Team communication and group processes are used by the team to maximize productivity.

This concept has been used successfully in the hospital setting over the past 10 years under the title of shared governance or professional practice model. It has recently been successfully implemented in the home care setting.[20] At Westhills Home Health Care in Massachusetts, nursing visits increased from about 350 to 900/month after the organization implemented a professional practice model in just 18 months.[21] Essential beliefs include the following:

1. Professionals can manage their own practice and function as part of a self-directed work team.
2. The role of management is to develop and support an organizational culture that fosters professional practice and establishes clear expectations via well-defined goals, position descriptions, and standards.
3. Total quality management (TQM) is based on people and service.
4. Everyone shares the values of honest communication, and respect and trust for each other's ideas.[22]

Rather than using the council or committee structure of shared governance programs in acute care, home care utilized a self-directed work team due to the geographic separation of the team members. These teams consist of employees who are in agreement on objectives, have the required resources, and are empowered to make their own decisions in meeting the goals of the agency.[23] Initially, teams take on the responsibility for daily operations and problem solving using agency standards to maintain consistency and the agency's defined level of quality. As the team develops and matures, additional responsibilities can be added such as hiring, performance evaluations, and disciplinary action.[24] The role of the supervisor moves away from the traditional planning, organizing, and directing of the staff's workload to growth promotion functions for both staff and the agency. These functions can encompass aspects of marketing and include budgeting, strategic planning, and program development.[25] Notice that one of the key elements for the successful implementation of this approach is well-defined agency standards.

RELATIONSHIP OF STANDARDS TO QUALITY

From the consumers' perspective, there are three levels of quality that are attached to a service or product: (1) expected quality, (2) established quality, and (3) unexpected quality.

Expected quality is a minimum or acceptable level of quality that is taken for granted, for example, quality that is defined by an RN license. A consumer expects a nurse to be able to perform techniques and skills that are defined by law and guaranteed by the professional license. The consumer is usually not able to technically measure this type of quality (e.g., whether a nurse correctly changes a catheter). On the other hand, the consumers do not usually concern themselves with this level of quality; they consider this level of quality a given.

Established quality is a level of quality that places a service or product above its competitors, for example, a home care agency that always makes the first visit the same day the patient is discharged or an agency caregiver who always arrives promptly on schedule. This type of quality can be measured by the consumer, and it is. Not only is it measured, but the consumer uses it as the basis for determining the quality level of the product or service. It is this level of quality that is being placed on scorecards that consumers can use to determine if they want to use a given agency or caregiver.

Unexpected quality is the level of quality is known as the "ah-ha" level because it is a surprise quality (i.e., it is reached when an agency does something that is not expected). For example, this level of quality occurs when an agency has a caregiver waiting at the house when a needy patient is discharged from the hospital. This type of quality is seen quite often after there has been a problem and the agency goes beyond what is necessary to remedy it. An example from the retail world would be receiving a replacement product, no questions asked, when one has had a problem with a similar model. Interestingly, as more companies adopt this type of policy, former aspects of unexpected quality become part of established quality, and the premium for unexpected quality is raised.

All levels of quality are important for an agency. Standards are the foundation for the first level, expected quality. In one sense, that seems to make standards very unexciting, especially in a consumer-driven era, because they are not reflected in consumer attitudes or responses. The minute that expected quality is not present, however, there is no quality at all. It is the foundation for the other two levels. It is the basis of consumer trust. There is a trust on the consumers' part that the agency will maintain a standard level of quality. Defining those standards is an important part of the trust. Just as an RN's license defines a minimal level of quality that consumers can expect from any professional nurse, standards define an expected level of quality for a given industry, profession, or agency. In fact, a license is a standard established by legislators (external to the profession) to protect the consumer (minimum standard). Professional standards, such as the standards of clinical practice, are the self-regulatory, competency-based standards developed by the profession.

Because standards are basic to quality, it behooves an agency to define all the external and internal standards that impact on the services it provides as part of its quality assurance program and to establish a mechanism to ensure that those standards are maintained. Notice that this is quality assurance, not quality improvement. As mentioned before, standards are relatively stable by definition. Of course standards can be changed or improved, but that is not their primary purpose. Standards are a defined level of competency (expected quality) that become the keystone for established and unexpected quality, and for trust.

Immediate questions are, How does one ensure that standards are met? How can one monitor the myriad standards to which one is beholden? Good questions. The first step is to identify all these standards. The second step is to eliminate the ones that are inappropriate or that have been labeled incorrectly as standards. Wrongly identified standards are a legal liability, a constraint to practice, a monitoring nightmare, and totally superfluous. They create problems, potentially cause harm, and have no redeeming value. If one views an agency as a system that interacts freely with its environment, which is what the authors have been professing, then an agency can be viewed as an open system. An open system, by definition, is one that is sensitive to changes in the external and internal environment. It is open to evolving opportunities and adapting its beliefs and behaviors as necessary. For such a system to maintain itself, it must be flexible. Too many standards make it rigid. All that is needed are a few pertinent statements to define performance. Standards are those statements. Keep them simple and at a minimum.

Standards are usually monitored through audits, statistical review, and performance evaluations. These are tools from the old paradigm, however. If these tools are used, it is important both to apply them and to use the resulting data within the belief structure of the new paradigm. Remember, data are for learning and not for punishment. If someone is not adhering to standards, it may be because he or she is not aware of the standards or is not able to comply. The environment needs to be one of support and learning.

Standards are a means of self-regulating an industry, a profession, or an agency. Therefore, there is a more supportive and appropriate way of maintaining standards. For example, an approach for maintaining agency standards is to orient new staff to all standards to which they are held accountable. Then, have staff self-report on their ability to meet these standards on an ongoing basis. If they report they were unable to meet a certain standard, have them explain why and offer suggestions on how the situation can be remedied. If they need more learning, support them in that endeavor. If they have found some system barriers, assist them in overcoming the barriers. Helping them overcome the barrier may mean altering the system or revising the standard. The more the responsibility for maintaining the standards is placed on the individual staff members, the more standards can be used to establish trust within an agency. The more the responsibility for maintaining standards is placed with management, the more the standards become a mechanism for control and constraint.

The same is true at the industry level. The more the industry of home care accepts responsibility for defining and maintaining standards, the less the need for outside (government) regulation and control. Too many ill-conceived standards, however, will prevent the industry from being able to adapt to the evolving health care system. In defining their standards, professions need to be aware of the same potential dilemma.

RELATIONSHIP TO COST

Many people believe it should be sufficient to examine only the quality aspects of standards. In today's competitive market, however, many others have determined that the cost of standards must be identified concurrently to ensure that standards are cost feasible. How does one know then, whether or not standards are affordable? The answer is: Know your standards; know what activities are involved to accomplish the standards; and know what labor hours are necessary to accomplish the defined activities. How the cost of those labor hours relates to the operating budget and the agency's priorities determines the affordability.

One way to document affordability is to determine the number of standard care hours needed to provide each unit of service (such as a visit or treatment). Standard care hours are determined by totaling all the activities and their associated times within the unit of service and then averaging the times (see Figure 7–3). This provides a common denominator for use in evaluation and comparison within the budget.

Defining the affordability of standards can be especially useful when associated with the flowcharts that address agency processes. A process can be costed by adding labor hours to the identified steps/activities. Once the cost for a process has been defined, that cost can be added to the cost of the care of a patient. This means of determining cost can be illustrated using the referral process diagrammed in Figure 7–2. In measuring the activities, it may be found that more labor hours are involved if disciplines are not assigned than if they are (e.g., comparing activity times of "refer to disciplines" to "assign to assignment coordinator"). This would make the referral of cases that have disciplines not assigned more expensive and charges could be made accordingly.

It is important to remember the law of diminishing returns. In the beginning, it is likely that the agency will benefit more from costing out actual service delivery processes, than from costing out standards. Emphasis should be placed first on those activities that are the most important aspects of care, or the most time-consuming activities. Since standards are a rigid level of activities required within an agency, however, it is important to know the impact on cost. This knowledge is especially important when trying to maintain the delicate cost/quality balance. Knowing how much labor time, and its associated cost, is needed to deliver a predetermined level of quality care that is based on defined required activities, has a great impact on productivity standards. As benchmarking becomes more popular and agencies compare productivity rates, the cost of agency standards will be significant. Those agencies that have similar outcomes but different productivity rates will have to look not only at the patient care guidelines used to reach the outcomes, but also at the agency standards that are in place.

$$\text{Standard care hour per unit of service} = \frac{\Sigma \text{ Activity costs per unit of service}}{\text{Number of activities}}$$

Figure 7–3 Determining Standard Care Hours

IMPLEMENTATION OF STANDARDS

The implementation of standards within an agency can be seen as a formidable activity for several reasons.

- Standards must be defined and identified.
- Standards may be perceived as threatening to those who feel insecure.
- Standards may be perceived as uninspiring and banal.
- The process of redefining what are standards, as opposed to guidelines, and rewriting standards appropriately is time-consuming, especially in light of other high-priority items on an agency's agenda.

For all these reasons, the job of implementing standards may meet with resistance. But since standards are an essential tool for quality, resistance must be overcome. Key strategies for implementing standards include:

1. Identify all the standards for which staff are to be held accountable. Involve everyone in this process. An important part of the process is getting staff to identify the standards they practice by. The variety and scope of the answers can be very enlightening, and a beginning point for establishing consistent agency standards.
2. Engage staff. Get staff involved wherever possible. Staff are the ones responsible for standard-based performance. It is a belief in the value of standards and the employees' ability to function at a standard level that provides the foundation for an agency's quality improvement program. Without staff's engagement in standards, there is no guarantee of expected quality.
3. Educate, educate, educate. Educate on the definition and role of standards. Standards are the basis of trust. Educate on the identification of relevant standards. Educate on the responsibility and accountability of each person (in upholding standards).
4. Develop a process for revising standards. Although standards are considered relatively stable, they still need to be reviewed periodically for efficiency, safety, effectiveness, and relevancy. Outdated standards become a liability.
5. Emphasize standard-based performance at time of hire, during orientation, and periodically thereafter. Set the expectation for standard-based performance at the time of interview and reinforce the integration wherever possible. Another method would be to use standard-based performance evaluations.
6. Reward staff for integrating standards into their performance. Make standard-based performance fun and rewarding. Demonstrate how the use of

standards establishes trust by giving staff more latitude when they produce standard-based performance. For example, when standards are well defined, instead of doing audits to determine compliance, have staff sign a contract to provide that level of performance. Then take them at their word.

CONCLUSION

Standards are the beginning for quality care and the establishment of trust. The challenge is to overcome the confusion over the term standard and how it is used. There are industry, professional, and agency standards. Agency standards include policies, flowcharts, and position descriptions. The following are the key characteristics of standards. Standards

- Are stable over time
- Reflect values and beliefs
- Focus on the agent
- Are rigidly followed with few, if any, exceptions
- Involve legal liability

From these characteristics, it can be seen that too many standards constrain growth and create additional liability. Too few agent-generated standards foster regulation from the environment. The balance comes from two perspectives: (1) have well-defined, essential standards to delineate expected performance behaviors, and (2) eliminate the nonessential standards in order to promote growth based on feedback from the external environment. Standards are a means for each entity (industry, professional, and agency) to establish a baseline of quality below which it will not go. In keeping that promise, these entities establish the basis for trust for all with whom they interact and with all to whom they provide service.

NOTES

1. S.L. Dean-Baar, Application of the New ANA Framework for Nursing Practice Standards and Guidelines, *Journal of Nursing Care Quality* 8, no. 1 (1993): 33–42.
2. American Nurses Association, *Standards of Clinical Nursing Practice* (Washington, DC: 1991).
3. S.L. Dean-Baar, Application of the New ANA Framework, 33–42.
4. S.F. Hoss, Standards—Setting Rules in the Game, *Caring* 16, no. 6 (1997): 56–60.
5. D.A. Gillies, *Nursing Management: A Systems Approach* (Philadelphia: W.B. Saunders Company, 1982), 444–445.

6. B.C. Vladeck, Quality Assurance through External Controls, *Inquiry* 25, no. 1 (1988): 100–107.

7. J. Marcus, ed., ORT: Coming to Your Neighborhood Soon? *Home Health Digest* 3, no. 3 (1997): 3, 6.

8. Vladeck, Quality Assurance, 100–107.

9. Hoss, Standards, 56–60.

10. Hoss, Standards, 56–60.

11. S. Davis, ed., *Home Health Data Quarterly* 1, no. 1 (1997): 25.

12. American Nurses Association, *Standards of Clinical Nursing Practice.*

13. J. Disch and D. Peters, *Getting Your Say: Help Mold the Standards of Clinical Nursing Practice* (Paper presented at the American Nurses Association Convention, Washington, DC, 1997.)

14. Dean-Baar, Application of the New ANA Framework, 33–42.

15. S. Rowland and B. Rowland, *Nursing Administration Handbook*, 3d ed. (Gaithersburg, MD: Aspen Publishers, 1992).

16. S.S. Poe and J.C. Will, Quality Nursing-Patient Outcomes: A Framework for Nursing Practice, *Journal of Nursing Quality Assurance* 2, no. 1 (1987), 29–37.

17. C.A. Garfield, *Peak Performers* (New York: Avon Books, 1987), 192.

18. Pew Health Professions Commission, *Health Professions Education for the Future: Schools in Service to the Nation* (San Francisco, CA: Pew Health Professions Commission, 1993).

19. D.A. Peters, Outcomes: The Mainstay of a Framework for Quality Care, *Journal of Nursing Care Quality* 10, no. 1 (1995): 61–69.

20. C.W. Ling, Performance of a Self-Directed Work Team in a Home Healthcare Agency, *Journal of Nursing Administration* 26, no. 9 (1996): 36–40.

21. D.B. Michaels, Home Health Nursing: Towards a Professional Practice Model, *Nursing Management* 25, no. 4 (1994): 68–72.

22. Michaels, Home Health Nursing, 68–72.

23. Michaels, Home Health Nursing, 68–72.

24. Ling, Performance of a Self-Directed Work Team, 36–40.

25. Michaels, Home Health Nursing, 68–72.

CHAPTER 8

Guidelines for Practice

Guidelines are second cousins to standards. In fact, guidelines are often included in the category of standards. Unfortunately, there is a danger to that inclusion, because then one is held legally accountable for following the defined guidelines. Guidelines are not meant to define a level of performance, but rather to recommend a course of action in the practice of health care. They are, as their name describes, activity guides, or courses, to follow. Using a practice guideline requires clinical judgment to evaluate the appropriateness of the guideline in meeting a client's need. As in any course, there can be changes, alterations, or detours made depending on progress, interest, new knowledge, or barriers placed in the way. Guideline development is still in its infancy; its challenges and benefits are still being discovered. This chapter deals with

- defining guidelines
- comparing guidelines to standards
- describing types of guidelines—procedures, protocols, clinical pathways, and disease state management
- relating guidelines to quality

DEFINITION

Clinical practice guidelines are systematically developed statements of recommended activities to assist practitioners and patients in making decisions for the health care that is provided in specific clinical circumstances. These decisions address the determination of how diseases, disorders, and other health conditions can most effectively be prevented, diagnosed, treated, and managed clinically.[1] Guidelines address care that can be rendered to defined groups in defined situations. They are less useful for unique or complex cases.

168

Development of guidelines is a relatively new concept driven by the need to reduce costs, provide standardization, and improve the effectiveness of care. Impetus was also given to guideline development by the Omnibus Budget Reconciliation Act (OBRA) of 1989, which called for the establishment of the Agency for Health Care Policy and Research (AHCPR). AHCPR was created to respond to concerns about the variability in health care practices and to the uncertainty about the effectiveness of those services. The mission of AHCPR is to improve the quality, appropriateness, and effectiveness of health care and im-prove access to health services.[2] The Office of the Forum for Quality and Effectiveness in Health Care (the Forum), one organizational component of AHCPR, is directed to arrange for the development, periodic review, and updating of clinically relevant guidelines, among other things. Currently, guidelines for the conditions listed in Exhibit 8–1 have been developed and disseminated.

One of the challenges faced by the Forum is how to keep guidelines current with the latest information, despite the rapid changes in health care practice. AHCPR has been criticized as being slow and too rigid in its prescriptions.[3]

Clinical practice guidelines are narrower in scope and intent than standards. In addition, guidelines are more flexible and focus on the patient; standards are rigid and focus on the caregiver. (See Chapter 7 for a full explanation of quality and financial standards.) Table 8–1 provides a comparison of the focus, scope, and

---

Exhibit 8–1 AHCPR Guidelines

Acute Pain Management
Acute and Chronic Incontinence
Pressure Ulcers in Adults: Prediction and Prevention
Cataract in Adults
Depression in Primary Care
Sickle Cell Disease
Benign Prostatic Hyperplasia
Management of Cancer Pain
Unstable Angina
Heart Failure
Otitis Media with Effusion in Young Children
Quality Mammography
Acute Low Back Problems in Adults
Pressure Ulcer Treatment
Post-Stroke Rehabilitation
Cardiac Rehabilitation
Smoking Cessation
Early Alzheimer's Disease

Source: Data from the Agency for Health Care Policy and Research.

Table 8–1 Comparing Standards and Guidelines

	Quality Standards	Financial Standards	Practice Guidelines
Focus	Agent responsibilities	Utilization (dollars and/or units)	Patient
Scope	Care provided to all consumers	Cost of care provided to consumers	Care provided in specific settings or to defined groups or for defined problems
Intent	Efficiency—doing things well	Affordability—doing things well within cost restraints	Effectiveness—doing the right things
Application	Rigid application toward a level of care; requires little or no judgment by the practitioner	Rigid application toward a level of cost; requires little or no judgment by the practitioner	Flexible application of activities of care; requires practitioner judgment

intent of clinical and financial standards and practice guidelines. It expands on Table 7–1 from the previous chapter.

Attributes that apply to the development of practice guidelines include:

- *Validity*. Guidelines are valid when they are derived from a synthesis of the best scientific evidence and expert opinion available and, when followed, lead to desired health and cost outcomes.
- *Reliability*. Guidelines are reliable if (1) given the same evidence and methods for development, the same recommendations would be produced by another group, and (2) given the same clinical circumstances, the guidelines would be interpreted and applied consistently by all who used them.
- *Applicability*. Guidelines must define the patient populations to which they apply. They should be as inclusive of the defined population as clinical evidence and expert judgment permit.
- *Multidisciplinary Participation*. Guidelines should be developed by a process that includes participation from all groups, including consumers, that are affected by the guideline. Input can take various forms such as survey responses, focus groups, and committee participation.
- *Clarity*. Guidelines should be written using precise and concise language, and clearly defined terms, in an easy-to-follow layout.[4]

Guidelines should also include documentation of the method and sources used in their development. Furthermore, a process must be established for periodic review to determine if new clinical evidence or changing viewpoints necessitate revisions.

In addition to the high-level guidelines developed at the national level to address certain conditions, different renderings of practice guidelines are also being developed within geographic regions, managed care networks, and individual agencies. These versions of guidelines are produced under a variety of names: procedures, protocols, clinical pathways, and health (versus disease state) management. Each of these will be addressed in this chapter.

PROCEDURES

Procedures are written step-by-step chronological outlines of the requirements to perform particular clinical tasks. They primarily focus on the psychomotor skills required to accomplish the given task. Procedures assist the practitioner in deciding the most effective way to perform a clinical task that requires both cognitive abilities and manual dexterity.[5] Examples of tasks include how to remove sutures or how to insert a Foley catheter. Directions that accompany the use of disposable equipment, such as a Foley insertion kit, can sometimes be found on the side of the box. They do not address the level of clinical skill needed to carry out the procedure. Professional procedures can be found in professional texts or manuals, which can be used as the basis for an agency's procedure book. Such procedures must be adapted to fit individual agency situations and needs.

PROTOCOLS

Protocols outline the steps to be taken in treating a certain condition and include both routine and emergency situations. In specific terms, they establish a course of action to be taken under defined conditions. They may also include expected outcomes. Protocols are usually discipline specific but may encompass delegated therapeutic or diagnostic steps from the physician. In nursing, the specific condition for a protocol may be delineated by a nursing diagnosis. Three types of protocols are defined based on the need to involve the physician. These types are (1) dependent, (2) interdependent, and (3) independent.[6]

Dependent. A dependent protocol is one that outlines the steps for a course of action that has been completely delegated by physicians. An example is any form of standing or perpetual orders.

Interdependent. An interdependent protocol is one that outlines the steps for a course of action that contains actions that are delegated by physicians and actions that are autonomous to the discipline. For example, Foley care may be an interdependent protocol dealing with the nursing diagnosis of "genitourinary functions: impairment," if it includes standing orders for how often to change the Foley. Notice that this protocol may also include, or refer to, the procedure for how to change a Foley catheter.

Independent. An independent protocol is one that outlines the steps for a course of action that is autonomous and contains only steps that can be independently carried out by the discipline. An example of an independent nursing protocol is the management of the nursing diagnosis, "emotional stability: impairment" or "grief: impairment." These protocols also may include procedures, such as how to refer a patient to a counselor or social worker.

CLINICAL PATHWAYS

A clinical pathway is an evolving concept/tool that has attracted a great deal of interest with the rise of managed care. The concept is to outline and schedule the best practice efforts to be rendered to defined patient groups by the health care team. Critical to the successful use of the concept is the belief structure that surrounds it. These beliefs need to be in concert with quality improvement as perceived in the new paradigm and managed care, and as depicted in Exhibit 1–1. One essential element is an environment of trust. Also critical are the beliefs that

- Quality is everyone's business
- Mistakes are tolerated
- There is room for innovation and creativity
- Employees are cocreators (collaborators)
- Learning is key to promoting continuous improvement
- Data are for learning, not for punishment

Thinking is directed toward, "Here are the outcomes we want for this type of patient; do your best to reach them" rather than, "Here are the rules, do your best to follow them."

From the context of these values, clinical pathways can be a useful tool, if the concept is understood. The following is a discussion of the definition of a pathway, the benefits from using pathways, the components of a pathway, the tracking of pathway variances, the development and implementation of a path, and the challenges of using pathways.

Definition

Clinical pathways are an outgrowth of critical paths or pathways. A critical pathway is the most appropriate trajectory to take toward a target; it is not a perfect path.[7] Along the path there is room for mistakes and corrections. A critical path is an outline of activities and times for a particular project or condition that are essential to the completion of the project (or the discharge of a patient) in the projected time period. A delay in any activity on the critical path could interfere with the timely completion of the project (or timely discharge of the patient) or adversely affect the achievement of an outcome. Critical paths were popularized during the early years of the space program. Although the people guiding the astronauts had to be precise and operate within strict accuracy limits, they did not insist upon perfectionism. In fact, the Apollo ships were off the "perfect" path 90 percent of the time. The spacecraft would wander off the path and the crew would correct, it would wander again and the crew would correct, and so on. The spacecraft still got to the moon and home again. Those results (outcomes) are what are important. There will always be the unpredictable, the ambiguous, the emergency, or the variance that requires a change.[8] The goal of the critical path is not to eliminate the variance (or changes in care) but to reduce and/or prepare for it.

When critical paths were adapted within the health care arena, a change was made in their use. Rather than simply outlining the critical activities required to complete the project on time, in health care they were used to outline *all* the activities required to care for the condition and discharge the patient on time (or achieve the milestones/outcomes). All the implications of this change are still not completely understood. In any event, its usage in health care has led to the term clinical paths or clinical pathways. The expected results of the pathway, or outcomes, are also included with the pathway.

Clinical pathways are guidelines that are largely tailored to the patterns and resources of care in the institutions where they are developed and refined over time by the clinicians within that institution. Clinical pathways can be defined as the predetermined, optimal sequencing and timing of clinical activities by the health care team that guide a patient through a course of care toward expected outcome(s). They are tools to assist with the effective management of clinical outcomes related to specific problems or conditions. They are also multidisciplinary and address groups of patients with a common condition. Adjunctive to the path may be protocols and procedures. For example, Exhibit 8–2 illustrates a pathway for pneumonia. Associated with the task of "assess condition" could be an independent protocol on assessing the condition of patients with the nursing diagnosis of "respiratory: impairment." Another protocol associated with the pathway could be for care of the patient with oxygen. There could also be a procedure for how to order oxygen equipment associated with the task of "Instruct: oxygen use and safety." The time frame for the expected outcomes at the beginning of the pathway is by visit 6, or at discharge if subsequent visits are scheduled.

A clinical pathway is not the same thing as a nursing care plan. There are several differences. First of all, interventions (a subclassification of activities) included in a

Exhibit 8–2 Home Care Clinical Pathway: Pneumonia

Expected Outcomes:
Temperature less than 99.6° F oral
Blood pressure within normal limits
Pulse within normal limits
Respirations within normal limits
Lung sounds clear in _____ lobe
Lung sounds clear in unaffected lobes
Nutritional intake adequate to support health
Skin warm and dry to touch

Visit 1	Visit 2	Visit 3	Visit 4	Visit 5	Visit 6	Subsequent Visits
1. Assess condition 2. Instruct: • pt. rights and responsibilities • pt. financial liability for home care • pt./home safety • expectations of home care • plan for care • written visit schedule • medication regimen • pertinent phone numbers • oxygen use and safety	1. Assess condition 2. Obtain recall from instruction completed during visit 1 3. Instruct regarding care and maintenance • timely notification of MD • preventive measures to avoid a relapse • energy conservation methods • breathing exercises 4. Instruct regarding medica-	1. Assess condition 2. Obtain recall from instruction completed during visit 2 3. Instruct regarding disease process: • definition • S & S 4. Instruct regarding medication 2	1. Assess condition 2. Obtain recall from instruction completed during visit 3 3. Instruct regarding causes and risk factors of pneumonia 4. Instruct regarding medication 3	1. Assess condition 2. Obtain recall from instruction completed during visit 4 3. Instruct regarding medications 4 and 5	1. Assess condition 2. Obtain recall from instruction completed during visit 5 3. Instruct regarding medications 6 and 7	1. Assess condition 2. Obtain recall from instruction completed during previous visit 3. Continue instruction as warranted by condition

Exhibit 8–2 continued

Visit 1	Visit 2	Visit 3	Visit 4	Visit 5	Visit 6	Subsequent Visits
OUTCOME(s): Patient is able to . . .	• notify MD in a timely manner • state preventive measures to avoid a relapse • describe energy-saving measures • demonstrate breathing exercises	• define pneumonia • state signs and symptoms of pneumonia	• state causes and risk factors of pneumonia			

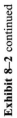

Source: Adapted from B.S. Gingerich and D.A. Ondeck, *Clinical Pathways for the Multidisciplinary Home Care Team,* Supplement 4, pp. 109–111, © 1997, Aspen Publishers, Inc.

care plan are not sequenced in time; in a clinical pathway they are. In addition, every patient has a care plan; not every patient has a clinical pathway. Pathways are not appropriate for all patients. Pathways address the course of action for a condition, or combination of conditions; therefore, pathways are appropriate for only those patients that can be grouped with patients in a similar set of circumstances. It has been found that clinical pathways (including home health pathways that are developed jointly with hospitals) are best suited to patients with surgical conditions because their care tends to be highly predictable and they all enter the path at a similar place (first-day postoperative). It is difficult to develop critical pathways for medical procedures and conditions because of their greater inherent variation. It is also difficult to "path" chronic care patients because the care of these patients is usually triggered by the presentation of various symptoms, not a similar time.

Clinical pathways are also different from case management. Case management deals with the course of care for one individual patient. This patient usually has a complex situation that does not permit him or her to be placed into a grouping required for utilizing a clinical path. Therefore, his or her care is planned and managed as an individual case. Activities may or may not be sequenced in time depending on the condition(s) being managed.

Benefits

Use of clinical pathways varies, but it is generally increasing throughout the health care arena. In a recent survey of hospitals, 81 percent of the respondents used clinical paths.[9] Usage in home health is not as extensive, but it is growing. The use of clinical pathways yields the following benefits.

Comprehensive Method of Planning, Delivering, and Monitoring Care

By definition clinical paths contain all the activities required for caring for a given group of patients. Therefore it is self-evident that they provide a comprehensive approach for planning and delivering care for this group of patients. All the activities are defined in advance. All that is required is for the practitioner(s) to individualize the path as necessary and begin delivering care. Monitoring and the necessary data collection can be done and tracked by documenting when the activities and outcomes were actually done. It is then easy to know when each intervention and outcome were completed. If an intervention or outcome is incomplete, a variance reason is given.

Standardized Care

Because clinical pathways outline a course of care for a given condition, they provide a uniform beginning point for providing care to this type of patient. Therefore, all those providing care to a given patient have access to the same beginning point, rather than relying solely on their own knowledge and past experience. Recall that it is this access to expert experience on providing care that is one of the main drivers of managed care. Because of the availability of this information, care to a given type of patient becomes more standardized or uniform. This is different from a "standard of care" because clinical pathways are guidelines or recommendations, not standards.

Guideline for Best Practice

Clinical pathways are developed by exploring current practice via chart reviews and past quality improvement studies, reviewing research findings in the literature, obtaining patient databases of treatments and outcomes, and seeking the input of experts. The synthesis of the information obtained represents the "best practice" for a given condition at the time of development. By monitoring the variance to the pathways as they are used, and determining which interventions best accomplish what outcomes, pathways can be updated. Revised pathways incorporate those interventions that work best, thereby constantly improving the quality of care and reflecting "best practice."

Resource Management

Clinical pathways by definition outline the course of care for a given condition, which includes all activities by all disciplines involved. The value in this is twofold. First, it delineates the role of each discipline so each knows its responsibility. This clearly defined role responsibility is helpful in resource management because it avoids duplication of activities and reduces the amount of missed instruction to the patient. The second advantage to having the interdisciplinary guide to care is that it assists with interdisciplinary coordination. From the beginning of care, each discipline knows the role of every team member in relation to the timeline. Knowing the who, what, and when facilitates teamwork, rather than a group of individuals duplicating or missing work on the same case.

Furthermore, because disciplines have overlapping roles (e.g., both a physical therapist and a professional nurse can do range of motion and other rehabilitative techniques), the interventions (as a subclassification of activities) can be assigned to different disciplines depending on availability, cost, or patient preference. The outcomes, variances (positive and negative), and cost of the different team configurations can be monitored to determine the best team mix for a given condition.

Educational Guide

Clinical pathways are useful in educating staff, and orienting new staff, on how to treat a given condition. They outline all the required steps but are also permissive, meaning they allow the practitioner to add steps that he or she feels may be helpful. The exciting thing about pathways is that when a practitioner does add an intervention because of patient preference or the clinician's previous success with it, that intervention is tracked. Thus, the success of the intervention is known (e.g., it shortened the length of time to meet the outcome; the outcome was achieved more frequently). Successful interventions can be added to the pathway for others to use, and unsuccessful ones can be eliminated from the clinician's practice. An intervention is eliminated not "because someone said so" but because data actually demonstrated that it was neither efficient nor effective.

Clinical pathways can also be used as teaching tools for patients. Sharing the pathway with them at the beginning of care informs them of what is involved in the course of treatment, reduces anxiety, and affords them the opportunity for input into their own care. A clinical pathway is in many ways a tool to assist in establishing a partnership with clients.

Components

There are six key components of a clinical pathway.[10] They are: (1) scope, (2) condition, (3) activity categories, (4) outcomes, (5) format, and (6) documentation.

Scope

The period of care for which the pathway is developed. It may be for a hospitalization, a home health care length of stay, or a complete episode of care.

Condition

The medical condition, nursing problem, or case type for which the pathway is developed and applied. Most clinical pathways have been developed for a medical condition or diagnosis. The challenge in home health care is that few, if any, patients have only one medical condition. Thus clinicians must follow multiple pathways for a single patient, which makes adherence difficult and documentation and revision almost impossible. There are some alternatives beginning to emerge with the advent of electronic documentation. Component pathways can be developed that deal with a medical condition, patient problem, or nursing diagnosis. The appropriate components can be selected for a patient and then merged electronically, eliminating duplicate interventions and producing one pathway for the patient, which can then be further individualized as needed.

Activity Categories

Activity categories represent a standard set of groups of activities within an agency to classify staff actions. The same categories are used consistently across pathways. For example, in the clinical pathway for pneumonia in Exhibit 8–2 the categories are direct care (assessment of condition) and instructions. Another example would be to start with the activities basic to home care—monitoring, instruction, coordination, and direct hands-on care. With the concept of patient partnership, the additional categories of psychological support and/or coaching also may be of assistance. Others feel that it is important to separate out items such as medications and lab studies. There is no set way to do it. The implications, however, can be far reaching. If the agency is involved in, or planning to do, activity-based cost management (ABCM), these activity labels are the ones used as the basis for costing. It is important then to ascribe activity labels that are consistent with the activities for which one wants to gather costing data. For example, if one wanted to find the cost of collecting the OASIS data, he or she would need to include an activity category of assessments since those data are collected during an assessment.

Outcomes

The outcomes that are included in clinical pathways are the expected outcomes for the patient and/or family. These expected clinical outcomes are included for the episode of care and for each visit. Using the terminology from Chapter 6 on outcomes, the visit outcomes are immediate or short term; the outcomes for the pathway are intermediate or long term, depending on the scope of the pathway.

Outcomes defined as "pure" outcomes (see Chapter 6) can also be included in the pathway. These outcomes, as the reader may recall, are the measurement of the change in a health indicator over two or more points in time indicating a change in health status. Therefore, requiring the assessment of a given health indicator on certain visits would allow for the comparison of the health indicator over time and thereby provide an outcome measure. For example, if an agency wanted to include elements from the OASIS-B data set, such as the questions on pain, in a clinical pathway for outcome measurement, the task on the pathway would be "assess pain status." Then there would be an agency procedure on "how to" assess the pain status. The procedure would incorporate having the clinician ask questions M0420 (frequency of pain interfering with patient's activity or movement) and M0430 (intractable pain) and provide the mandated choices. The procedure may be provided on a separate assessment form or incorporated into the pathway form itself, depending on agency format and preference.

Format

Format is the way the clinical pathway activities are presented for use. For example, all the activities may be laid out as a matrix over the entire episode of care as in Exhibit 8–2, or there could be a separate sheet for every day that listed only the tasks for that day. (See Exhibit 8–3.) Format can also differ in the amount of detail shown on the pathway (e.g., whether it lists only activities or tasks, or includes protocols and procedures). Format can be paper-based or electronic. An electronic format allows for more flexibility in presentation since there can be hidden screens behind an intervention to show a protocol or procedure. An electronic system also allows for a rescheduled intervention to be inserted under the appropriate new visit.

Documentation

A clinical pathway may or may not be used as part of the patient's permanent medical record. In acute care, pathways (or the variance sheets) are often kept separate. In home care, pathways are often used as a visit documentation tool incorporating various codes to indicate whether or not the task was completed and/or rescheduled. There are pros and cons to both methods. Keeping the pathway separate may mean more documentation; incorporating the pathway into the patient's record means it does not maintain its exclusiveness as a quality improvement document (i.e., it is subject to legal subpoena).

Tracking Variances

Variances are simply deviations or departures from the defined pathway. These variances can be positive or negative. Positive variances exist when an item is accomplished sooner than planned and/or produces a result better than antici-pated. Negative variances exist when interventions are delayed or produce suboptimal outcomes. Variance tracking is comparing the actual care delivered with the planned care and explaining why care differed, either positively or negatively. Feedback from the tracking will provide data regarding what is the waste in the current pathway and what items are responsible for the waste. Waste refers to noncontributing interventions or treatments, for example, including an intervention for teaching insulin injection in a pathway for *established* insulin-dependent diabetics. Variance reasons are usually set up in categories such as patient/family, environment or external, internal or agency system, and caregiver.

Variance tracking analysis can be both prospective and retrospective.[11] Pro-spective variance analysis is the rapid identification of negative variances or unexpected patient needs. This allows for the implementation of clinical interven-

Exhibit 8–3 Clinical Pathway: Pneumonia

VISIT 2	
Actions	*Date*
DIRECT CARE:	
Assess condition	
Vital signs:	
Temperature	
BP (R)	
BP (L)	
Apical pulse	
Respiration rate	
Lung sounds:	
Nutritional intake:	
Skin color:	
Skin integrity:	
Effectiveness of medications:	
Untoward side effect of medications:	
Other direct care: (specify)	
INSTRUCTION:	
Instruct re: care and maintenance	
Timely notification of the physician	
Preventive measures to avoid a relapse	
Energy-conservation methods	
Breathing exercises	
Instruct re: medication #1	
Obtain recall from instruction completed during visit 1:	
Patient rights and responsibilities	
Patient financial liability for home care	
Patient/home safety	
Expectations of home care:	
Use of clinical pathway	
Role of patient	
Role of significant other	
Role of home care staff	
Payer criteria/discharge plans	
Plan for care (discuss/collaborate)	
Written visit schedule	
Medication regimen	
Pertinent telephone numbers	
Physician	
Agency	

continues

Exhibit 8–3 continued

> Department of Health hotline
> Pharmacy
> Durable medical equipment
> Oxygen use and safety
> Other instructions: (specify)
>
> VISIT OUTCOMES:
>
> Patient able to notify MD in a timely manner
> Patient able to state preventive measures to avoid a relapse
> Patient able to describe energy-saving measures
> Patient able to demonstrate breathing exercises
> Other outcomes: (specify)
>
> Codes: x=Done; I=Instruction/Reinstruction; N/A=Not Applicable; V=Variance; A=Achieved; R=Return Recitation/Demonstration
>
> Variance Key: Variance occurred due to: A=Patient condition; B=Cognitive deficits; C=Patient disinterest; D=Other (specify)
>
> *Source:* Adapted from B.S. Gingerich and D.A. Ondeck, *Clinical Pathways for the Multidisciplinary Home Care Team,* Supplement 4, pp. 109–111, © 1997, Aspen Publishers, Inc.

tions to preclude the deterioration of the condition and avoid undesirable outcomes. Prospective variance should automatically trigger a reassessment of the patient's condition and corrective action, where appropriate. It also may be appropriate to require a supervisor or clinical care consult on cases where the variance is not correctable within a specified period of time.[12]

Retrospective analysis is the aggregation of variances across patients on the same pathway in order to identify trends and patterns that may be useful in improving the pathway and/or the system of care. For example, if it is discovered that on a pathway requiring supplies, such as wound care, the hands-on care was never provided on the first visit as planned, it may be because the required supplies were not available. Improving the pathway would then require improving the system for getting the supplies to the homes in a timely fashion. It is through retrospective analysis that those pathway items that are value-added (contribute to the outcomes in the pathway) can be assessed and retained, and those items that offer little or no value can be revised or deleted. The consolidated pathway that results is closer to the original concept of critical pathways.

In order to make retrospective analysis meaningful, three elements are required: (1) an understanding of common cause and special cause variation, (2) statistical guidelines to differentiate common cause and special cause variation, and (3) a formalized tracking system.

Common cause variation is also known as random or unassignable variation. It is part of the random variation inherent in the process (clinical pathway) itself. It is due to regular, natural, or ordinary causes. Because the variation is predicable, it results in a "stable," although not necessarily acceptable, process (pathway). When common cause variation exists, revision strategies focus on changing the process to be improved (the pathway). It should be noted, however, that every process (pathway) has common cause variation. Most variation is common cause variation. Once it is identified, it requires professional management—continuous quality improvement (CQI)—to determine if the pathway should be improved. If, on the other hand, common cause variation is treated as special cause variation, the result will be distorted data and increased variation.[13] See Figure 8–1.

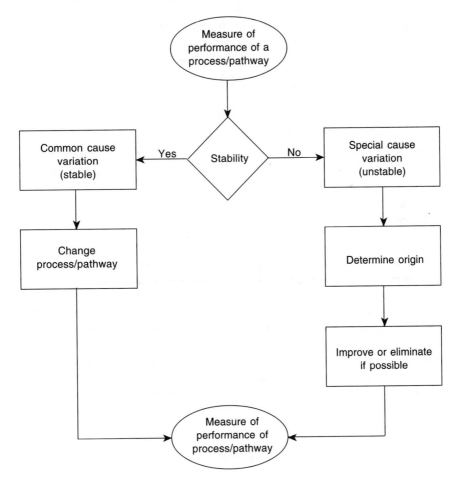

Figure 8–1 Using Variation for Improvement

An example of common cause variation is the use of different protocols for pain management by different practitioners. If pain is controlled equally well with either of the two protocols (e.g., the outcome is the same) and one is less costly and/or more efficient, then the less costly protocol should be encouraged. This can be done by presenting the cost/efficiency evidence to those practitioners using other protocols and requesting that they change. Once the change is made, data again need to be collected to determine if the change has been effective and the variation reduced. If there is no value in changing the protocol (no cost or time savings), then both protocols should be allowed.

Special cause variation is also known as nonrandom or assignable causes of variation. It is intermittent and due to irregular or unnatural causes that are not inherent in the pathway or process. Because it is not predictable, it results in an unstable process (pathway). When special cause variation exists, improvement strategies focus on finding the origin. It may or may not be possible to improve or eliminate the situation depending on where it is coming from. The consequences of treating special cause variation as common cause variation are unnecessary rework and cost (wasted resources).[14] In addition, using common cause approaches to special cause variation rarely eliminates the reason for the special cause. In Figure 8–1 the process depicted applies to all types of measures, such as cost, customer satisfaction, utilization, and/or clinical outcomes.

A second element needed to make retrospective analysis meaningful are statistical guidelines to differentiate common cause and special cause variation. There are two statistical guidelines that can be used to differentiate common cause and special cause variation depending on the type of data that are collected. If the measures are dichotomous (e.g., met/unmet), then a targeted proportion achieved should be determined with an expected variation associated with each measure. The expected proportion (p) would be equal to the sample proportion plus or minus two standard errors (SE) of the proportion. Standard error (SE) = the square root of $[p \times (1-p)/n]$ where n represents the number in the sample.[15]

If the measures are interval or ratio-scaled, then a confidence interval can be established for the measure based on the standard deviation (SD) of the variable. For a 95 percent confidence interval, the variation is plus or minus two SEs of the average score based on past data. In this case, SE = SD × the square root of n.[16] Variations that fall outside of the confidence interval are special cause variations.

The third, and final, element that makes retrospective analysis meaningful is a formalized tracking system. In order to get useful information, data must be collected, analyzed, and reported. The following questions need to be answered in order to establish such a system:

- Is everyone committed to collecting data routinely and efficiently on all pathway patients?

- What variances will be tracked for each pathway?
- What instrument will be used to document the variances?
- Where will the document be placed once it is completed?
- Who enters the variables into the database?
- What database system will be used?
- How will the completeness, accuracy, and consistency of the data be ensured?
- What information is needed on variance reports?
- What are the staffing needs for variance tracking?
- Who is responsible for correcting the variance, if it is correctable?[17]

Implementing Clinical Pathways

Crucial to the successful development and implementation of clinical pathways is a steering committee that provides oversight. This committee includes representatives from senior management, nursing, rehabilitation therapies, physicians, quality improvement, information services, and finance. Responsibilities of the steering committee include

- developing and approving definitions for clinical pathways and variances
- developing the criteria for selection of case types for clinical pathways
- developing the format and activity categories
- developing and approving the method for collecting variances
- developing the documentation
- identifying the educational needs of the staff
- providing guidance and support to the pathway teams through development and approval of procedures, education, and resources
- receiving and reviewing information from the teams including updates, reports, and minutes
- identifying barriers and strategies to enhance the system
- evaluating the impact and outcomes of clinical pathways, including enhanced quality and cost effectiveness[18]

Also crucial to the successful development of clinical pathways is an environment that supports experimentation and mistakes. Clinical pathways are guidelines to grow from, not gold standards that mandate adherence. Commitment to success starts at the top and proceeds from there. Everyone must be involved. Each pathway should be developed by a project team consisting of a member from each discipline represented on the pathway, including physicians and support staff, and someone from quality improvement, finance, information services, and form development. The flowchart depicting the basic implementation process is presented in Figure 8–2.

Challenges and/or Failures in Implementing Clinical Pathways

As exciting and beneficial as clinical pathways are, there are several serious pitfalls that home care agencies face. Unfortunately, falling into one of these

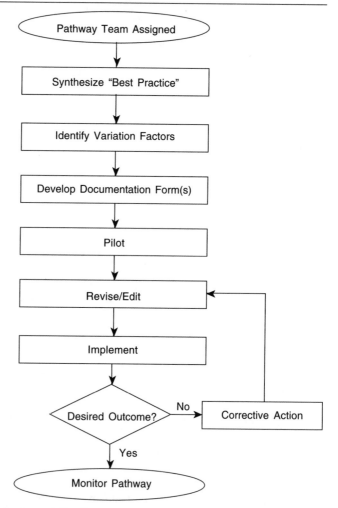

Figure 8–2 Pathway Implementation Process

"pits" diminishes the benefits of using the pathways and reduces the agency's return on investment of this resource-intense project. Pitfalls to avoid include

- Failure to include the implementation of a correction action plan(s) to address concurrent variances.
- Inadequate or no integration of clinical pathways into the overall agency quality improvement program such as insufficient retrospective variance tracking and analysis. If the pathway program is poorly designed, it may lead to incorrect decisions based on faulty information.
- Setting up barriers for staff to revise care. The format of pathways often makes it difficult to revise them, so they are treated as a gold standard rather than a guideline. Unfortunately, this stifles creativity in providing care and reduces customization for the individual client.
- Forgetting to include the client in care. Sharing the pathway with the client is an excellent way to get the client involved in care and to establish realistic expectations for the episode of care.
- Goal displacement from client goals to utilization goals. Many agencies focus on getting the care done in x visits to match a managed care contract rather than providing the patient with what he or she needs and measuring variance.
- There is no standardization to pathway development or design within the home care and health care industries, thus limiting the value of the data to the agency level.

DISEASE STATE AND HEALTH MANAGEMENT

Disease state management is an extension of clinical pathways. It integrates clinical pathways and protocols from every possible setting in order to manage a patient's treatment of a given disease. This integration spans the continuum of care, not just in the hospital or home care setting. Furthermore, its intent is to keep people out of health institutions and agencies by managing chronic conditions so that these consumers enjoy the best possible health and consume the most appropriate and effective health care resources.[19] Consumers under disease state management are never thought of as patients that should be "discharged" but rather as individuals who will always need monitoring, changes in medication, equipment, and/or ongoing medical supervision.[20] The following is a discussion of the definitions of disease state management, a comparison of disease state management to health management, the required components of disease state management, and the implementation of a disease state management partnership.

Definition

Disease state management is a comprehensive, integrated, multidisciplinary set of interventions that coordinates resources across the health services continuum for a group of patients with particular diseases with the intent of altering the course of the disease, preventing exacerbations, and improving the consumers' quality of life.[21] The term was originally conceived in 1993 by the Boston Consulting Group for the pharmaceutical industry.[22] The cornerstone of the concept started as drug therapy—educating patients to manage their own drugs in the outpatient setting in order to improve disease control and result in a better quality of life.[23] Disease state management programs target two types of chronic diseases:

1. Costly and relatively rare diseases such as hemophilia. Hemophilia is a very expensive disease that is present in only 4 to 6 people out of a population of 200,000 to 300,000.[24] Because of the combination of expense and rarity, it is difficult for providers to manage, thus making it a good candidate for disease state management.
2. Common chronic diseases that affect a large population for which proper monitoring and management can prevent costly acute care episodes and improve the patient's quality of life. Examples include diabetes, asthma, hypertension, congestive heart failure, HIV/AIDS, and depression.

The health care cost of diabetes, for example, is roughly $92 billion per year with an additional lost work time of $41 billion. Approximately 1 of every 17 people in the general population is afflicted. Complications include heart disease, stroke, kidney failure, blindness, and amputations.[25] If providers had timely information upon which to act, however, many of these complications could be avoided. For example, 90 percent of the time blindness would be avoided; 50 percent of the time lower extremity amputation would be avoided; and 50 percent of the time kidney dialysis would be avoided.[26] All of these eliminated complications promote great savings and are the reasoning behind disease state management.

At the center of any disease state management strategy are outcomes. In fact, the term has been used synonymously with outcome management.[27] Outcome management works best with a homogeneous population. (See Chapter 6.) Therefore, it is important to identify clinically significant subpopulations. For example, in dealing with the population of diabetics, the Group Health Cooperative of Puget Sound defined a subpopulation of Type 2 diabetics who were 30 years of age and older and met one or more of the following criteria:

- have a prescription for insulin or an oral agent
- glycohemoglobin > 7.5%

- fasting blood glucose > 140
- random blood glucose > 200[28]

Once this subpopulation was identified, Group Health was able to define key outcomes, measure the performance of its diabetic program using the outcomes, identify gaps between optimal performance (obtained by benchmarking) and its own system, and then design improvement strategies.

Health Management

Certain "nondisease" areas can also benefit, both in terms of improved quality of life and reduced costs, from an integrated management approach. Examples include pregnancy and childbirth and smoking cessation. In addition, one of the prime components of a disease state management program is preventive care and wellness. Therefore, this extension into wellness areas has broadened the thinking of some to expand disease state management into health management. The concept is carried even further by the futuristic thinking into life paths that would answer the consumer question of "How are you working with me to manage my health and wellness?"[29]

Components of a Disease State Management Program

One of the values of disease state management is the richness of the multidisciplinary team. This team can include not only clinicians from diverse backgrounds such as physicians, nurses, and therapists, but also clinical researchers, data analysts, quality control experts, and payers. The corollary of the team expertise is the wide and diversified components of a disease state management program. Key components include

- coordination and balance of primary and specialty care
- practice guidelines, including procedures, protocols, and pathways
- patient education in self-care management and empowerment to take control over the condition
- preventive care/wellness for at-risk individuals
- compliance with appropriate drug therapy (e.g., providers are prescribing the most appropriate drug therapy and patients understand the importance of adhering to the prescribed regimen)
- information technology for ongoing assessment of data, outcomes research, and database analysis[30]

Implementing a Disease State Management Partnership

As delivering care continues to move toward alternative and community settings, home care finds itself well placed to be a key player in disease state management. In addition to the provision of care, it has much to offer. The home care industry has historically worked toward improving quality care, promoting wellness, enhancing the role of the patient in self-care management, and coordinating the many facets of the fragmented health care industry to offer the patient some sort of "seamless care." Taking on such a challenge, however, is not to be taken lightly. Issues to be considered include

- How does it fit into the agency's strategic plan?
- What is the agency's financial and human resource capacity for the initiative?
- What disease(s) are prevalent in the community that could be managed effectively?
- Are the resources available to conduct the high-quality research that would be required?
- Is the agency prepared to navigate through the community politics?
- Will it be possible to standardize the clinical data from multiple sources so they can be analyzed?

A first step would be to integrate pathways with other providers, each defining areas of responsibility. A bigger step would be to initiate or participate in implementing a disease management partnership with the community. An outline of the process for such an undertaking is depicted in Figure 8–3.

RELATIONSHIP OF GUIDELINES TO QUALITY AND COST

In quality improvement, processes are proactively evaluated for their ability to (1) reliably and predictably achieve desired outcomes, and (2) achieve results within time and cost parameters. Guidelines contribute to both of these goals.

Reliably and Predictably Achieve Outcomes

One of the essential contributions of guidelines is the standardization of care. Standardization promotes quality because it provides the same information for all to follow, thus improving reliability and predictability and allowing for comparison and analysis of data. Guidelines offer the "best practice" information. Through a CQI program, those best practice guidelines are continually updated, which

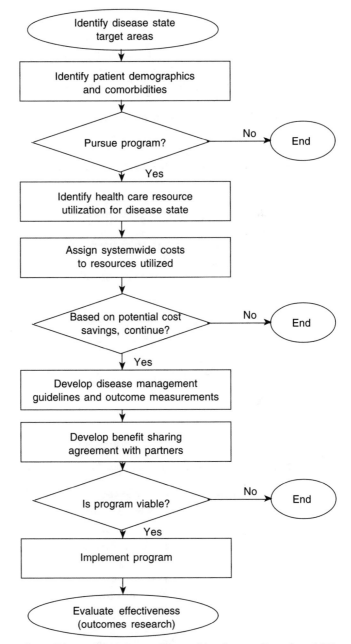

Figure 8–3 Implementing a Disease Management Partnership. *Source:* Data from M.F. Sylvestri and E.P. Marro, Disease Management: Partnering for Better Patient Care, *The Remington Report*, Vol. 5, No. 4, p. 28, © 1997.

should provide for more effective care. Similarly, guidelines should provide for more efficient care by eliminating those interventions that are not adding value to the outcome. The concern is that standardization can also reduce autonomy and ability to make independent decisions. Therefore, it is important that the surrounding agency environment be one that allows for creativity and the opportunity to try new things.

Figure 8–4 depicts the relationship of guidelines (pathways, protocols, and procedures) to the agency system and the patient-focused care process, including the associated outcomes. Procedures, protocols, interventions, and activities may be separate entities or components inside a clinical pathway.

Achieve Results within Time and Cost Parameters

Guidelines help determine the achievement of results within time and cost parameters by fostering standardization so that cost of care can be measured and compared. It is of little value to measure cost of care by visit since visits are not

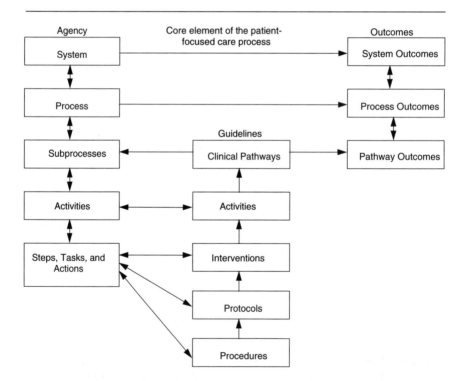

Figure 8–4 Relationship of Guidelines to Agency System, Processes, and Outcomes

homogeneous and vary in length of time. It is too difficult to measure costs at the intervention, procedure, or protocol level. The measurement variation at that level is too great and depends on the level of expertise and competency of the practitioner and how many interventions are being done at once (e.g., the dressing change and wound care teaching could be done simultaneously or separately depending on the experience/dexterity of the clinician and the comprehension of the client). Thus, the return value on costing these levels of guidelines is below the value of the time required to do the measurement. Determining cost, therefore, begins at the activity level (see Figure 8–5). Although variations still exist, it is easier to accommodate them at this higher level. The existence of standardized guidelines helps reduce unnecessary variation created by multiple, individual practitioner interventions, and a more consistent, reliable cost can be determined for different conditions. Figure 8–5 reflects the relationship of guidelines to costing. It presents a visual demonstration that the activity level is the lowest level

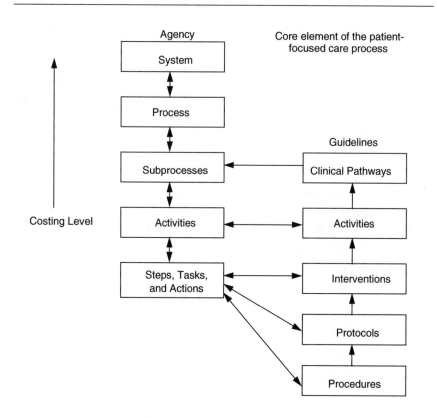

Figure 8–5 Relationship of Guidelines to Costing

at which costing occurs, and then is rolled up into subprocesses, processes, and the system.

CONCLUSION

Guidelines are essential to managed care. They offer the expertise of many to provide a recommended course of action for a practitioner to use in the care of a given patient or condition. This means that the practitioner has available the benefit of others' experiences and knowledge, not just his or her own. Guidelines offer guidance, however. They are not gold standards and need to be modified for particular clients or situations. They do not replace professional judgment or common sense. The use of guidelines also requires a built-in system that makes it easy to incorporate and integrate improvements to the guidelines as new knowledge is obtained, and to communicate these changes readily to agency clinicians.

Guidelines take many forms. Table 8–2 lists the different types of guidelines and compares their applicability, focus, and level.

By understanding the relationship of guidelines to standards, cost, and quality, clinicians have the opportunity to use them to advance their practice rather than constrain their care through misunderstanding of standardization or fear of practicing cookbook health care. It is important to clarify the use of the terms standards and guidelines. Standards are the letter of the law to which practitioners are held accountable. Guidelines are suggested guides for care; they are more flexible in their application. Confusing guidelines with standards removes a lot of the professional latitude from the provision of care and restricts creativity and the use of new knowledge; standards are cumbersome to change. Labeling and using guidelines appropriately, on the other hand, promotes "best practices" from all clinicians and gives them the opportunity to apply professional judgment as

---

Table 8–2 Guidelines

	Procedures	Protocols	Clinical Pathways	Disease Management
Applicability	Discipline neutral	Discipline specific	Multidisciplinary	Multidisciplinary
Focus	Clinical task	Clinical condition	Clinical condition	Healthy state
Levels		May contain procedure	May contain protocols and procedures	May contain clinical pathways, protocols, and procedures

needed. They are valuable in expanding practice parameters and supporting quality care.

NOTES

1. Agency for Health Care Policy and Research, *Using Clinical Practice Guidelines to Evaluate Quality of Care, Volume 1: Issues,* AHCPR Pub. No. 95–0045 (Rockville, MD: 1995).

2. Agency for Health Care Policy and Research, *Using Clinical Practice Guidelines.*

3. C. Havighurst, What's at the End of the Path? *Health Systems Review* (Jan/Feb 1996): 49–54.

4. AHCPR. As reported from the Institute of Medicine, Committee on Clinical Practice Guidelines, *Clinical Practice Guidelines: Directions for a New Program,* eds. M.J. Field and K.N. Lohr (Washington, DC: National Academy Press, 1990).

5. S.S. Poe and J.C. Will, Quality Nursing-Patient Outcomes: A Framework for Nursing Practice, *Journal of Nursing Quality Assurance* 2 (1987): 29–37.

6. Poe and Will, Quality Nursing-Patient Outcomes, 29–37.

7. C. Garfield, *Peak Performers* (New York: Avon Books, 1986).

8. Garfield, *Peak Performers.*

9. C. Havighurst, ed., The Prognosis for Pathways: A Study of Clinical Path Trends in Health Care, *Health Systems Review* (Jan/Feb 1996): 48–54.

10. J.F. Preston and E. Sugrue-McElearney, *Pathways for Care Management* (Paper presented at the Associated Home Health Industries of Florida, Inc., Annual Conference, 1994).

11. T.W. Whipple and A.B. Little, Variance Analysis for Care Path Outcomes Management, *Journal of Nursing Care Quality* 12, no. 1 (1997): 20–25.

12. Whipple and Little, Variance Analysis, 20–25.

13. R. Carey, Measuring Quality Improvement in Healthcare: A Guide to Statistical Process Control Applications (Paper presented at the Disease Management Congress, Phoenix, AZ, March 4, 1997).

14. Carey, Measuring Quality Improvement in Healthcare.

15. Whipple and Little, Variance Analysis, 20–25.

16. Whipple and Little, Variance Analysis, 20–25.

17. K. Keech-Hunsicker, Managing Clinical Utilization through Total Quality Management, in *Clinical Pathways for the Multidisciplinary Care Team,* eds. B.S. Gingerich and D.A. Ondeck (Gaithersburg, MD: Aspen Publishers, 1997), 3.1–3.5.

18. Havighurst, ed., The Prognosis for Pathways, 49.

19. F. Bazzoli, Putting the Pieces Together, *Health Data Management* (January 1996): 29–37.

20. E. Sampson, Disease State Management: New Models for Case Management, *The Remington Report* 4, no. 5 (1996): 21–25.

21. Bazzoli, Putting the Pieces Together, 29–37.

22. S.S. Lee, A Primer on Disease Management, *The Remington Report* 4, no. 5 (1996): 30–33.

23. B. McKinnon, Is Disease State Management a Strategy for Success, or Just Another Industry Buzzword? *The Remington Report* 4, no. 5 (1996): 26–29.

24. Sampson, Disease State Management, 22.

25. C. Stolte, Nurses' Role in Disease Case Management, *Journal of Healthcare Resource Management* 15, no. 10 (1996): 21–23.

26. M. Daniels (Presentation at SMS marketing meeting, Malvern, PA, October 3, 1997).

27. Bazzoli, Putting the Pieces Together, 29–37.

28. E.H. Wagner, A Successful Model for Coordinating Outcomes Management and Quality Improvement (Paper presented at the Disease Management Congress, Phoenix, AZ, March 6, 1997).

29. Havighurst, What's at the End of the Path? 52.

30. M.F. Sylvestri and E.P. Marro, Disease Management: Partnering for Better Patient Care, *The Remington Report* 5, no. 4 (1997): 29.

CHAPTER 9

Activity-Based Cost Management

The preceding chapters have painted a picture of changing perspectives about an agency's relationship to information management. Information takes many forms, and one of them is conveyed through the concept of cost. Traditionally, cost-oriented management information has been provided by means of a profit and loss statement, which identifies total dollars spent by category. The profit and loss may have been presented as a stand-alone statement or used to compare actual expenditures to budget, or a prior period. This type of reporting helped to keep management informed of revenue and expenses for a given period, provided a control vehicle in an attempt to force accountability, and has become a generally accepted yardstick of agency operations. The only problem is that the traditional profit and loss statement is usually compared against a budget that is outdated moments after it is published or is produced so far after the month has ended that its relevance has diminished dramatically.

Proponents of traditional financial reporting would argue that closing the books faster and producing a profit and loss statement several days after the month has ended will provide more value to management than a slow monthly close. This perspective says that if we can reduce the cycle time associated with producing the monthly financial statement, then we have increased the value to those who use the financial statements. Or, if we transition from an annual or semiannual budget to a rolling budget, then we will be able to compare actual expenditures against a budget that reflects current thinking.

Although both of the above approaches would increase the value of the traditional financial reporting process, financial reporting is an old paradigm process. It is compliance oriented and provides little value to the management of an agency. Yes, financial reporting does identify whether an agency is making money. Yes, financial reporting will still be required for external purposes such as providing information to lending institutions, the Internal Revenue Service (IRS), and fiscal intermediaries. Agencies need a tool, however, that can satisfy the information requirements of their internal management teams.

An approach to meeting the growing information requirements of internal managers is activity-based cost management (ABCM). ABCM is a language, a philosophy, and an approach to transition from reporting total expenditures to understanding the causes of resource consumption. It is this shift in philosophy that makes ABCM a tool for clinicians and administrators instead of being a tool solely for financial practitioners.

This chapter is about activity-based cost management and its application to the home care setting. This chapter looks at

- the changing environment dictating a move to ABCM
- the ABCM model
- activity-based costing
- activity-based management
- costing clinical pathways
- prospective payment

It is the combination of activity-based costing and activity-based management that provides a powerful framework for aligning and quantifying organizational strategies as management positions the agency for survival within the evolving health care delivery system.

THE CHANGING ENVIRONMENT

Life appeared good before managed care began to make inroads and reshape the health care delivery system. Albeit, there were rumblings of prospective payment, bundling of costs, copayments, and shifting services from Medicare Part A to Part B. But for the most part, if an agency followed the Medicare rules for reimbursement, abided by the Conditions of Participation (COPs), and satisfied the regulatory or accrediting agencies, business proceeded as usual perhaps with an occasional audit. Home care, unlike most industries, had minimal business risk because the federal government has been reimbursing Medicare-certified providers for reasonable costs incurred in providing patient care. This minimal risk has increased significantly with the federal government's introduction of the interim payment system (IPS) for Medicare providers. This system is intended to control utilization through restructuring the cost reimbursement formula to be the lower of costs, limits, or the per-beneficiary cap. Still, if structured properly, a Medicare-certified agency can provide an opportunity to offer community-based programs whose cost can be rolled into the aggregate cost reimbursement (i.e., flu shots and diabetes screening aggregated under the cost of the Medicare program) or whose cost could be shifted among product lines.

Managed care, however, is changing the health care delivery system. Managed care plans are enticing purchasers of health plans away from traditional indemnity policies to those plans offered by managed care organizations (MCOs). Patients who had once been Medicare beneficiaries are now shifting to managed health plans. It is projected that, by the year 2000, 80 percent of all Americans will be covered by managed care plans.[1] As the number of members participating in managed care plans swells, these plans are negotiating with providers to care for their members in a cost-effective way while demonstrating to their accrediting bodies that their members are satisfied with the care they receive.

As managed care continues to increase the financial risk associated with providing care, many providers are seeking ways to reduce the cost of providing care. One of the tools for risk diversification, from a hospital's perspective, is through integrating home health services into its service continuum. With this change in perspective, home care is no longer the forgotten stepsister within the health care delivery system. Many providers who historically wanted no part of home care now want to be involved. Home care is now being recognized as a low-cost solution to a capital- and labor-intensive industry.[2] This translates into competition for home care agencies. The competition is for referral streams that once came freely from hospitals, physicians, nursing homes, and the community, or in competing for contracts that would guarantee a steady stream of patients.

Concurrently, MCOs are contracting directly with home health agencies. Their approach is similar to the strong-arm approach that they use when contracting with providers that have deep pockets. Their approach has been to offer contracts that have deeply discounted per-visit rates, episodic payment scenarios, or capitated contracts.[3] Unfortunately, cost reimbursement never provided home health agencies the opportunity to develop deep pockets. Furthermore, many of the processes, procedures, and protocols under which a home health agency operates have been developed under a system and philosophy of cost reimbursement.

Specifically, transitioning to a competitive environment requires the adoption of new tools and approaches for critically viewing and understanding agency operations. Otherwise, if one were to rely solely upon the numbers generated through the Medicare cost-finding process for negotiating with MCOs, one could potentially destroy an agency financially through either under- or overpricing services.

The Medicare cost report was developed to determine the reimbursable cost and not the "true" cost of a visit. It employs an average cost methodology that combines all types of visits into a common pool and treats them as a homogeneous group, when in reality they are not. In addition to collapsing all visits into a common pool, the cost-finding process ignores the nuances related to patient care such as the amount of travel, documentation requirements, telephone support, conferences on the patient's behalf, and patient-specific supplies. Beyond costs that can be directly attributable to a specific patient are all of the other costs associated with bringing the patient onto service: the cost of billing, recordkeeping, and administrative activities. These other costs have no direct bearing upon a specific patient but are critical to supporting the agency as an ongoing entity.

Many agencies have recognized that their costs differ by product line, program, and payer and they have developed financial reporting formats to capture these differing costs. Some have even expanded their reporting to include differences in revenue and expenditures by branch office or service location. But differentiating patient support services such as intake and supervision, billing, records management, and administrative costs still tends to distort true patient costs. Costs end up being charged or allocated based upon some predetermined formula. The difficulty is that there is usually no relationship between the basis for allocation and the reason the costs were incurred by the agency. The good news is that these "hybrid" systems provide a better understanding of product line, program, and payer profitability. They can identify the amount of resources that came into the agency in the form of revenue. They can also identify the amount of resources that were consumed by the agency by listing total expenditures by category. These hybrid systems, however, still do not answer a very basic question: "What caused the resources to be consumed?"

Answering this question is the contribution that ABCM can make to the workplace. By understanding the underlying activities that were performed by staff, it is possible to understand how to improve the workplace, to enhance individual and organizational efficiency, to pursue organizational effectiveness, and to manage the drivers of cost, or its root causes.

Traditional systems captured total dollars for payroll expenditures. Capturing these dollars quantified how much money was spent on staff and staff-related benefits. It did not explain what actions, tasks, or steps staff completed or performed while earning their compensation. Figure 9–1 illustrates the concept of going below the outer layer of payroll information to seek additional information. Similar to peeling an onion, as each subsequent layer of Figure 9–1 is removed, there is new information that can be used to understand agency operations. For instance, understanding the activities that were performed provides a basis for developing a better understanding of product line, program, and payer profitability; provides the potential to develop better pricing strategies; and creates a significant competitive advantage for those who adopt a proactive management tool.

The real power is not in the costing applications. The real power is in understanding the cost drivers or the root causes that explain why work was done and what caused resources to be consumed. This is where the concepts of ABCM transition from a sophisticated tool for accountants and financial managers into a

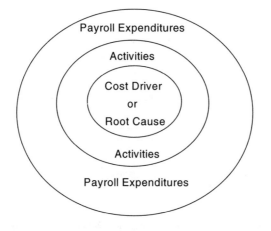

Figure 9–1 Information Core

---

process-improving, customer-oriented management tool that can be utilized by all facets of management.

THE ACTIVITY-BASED COST MANAGEMENT MODEL

The ABCM model was initially developed in the 1980s by Peter B. B. Turney and Norman Raffish in response to the emerging needs of the manufacturing industry as it struggled with increased competition from overseas.[4] The ABCM model consists of two components and is illustrated as a cross with the vertical element representing the costing component and the horizontal element representing the management component. Both the vertical and horizontal elements share one common theme and that is activities. The ABCM model is illustrated in Figure 9–2.

One of the core concepts of the ABCM model is that costs are incurred by an organization that has different relationships to the product that it is producing. From the perspective of home health, this means that it is possible to identify costs based upon its relationship to the patient. Understanding the relationship of costs to the patient provides the basis for beginning the costing process. Stated differently, there are activities that are performed that have a direct correlation to the patient, an indirect correlation to the patient, and no correlation to the patient. Home health services revolve around the patient. It is through understanding the relationship of cost to the patient that one is able to make a smooth transition into the foundational principles of activity-based costing. It is the same foundation that provides a methodology for costing cross-functional processes.

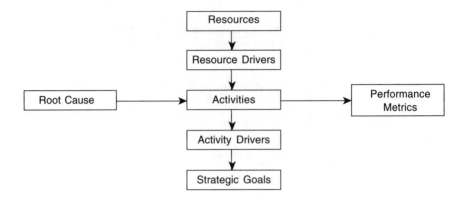

Figure 9–2 The Activity-Based Cost Management Model. *Source:* Adapted with permission from G. Cokins, A. Stratton, and J. Helding, *An ABC Manager's Primer,* © 1993, Institute of Management Accounts.

ACTIVITY-BASED COSTING

What is activity-based costing? It is a two-step cost assignment process that begins with the valuation of activities. Once activities have been valued, activity cost is assigned to strategic costing objectives. This process is explained though the use of an illustration. Table 9–1 is an example of how an activity-based costing system would apply to a field clinician's annual salary. In this example, the agency had decided that its primary objective for its cost management system (its strategic goal) is to understand cost by product line and payer. Therefore, the goal of the costing system is to capture and report all cost by product line (e.g., skilled intermittent care, private duty, and hospice), and then differentiate payer-specific results for each product line. In the example illustrated by Table 9–1, the clinician provided services to only one of the agency's three product lines (skilled intermittent care); however, she saw patients from three different payers. Payroll costs associated with the clinician are used to value activities, and then the valued activities are charged to each of the three payers using activity drivers specific to each of the activities that were performed.

The first step is to accumulate resources. Table 9–1 lists a total of $45,474 in payroll-related costs for this individual. This example addresses only payroll-related costs but could include travel reimbursement, educational reimbursement, and additional benefit costs such as pension contributions and paid time off. Once all resources (costs) have been determined, either on an individual or departmental basis, then there is a need to understand the activities that the individual or department performed.

Table 9–1 The Cost Assignment Process: A Clinical Example

ABCM: A Field Clinician's Salary for Fiscal Year 19XX

Accumulate Resources

Salary	$38,000
Payroll Taxes	3,724
Workers' Compensation	1,900
Health Insurance	1,850
	$45,474

Determine Resource Driver and Activity Cost

	Resource Driver (% of time)	Activity Cost
Documentation	5%	2,274
Travel	25%	11,368
Care Coordination	5%	2,274
Direct Care	60%	27,284
Staff Meetings	5%	2,274
		$45,474

Assignment of Activity Cost to Cost Objectives

	Number of Visits	Cost of Documentation Activity
Payer A	425	859
Payer B	500	1,011
Payer C	200	404
	1,125	$2,274

	Miles	Cost of Travel Activity
Payer A	5,623	5,188
Payer B	3,829	3,533
Payer C	2,869	2,647
	12,321	$ 11,368

	Time (Est.)	Cost of Coordination Activity
Payer A	30%	682
Payer B	20%	455
Payer C	50%	1,137
	100%	$2,274

continues

Table 9–1 continued

	Actual Time (hours)	Cost of Direct Care Activity
Payer A	398	10,730
Payer B	383	10,326
Payer C	231	6,228
	1,012	$ 27,284
Staff Meetings		$ 2,274

Activities are action oriented. They should be broad enough to describe a general sequence of steps, tasks, interventions, and protocols that are performed. The challenge, however, is not to get caught up in the actual measurement of the steps, tasks, interventions, and protocols, but to stay focused on the activity level. (Refer to Figure 8–5.) For example, in Table 9–1 five activities are identified. It is possible to look at any of the activities and describe a subset of tasks, steps, or protocols that would support the activity. For instance, let's look at the activity of direct care. Direct care has many steps, tasks, and protocols that support this activity. Some of the steps could include dressing changes, teaching wound care, and nutritional evaluation. From a measurement perspective, multiple tasks, actions, and protocols could occur simultaneously, making it impossible to provide a meaningful measurement for costing purposes. Therefore, costing occurs at the activity level and not at the task, action, or protocol level.

Referring back to Figure 9–2 it can be seen that understanding the activities is accomplished by using a resource driver. In a service environment, such as home health, the best resource driver to use is time. Time can be tracked using time sheets or some other tracking mechanism. The goal is to account for all of an individual's time and then associate it with the various activities that he or she was involved with during the course of the day, month, and year.

Table 9–1 indicates that this individual spent all of her time on five activities: documentation, travel, care coordination, direct care, and staff meetings. Using the time percentages associated with each activity, it is possible to prorate accumulated resource cost to each activity that has been identified. The prorating of resource cost to each activity needs to be consistent with the time periods being analyzed. In this example, the time period is fiscal year 19XX. Prorating of resource costs were for costs that occurred during this time period.

Once each activity has been valued, it is necessary to determine its activity driver in order to assign the activity cost to the appropriate product line and payer. Refer to Figure 9–2. An activity driver is a factor or indicator that provides a causal understanding of why activities were performed and their relationship to the costing objective. Table 9–1 illustrates that four of the five activities have been associated with an activity driver. In this example, the four activity drivers are: number of visits, actual mileage driven to the patient's home, estimated time spent on coordination of care, and the number of hours spent providing direct care. These activity drivers will be used to assign activity cost to each payer. The fifth activity, staff meetings, has no activity driver that relates to a specific payer; therefore, it would be listed as an administrative cost.

Table 9–1 illustrates that there were 1,125 visits by this individual and that the largest number of visits was for Payer B. Patient visits are the activity driver that is used to identify documentation activity cost for each payer in this example. It is important, however, to note that activity drivers are not static. Activities and their related drivers should be reviewed to determine whether the activity drivers selected for a particular activity are the most appropriate for generating the required information. For instance, time may be a better indicator for assigning activity cost for documentation if there are different documentation requirements between payers.

Travel, on the other hand, uses an activity driver of actual mileage to the patient's home to assign the activity cost associated with travel to each payer. Although Payer B has the greatest amount of visits, Payer A required the greatest amount of travel. This may be the result of the location of the referral source or the geographic location of the patients who have that particular insurance. This result also highlights an opportunity for the agency to improve its scheduling system. Improvements can be quantified through changes in travel cost related to Payer A.

Coordination of care uses an estimate of time for its activity driver. Payer C had the least amount of patients; however, Payer C required the most amount of time for the coordination of patient care. This could be because Payer C's patients were discharged from the hospital sooner and sicker than other patients and thus required multiple service interventions or because these patients were frail and required more interdisciplinary support.

Direct care uses actual time, in hours, as its activity driver. Payer C patients require more time or longer visits than either Payer A or Payer B. This is consistent with the results of the preceding activity analysis as shown in Table 9–1. For example, actual time in hours for Payer C is 231. Although this is the lowest number of hours of the three payers, Payer C also has the lowest number of visits (200), resulting in the longest time per visit (1.155 hours).

The vertical element of the ABCM model (see Figure 9–2) enables agencies to arrive at better costing than using a Medicare or hybrid costing model. This is illustrated in Table 9–2 by the differences in cost per visit by payer. The Medicare model spreads cost evenly among payers. Using an ABCM model, however, it is clear that there are significant cost differences among payers. This example does not include any costs other than those illustrated for one clinician in Table 9–1, however it still is useful to demonstrate the problems that over- and undercosting can cause. If the average cost of $40.42 was used to bid on a managed care contract

Table 9–2 Assignment of Cost: Traditional vs. Activity-Based

Medicare Assignment of Payroll Cost

	Visits	Cost	Cost/Visit
Payer A	425	17,179	40.42
Payer B	500	20,211	40.42
Payer C	200	8,084	40.42
	1,125	45,474	40.42

Assignment of Activity Cost

	Visits	Cost	Cost/Visit
Payer A	425	18,318	43.10
Payer B	500	16,336	32.67
Payer C	200	10,820	54.10
	1,125	45,474	40.42

that produced 10,000 nursing visits, then the agency would have made a lot of money if the MCO was in reality Payer B. If, on the other hand, the MCO was Payer C, then the agency would have had some serious financial difficulties. The financial impact of both of these scenarios is illustrated in Table 9–3.

The bottom line is that as more business shifts away from cost-reimbursed Medicare services, there is a need to have a better understanding of what it costs to provide services. Better costing will be a necessity for survival under IPS and the episodic payment system slated for 1999. An ABCM system is a tool to identify an agency's cost structure. Once a cost structure is understood, an agency is in a much stronger position to bid on managed care contracts or to offer discounted fee-for-service arrangements because it knows what its cost structure is, what profit is necessary to remain viable, and what resources will be required to invest in its future.

ACTIVITY-BASED MANAGEMENT STATEMENTS

The concepts of ABCM lend themselves to another tool that is beneficial to the management of agency operations. In fact, the expansion of the earlier example of

Table 9–3 Undercosting/Overcosting Dilemma

	Bid	Actual	Difference	Volume	Profit/Loss
Payer B	40.42	32.67	7.75	10,000	77,500
Payer C	40.42	54.10	−13.68	10,000	(136,800)

cost as having a direct, an indirect, or no correlation to the patient, provides a tool for developing a multilevel, activity-based, contribution margin–oriented profit and loss statement. Activity cost tends to follow a process orientation as opposed to the traditional department structure.

In Chapter 3, the basic model of a system was identified. (See Figure 3–1.) A system, or an agency, is made up of several interrelated processes, which in turn are composed of activities, steps, tasks, and actions. Figure 9–3 expands upon this concept by identifying two major groups of processes (patient-focused care and support) and their related subprocesses. Patient-focused care processes are an agency's reason for being. It is through these processes that revenue is produced and value is provided to the primary customer group, the patient. The patient-focused care process is made up of an upstream element, core process, and downstream element. The upstream element is where the activities of intake, insurance verification, and initial visit are performed. Once the patient is admitted onto service, the core processes section takes over. Core processes include all activities related to patient care, logistics or scheduling, and case management. The downstream element of the patient-focused care process is where the activities of record management, billing, and collections are performed. Together these three interrelated processes enable a patient to come into the system, receive care, and be discharged; then the agency closes out or completes the process by collecting payment for services provided. When viewed from this perspective, management can begin to think in terms of complete episodes of cost and care, instead of fragmented services, visits, and costs.

From a costing perspective, the core process contains activities that exhibit a one-to-one correlation with the patient. As described above, the amount of activities depends upon the intensity of patient problems. Activities in both the upstream and downstream processes exhibit an indirect relationship to the patient.

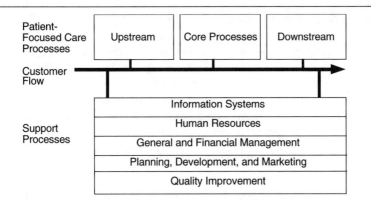

Figure 9–3 A Process Model. *Source:* Courtesy of Gemini Home Health Services Case Study, Malcolm Baldrige National Quality Award, 1998.

The reason that these activities exhibit an indirect relationship is that they are characteristic of a one-to-many relationship. For instance, the *one* is an activity such as invoicing or billing and the relationship is *many* invoices or bills. Therefore, from a cost assignment perspective, it is more beneficial to track the nuances in activity consumption using a driver that reflects the number of invoices or bills by payer.

Support processes on the other hand should be designed to support the agency's reason for being—providing patient care. Support processes are enablers. They need to support operational and business endeavors. Table 9–4 illustrates the different activities that occur within the patient-focused care and support process categories. Listed next to each activity is a bullet that corresponds to a specific customer group. The challenge, as described in Chapter 4, is to focus process owners on meeting the needs of the internal customers, patients, and payers, instead of meeting the needs of regulatory bodies and accreditation agencies. Table 9–4 illustrates that activities may be serving many customers and it is management's job to focus all activities toward common goals in order to serve the customers who pay the bills.

From a costing perspective, the activities associated with support processes have no direct or indirect correlation to the patient. They do have a relationship to a specific product line. As mentioned above, these preceding processes support the business operations of the agency; therefore, their activities should be assignable based upon the product or service lines that they support, or identified as supporting the entire agency infrastructure. For instance, accounting activities can be differentiated by product or service lines and any residual would be incurred to support the agency as a whole. "One rule to remember is that 99 times out of 100, an imprecise estimate using some logical basis is better than a general distribution using an irrelevant, but available basis. For example, it is better to estimate in what proportions electricity is consumed than to distribute it on an irrelevant basis, such as square footage or direct labor."[5] (p.56)

The development of a multilevel, activity-based, contribution margin–oriented profit and loss statement uses the preceding concepts. (See Table 9–5.) First, unit-level costs, or costs that have a direct correlation to the patient, are easily identified as occurring in the core process section of Figure 9–3. Activities with the upstream and downstream sections of the core process in Figure 9–3 generally have a *one-to-many* relationship with the patient. Typically, they are found in the upstream and downstream sections of Figure 9–3. The support process section of Figure 9–3 includes activities that are critical to supporting a specific product or service line, the agency or business entity, and the patient-focused care processes. There is usually no relationship to a specific patient in any of these support activities. Finally, there are costs that do not take the form of activities. These are enterprise-level costs and are incurred to support the entire agency regardless of the number of product lines, payers, or programs the agency has developed.[6]

Activity-Based Cost Management   209

Table 9–4 Customers and Activities by Process Category

Process	Activities	Patient	Internal Customer	MCO Customer	Agency	Regulatory
Upstream	Intake	•	•			
	Data Entry		•		•	
	Ins. Verification		•		•	
	Scheduling	•	•			•
	Assessment	•	•	•	•	•
Core Process	Scheduling	•	•			•
	Care Coordination	•	•			•
	Hands-On Care	•	•	•		
	Case Conference	•	•	•		•
	Travel—Patient	•		•		
	Travel—Lab			•		
	Documentation		•	•		•
Downstream	Data Entry				•	
	Records Management		•	•	•	•
	Invoicing	•		•	•	
	Collections				•	
	Cash Applications				•	
Information Systems	Info. System Planning		•		•	
	Training		•		•	
	Maintenance		•		•	
	Reporting		•	•	•	•
Human Resources	Resource Planning		•		•	
	Training	•	•		•	
	Recruitment	•	•		•	•
	Benefits & Comp. Mgt.				•	•
	Personnel Mgt.				•	
General Management & Finance	Plan & Strategy Devlp.				•	
	Fin'l., Cost, & Tax Rept.		•		•	•
	Coord. & Deployment		•		•	
	Accounting, AP, PR		•		•	•
	Process & Opts. Mgt.	•	•	•	•	
	Supplier Management	•	•	•	•	
Planning, Development, & Marketing	Market Analysis				•	
	Cust. Svc. & Reception	•		•	•	
	Coordinators/Liaison			•	•	
	Community Education	•		•	•	
	Contract Development		•	•	•	
Quality Improvement	Quality Assur./Inspect.		•	•	•	•
	Training		•		•	•
	Process Improvement	•	•	•	•	•

Table 9–5 Multilevel, Activity-Based, Contribution Margin–Oriented Profit and Loss Statement

Revenue	$337,500	100%
Direct Care	95,250	
Travel	10,500	
Care Coordination	1,250	
Documentation	3,500	
Scheduling	5,000	
Staff Meetings	2,700	
Core Process	118,200	35%
Intake	18,230	
Assessment	7,500	
Data Entry	13,260	
Insurance Verification	3,280	
Records Management	3,250	
Billing	16,500	
Collections	5,200	
Upstream & Downstream	67,220	20%
Information Systems	23,560	
Human Resources	32,600	
General Management & Finance	41,600	
Planning, Development, & Marketing	21,600	
Quality Improvement	18,690	
Support Processes	138,050	41%
Enterprise Cost	8,650	3%
Net Income	$5,380	2%

The purpose behind using a multilevel, activity-based, contribution margin–oriented profit and loss statement is twofold. First, activities can be classified as value-adding or non-value-adding. Value-adding activities are those activities that provide value to the customer or to the business. It is important to note, however, that the emphasis should be placed on those activities that add value to the customer. Non-value-adding activities are activities that only add cost to the agency. For instance, using the activities identified in Table 9–1, two of the five activities add value to the customer. They are direct care and the coordination of care. One could argue that travel should be included as a value-adding activity. Travel, however, is a dimension of service that is an expectation from the patients' perspective and a requirement from the payer's perspective; if minimized through efficient scheduling, travel cost will not impact customer satisfaction. Non-value-adding activities would be travel, staff meetings, and documentation. The goal is to reduce or minimize non-value-adding activities. This could be accomplished through the following:

- the use of e-mail or other electronic communications to reduce the frequency and/or length or staff meetings
- the purchase of an electronic documentation system that reduces the amount of duplication in charting and saves documentation time
- the utilization of teams based upon geographic area to reduce travel-related costs

The goal is to continually increase the amount of value-adding activities while decreasing the amount of non-value-adding activities. Table 9–6 has summarized the expenses identified in Table 9–5 into a format that differentiates between value-adding and non-value-adding activities. Actual results are compared against a two-year goal.

The second reason a multilevel, contribution-oriented profit and loss statement makes sense is for negotiating with MCOs. Many MCOs are negotiating a discounted fee-for-service with home care agencies. MCOs promise a certain amount of volume and the management and financial teams together determine what price they can offer given volume estimates.

Using a format such as Table 9–5 allows management and financial teams to develop different pricing scenarios. For instance, at each level of the contribution margin statement there is another level of incremental cost. By understanding the activity drivers associated with each level it is possible to determine pricing for a one-time episodic case versus low-volume or high-volume contracts. Ultimately, enough of a margin needs to be generated to cover all four layers of activity cost and produce a profit; otherwise there will be no opportunity for long-term viability. There may be situations, however, where a price needs to be determined based upon levels of service or volume. Understanding how cost fluctuates on an incremental basis provides the astute manager with one more tool to survive in a highly competitive environment.

Another way to look at it is through the patient-focused care process, illustrated in Figure 9–3. This process includes activity costs that are incurred getting the patient onto service, during the patient's time on service, and after the patient has been discharged. From a political perspective, an agency may decide to offer a single pricing that covers core process cost only, or it may decide that pricing

Table 9–6 Activity Analysis and Comparison against a Two-Year Goal

	Actual Results		*Two-Year Goal*
Value-Adding Activities	216,260	65%	75%
Non-Value-Adding Activities	115,860	35%	25%
	332,120		

needs to cover all patient-focused care costs (upstream, core, downstream). If the decision is purely financial, then episodic revenue will need to cover all patient-focused care activity cost plus make a contribution toward support service overhead and profit generation. The size of the overhead contribution will depend upon volume. If the decision is political, then negotiate the best deal possible, but attempt to get as much of the patient-focused care cost covered as possible.

The methodology described above for episodic pricing can be used to determine which patients to accept under IPS. Substitute the agency's per-beneficiary cap as the episodic payment amount. Then determine what mix of patients is necessary to remain below the aggregate per-beneficiary cap. Prospective assessment systems will need to be developed that manage the mix of patients to ensure that there is a sufficient amount of short-term, low-resource-consuming patients to offset those patients with chronic needs who consume large amount of resources.

IMPROVING YOUR ACTIVITY-BASED COSTING SYSTEM

An ABCM system can be complex or designed to meet basic needs. Figure 9–4 illustrates the Plan-Do-Check-Act (PDCA) cycle that was initially developed by Walter Shewhart and has gained respect and popularity as a result of the work of W. Edwards Deming.[7] The PDCA cycle is used to outline an approach to implementing an ABCM system. Developing an ABCM system requires understanding the strategic requirements of your agency's costing system. It requires understanding what resources will be needed to develop or purchase an ABCM system, who will be responsible for training and maintaining the system, and, most important, the support and leadership of senior management.[8] Planning is a critical element and is necessary to determine the project scope, the activities to be analyzed, the drivers to be used for assignment of costs, and costing objectives. For instance, an agency may decide to cost out visits only by type and assign them to specific payers. This would provide a better understanding of activity cost as it relates to actual visits and of profitability by payer. This approach does not capture a great deal of activity-related cost; however, an initial start is better than no form of activity-based costing.

More adventurous agencies may want to consider developing a costing structure that provides a framework for costing clinical pathways, evaluating process improvements, maximizing human resources through capacity analysis, or quantifying decreases in process cost (e.g., related to cycle time reductions and customer satisfaction). Furthermore, by strategizing what data are critical to collect and measure it is possible to create a competitive advantage for the agency by using information provided by the ABCM system. For instance, patient data could include the patient's name, medical diagnosis, nursing diagnosis, presence of another caregiver, OASIS data, and physician information. Analyzing subse-

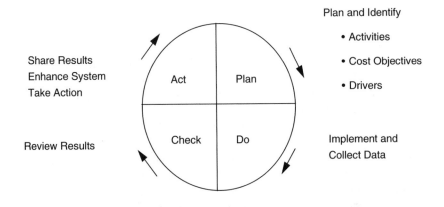

Figure 9–4 Using the PDCA Cycle To Enhance Your ABCM System

---

quent data may indicate that a 10 percent increase in functional improvement for patients with severe problems with activities of daily living (ADLs) may cost $300 to achieve. The point is that in the planning stage, it is important to understand the system requirements and objectives, identify how the data will be collected and by whom, and then focus on the improvement of the underlying processes.

One of the most important parts of the cycle is the action step. This is where results are reviewed and action is taken to either correct the process or improve the ABCM system. An ABCM system should continue to evolve and not become static. Activity drivers can be improved, cost objectives refined, and additional activities added. The point is that ABCM is a tool for continuous improvement of agency operations, and the tool should not be excluded from continuous improvement.

COSTING OF CLINICAL PATHWAYS

Why worry about pricing clinical pathways? Clinical pathways are being used as tools to manage the utilization of resources. It is the industry's response to managed care's focus on controlling utilization. It is also a solution to managing utilization under the IPS that will reimburse cost at the lower of cost, the limits, or the per-beneficiary cap. In a per-visit payment environment it is critical that the negotiated per-visit rate exceed all activity cost related to the agency's patient-focused care process (see Figure 9–3) and that this excess contribute to the support service cost associated with that contract. Conducting a break-even analysis using realistic volume estimates will identify whether contract pricing is adequate to meet agency needs. In an episodic pricing scenario, managed care and eventually the Health Care Financing Administration (HCFA) will identify a fixed payment up front, and it will be the agency's responsibility to control utilization and costs. The agency will need to assess whether the referral will result in a profit or loss to the agency and whether to accept the referral. The decision to accept the referral also will need to consider the agency's relationship with the MCO, its objectives for profitability, and the volume of referrals associated with episodic payments.

Understanding clinical pathway requirements helps an agency determine whether it is financially prudent to accept a referral. Depending upon the relationship with the MCO or referral source, it may be politically correct to accept one referral and lose money, if the hope is that profitable business will be forthcoming. If, however, the episodic pricing creates a loss for the agency or a large volume of the referrals require care in excess of the per-beneficiary cap, then that decision could seriously impact the organization's long-term financial viability.

There are several factors to consider when costing a clinical pathway. The best way to illustrate them is with an example. Table 9–7 illustrates the activities that could be associated with the clinical pathway for pneumonia described in Chapter 8. (See Exhibit 8–2.)

As mentioned previously, the definition of what constitutes an activity is agency dependent. So are the frequency and placement of activities. For instance, records management may occur daily if field staff document patient care using a paper system and forward notes to the office upon completion of the visit. Then, once the note has arrived at the office, a clerk locates the appropriate record and inserts the document in the patient's file. Field staff paperwork could also be used for daily data entry into the agency's information system. In this case there would be an "X" in each visit block in Table 9–7 for records management and data entry.

Table 9–7 Activities Associated with the Clinical Pathway for Pneumonia

	Clinical Pathway—Pneumonia							
Activity	Pre	One	Two	Three	Four	Five	Six	Post
Instruction		x	x	x	x	x	x	
Assessment		x	x	x	x	x	x	
Direct Care								
Travel		x	x	x	x	x	x	
Documentation		x	x	x	x	x	x	
Scheduling		x						
Intake	x							
Assessment	x							
Data Entry	x							x
Ins./Utilization Verification	x							
Billing								x
Records Management								x

If an electronic system is used and documentation is downloaded daily within the system, the activities of manual records management and data entry are minimized and may only occur when the patient has been discharged. The purpose of Table 9–7 is to illustrate the types of activities that should be considered within the clinical pathway. Consideration also should be given to eliminating redundant activities. In the preceding example, if redundant activity cost can be eliminated through point of care automation and the benefit exceeds the cost of automation, then the cost associated with a clinical pathway has decreased.

Automation has the potential to reduce activity cost associated with daily documentation, data entry, and records management.[9,10] Table 9–7 illustrated the importance of using activity cost when developing clinical pathway costs. There are many activities that occur before, during, and after the clinical pathway has been implemented. Consideration of all supporting activities must be included in pricing of services. Clinical pathway cost should also consider supplies, equipment, and IV therapies.

Another consideration for the costing of clinical pathways is that activity cost may vary in the amount of time required to complete the activities associated with patient care. Typical activities that occur within a patient's home are the assessment of the patient's condition or progress, providing instruction or education, and direct, hands-on care that may require the dressing of a wound, the care of a Foley catheter, or the performance of other skilled interventions. The length of time in the patient's home will depend upon the patient's problems and the amount of required interventions that must be performed. From a clinical pathway perspective, this may translate into longer activity time requirements associated with initial visits and shorter time requirements with subsequent visits.

Once inside the patient's home, multiple activities could occur such as instruction, assessment of patient condition, or provision of direct care. The challenge from a costing perspective is that these activities could occur simultaneously. A solution to this dilemma is illustrated in Exhibit 9–1, which lists the various interventions for the pneumonia pathway identified in Chapter 8 (Exhibit 8–2) and then categorizes them into agency-defined activity categories. Remember that activities are comprised of interventions, protocols, and procedures (Figure 8–5). Only the core processes are considered in this example, not the upstream or downstream processes.

In this example, there are a total of 12 possible interventions that could occur for the activity of instruction and 6 interventions for the activity of assessment. For calculating cost, however, the total times an intervention is utilized is the number used. For example, if care for the patient is given in concert with the planned clinical pathway, then 9 of the 12 instruction interventions and 1 of the 6 assessment interventions would be performed on the first visit. In looking at this pathway from the perspective of an episode, there would be 17 interventions that were instruction, and 15 interventions that belonged to the activity category of assessment.

Exhibit 9–1 Interventions and Their Relationship to Activities

Activity = Instruction or Education						
Interventions	1	2	3	4	5	6
1. Patient rights and responsibilities	x					
2. Patient financial liability for home care	x					
3. Patient/home safety	x					
4. Expectations of home care	x					
5. Plan for care	x					
6. Written visit schedule	x					
7. Medication regimen	x	x	x	x	x	x
8. Pertinent phone numbers	x					
9. Oxygen use and safety	x					
10. Instruct re: disease process/definition		x				
11. Instruct re: disease process/S&S		x				
12. Instruct regarding causes and risk factors of pneumonia			x			
Activity = Assessment						
Interventions	1	2	3	4	5	6
1. Assess condition	x	x	x	x	x	x
2. Obtain recall from instruction completed during visit one		x	x	x	x	x
3. Instruct re: care & maintenance/timely notification of MD		x				
4. Instruct re: care & maintenance/preventive measures		x				
5. Instruct re: care & maintenance/energy conservation methods		x				
6. Instruct re: care & maintenance/breathing exercises		x				
Number of interventions within activities						
Instruction	9	1	3	2	1	1
Assessment	1	6	2	2	2	2
Total interventions/visit	10	7	5	4	3	3
Percent cost attributable to each activity	%	%	%	%	%	%
Instruction	90	14	60	50	33	33
Assessment	10	86	40	50	67	67

Understanding the number of performed interventions by activity classification provides a methodology for costing the activities. The first step is to calculate the total number of interventions and the number of interventions within each activity category. The number of interventions in each category is then divided by the total to obtain the percentage for each activity category. In the preceding example, in the first visit the activity of instruction would receive 90 percent of the cost associated with the initial nursing visit. The balance of 10 percent would be charged to the activity of assessment. Exhibit 9–1 also illustrates how the balance of the pathway's activities would be calculated for the remaining nursing visits. For the entire episode, 53 percent of the interventions would be instruction and 47 percent would be in the activity category of assessment.

The second step to calculating activity cost is to calculate the total time that was associated with the clinical pathway. Table 9–8 shows the average time for each visit for the clinical pathway of pneumonia. These figures can be obtained through a time study or from the clinician's daily reports.

The third step is to calculate activity cost. The first piece of needed data is the number of direct care hours. This can be obtained from the clinician's salary report (Table 9–1). For this example, it is determined that the pneumonia pathway was utilized for those who had insurance coverage from Payer A. The direct care hours provided to Payer A patients for this clinician were 398 hours. Therefore, 6/398, or .01508 of this clinician's total visit time for Payer A would then be associated with the clinical pathway for pneumonia. This also assumes that this clinician made all the visits in this episode of care. To determine the direct cost, the previous percentage (.01508) would be multiplied against total direct cost attributable to Payer A ($10,730). This would result in a direct care activity cost attributable to the pneumonia pathway of $161.80/patient as illustrated in Table 9–9. The activity of direct care can be further refined using the ratio of total interventions as illustrated in Exhibit 9–1, which identifies that there were 17 instructional and 15 assessment interventions performed over the course of the clinical pathway. The ratio of instructional interventions to total interventions will provide that basis for the identification of activity cost for the activity of instruction. The ratio of assessment interventions to total interventions will provide the basis for the identification of assessment activity cost. Table 9–9 illustrates the actual activity cost for instruction and assessment. Remember this is the activity cost for direct care only. It does not include documentation, travel, care coordination, or any upstream or downstream activity cost.

Table 9–8 Total Visit Time Associated with the Clinical Pathway for Pneumonia

Visit	Average Time
One	1.5 hours
Two	1.0 hours
Three	1.0 hours
Four	1.0 hours
Five	0.75 hours
Six	0.75 hours
Total Visit Time	6.0 hours

Table 9–9 Calculation of Assessment and Instruction Activity Cost for a Pneumonia Clinical Pathway

Direct Care Hours—Pneumonia		6
Direct Care Hours Associated with Payer A (Table 9–1)		398
Percent Attributable to Pneumonia		1.508%
Total Payer A Direct Care Cost (Table 9–1)		$10,730
Direct Care Cost—Pneumonia		$161.80
Instruction Interventions	17	53%
Assessments Interventions (Exhibit 9–1)	15	47%
Total Interventions	32	100%
Direct Cost Attributable to:		
Instruction		85.76
Assessments		76.04
		$161.80

This methodology also provides a format for identification of activity cost on a visit-by-visit basis using the ratio of interventions identified in Exhibit 9–1 for each visit. For example, the activity of instruction would receive 90 percent of the cost associated with the nurse being in the patient's home for the first visit (1.5 hours). The balance of 10 percent would be charged to the activity of assessment for the first visit. This process could be repeated for each visit.

Associating interventions with activities provides a tool to quantify activity cost within pathways. Understanding clinical pathway cost provides agencies with a tool to quantify improvements to clinical pathways and to enter into episodic pricing negotiations. Through the use of statistics and control charts, clinical pathways also can be monitored for variation from standards. As improvements are implemented, the costs of those changes can be monitored. Once pathways are stabilized and are producing desired outcomes, they can be used for forecasting resource consumption by specific patient problem.

Understanding resource consumption from the perspective of patient problems will enable agencies to make prudent decisions regarding which episodic cases to accept, and which mix of patient problems they can handle, and provide a vehicle for maximizing profitability under HCFA's proposed Home Health Utilization Groups (HHUGs).[11]

ACTIVITY-BASED COST MANAGEMENT

As mentioned earlier, there are two elements of the ABCM model identified in Figure 9–2. The vertical element deals with costing an agency's services. The horizontal element deals with the management of activities. It is the horizontal element that creates a powerful opportunity for managers to begin to quantify process cost. The quantification of cost has far-reaching implications for today's environment. The integration of cost, outcomes, and quality is a concept whose time has not only come, but is a necessity as competition increases.

In an attempt to force accountability, traditional costing methodologies have identified how much money has been spent on a departmental basis. The problem is that an agency's processes are cross-functional and may begin in one department, cross into another's domain, and then conclude in a third department. This scenario can be illustrated by looking at the traditional flow of data through an agency. In this example, a referral comes in, a patient is admitted onto service, service is provided, and then attempts are made to collect moneys for services provided. If there are problems with the gathering of insurance information, timely receipt of documentation, or proper authorization, there could be a collections delay on the back end. The traditional department orientation allowed staff and managers to look the other way and proclaim that it was not their problem. Shifting to a process orientation enables management to leave their functional domains and look at a process from beginning to end. ABCM provides a tool to quantify each of the activities. More important, activity analysis provides a vehicle to understand internal customer relationships, identify activity output (products), financially quantify care processes and outcomes, and provide an additional format for key metric identification.

A performance measure hierarchy was presented in Chapter 3 (see Figure 3–3). At the top of the pyramid are agencywide performance measures that are rooted in strategic objectives. For example, these measures could include indicators of cost, quality, process improvement, and customer satisfaction. These are aggregate measures, however, that need to be cascaded down to the process and work unit level.

For example, if an agency's strategic initiative is to decrease its cost per visit from its current level of $70.35 down to $61.00 and it has developed a process orientation (see Figure 9–3), it would be possible to identify specific goals by process, associate those goals with process-dependent activities, and develop activity-oriented goals to support the larger process-oriented goal. If this were the case, process owners would have a format to identify whether activities were adding value to the customers they serve or whether activities were actually residual activities that no longer provided value to the customer in a managed care–dominated marketplace. Table 9–10 illustrates how the strategic cost initiative (e.g., decreasing cost per visit) could be cascaded downward to link strategic goals into specific process goals (e.g., two-year goal for the upstream process is $3.00, for the core process the goal is $34.00, and so on).

Table 9–11 identifies the activities that comprise the process cost for the upstream process. In this example, five activities are illustrated. Activity cost is divided by total annual visits. In this example, the objective will be to lower the cost of the upstream process from $3.65 to $3.00. The majority of the cost savings

Table 9–10 Cost per Visit by Process Category

	Process	Actual	Two-Year Goal
Patient-Focused Care Processes	Upstream	$ 3.65	$ 3.00
	Core Processes	38.50	34.00
	Downstream	2.95	2.50
	Information Systems	2.15	2.00
	Human Resources	2.25	2.00
Support Processes	General & Financial Management	16.25	13.50
	Plan, Develop, & Market	2.45	2.00
	Quality Improvement	2.15	2.00
	Aggregate Cost	$70.35	$61.00

will be attributable to the process of intake. In this example, the organization is looking at substituting RNs with LPNs and clerical help to reduce the cost associated with the intake process. Another way of reducing that cost could be through automation of the process.

This same approach could be used to evaluate internal and external customer satisfaction at a process level. Table 9–12 illustrates current results of an internal customer survey in comparison to specific growth objectives (two-year goals). Table 9–13 illustrates the activities that comprise the process of intake. Results are reflective of external and internal surveys and the predetermined valuation or weighting of activity contribution to process goals.

These illustrations provide an objective way to evaluate specific processes and illustrate how process measures could roll up to become part of an aggregate measurement system.

These examples also illustrate that to cascade aggregate measures down another level requires an understanding of the underlying activities that are performed within the agency. Refer to Table 9–4 for different activities that could be included in each process. Table 9–14 illustrates activity output or product.

Table 9–11 Composition of Process Cost for the Upstream Process

	Cost/Visit	
Upstream Process Activities	Actual	Two-Year Goal
Intake	1.85	1.35
Data Entry	.20	.15
Insurance Verification	.35	.30
Scheduling	.50	.45
Assessment	.75	.75
Total	3.65	3.00

Table 9–12 Internal Customer Satisfaction Levels

		Customer Satisfaction	
	Process	Current	Two-Year Goal
Patient-Focused Care Processes	Upstream	75%	91%
	Core Processes	75%	90%
	Downstream	63%	85%
	Information Systems	50%	80%
	Human Resources	40%	80%
Support Processes	General & Financial Management	60%	80%
	Plan, Develop, & Market	30%	80%
	Quality Improvement	50%	80%

Evaluating activity output from the perspective of a customer allows individual work units or teams to identify specific measures for improving their operating effectiveness and efficiency, thereby contributing to the larger goals of the agency.

The previous examples identified two specific agency goals: (1) to increase internal and external customer satisfaction, and (2) to decrease cost. Combining the two goals creates a multidimensional approach to process improvement. These goals are not mutually exclusive. The challenge is to accomplish both goals at the same time. For instance, indiscriminately reducing full-time equivalents, slashing programs, or eliminating benefits are all ways of decreasing cost; however, these measures do little to enhance employee satisfaction. They may represent necessary steps, however. Involving employees, explaining why cost reduction is necessary for survival, and soliciting their input for accomplishing

Table 9–13 Composition of Internal Weighting System for Process-Oriented Satisfaction Indicators

	Customer Satisfaction			
Upstream Process Activities	Weight	Actual	Weighted Average	Two-Year Goal
External Customer Satisfaction				
Intake	40%	90%	32%	40%
Internal Customer Satisfaction				
Data Entry	15%	60%	9%	12%
Insurance Verification	30%	80%	24%	27%
Scheduling	5%	60%	3%	4%
Assessment	10%	70%	7%	8%
Total			75%	91%

Table 9–14 Activity Output or Product

Process	Activities	Product
Upstream	Intake	Identify and gather relevant patient data and history
	Data Entry	Information transfer—automated, manual, verbal
	Insurance Verification	Visit and service authorization (units, dollars, expectations)
	Scheduling	Matching of appropriate team or individual to patient requirements
	Assessment	Assess patient problems, verify homebound, and need for home health services
Core Process	Scheduling	Matching & coordination of appropriate disciplines, teams, & services
	Care Coordination	Seamless service delivery, effective communication, & knowledge transfer
	Hands-On Care	Accomplish visit objective (may be related to milestone)
	Case Conference	Multidisciplinary status review (may include multiple service lines)
	Travel—Patient	Staff arrive on time and as scheduled
	Travel—Lab	Sample delivered
	Documentation	Information transfer—patient progress assessment
Downstream	Data Entry	Information transfer—automated and/or manual
	Records Management	Accurate filing/retrieval
	Invoicing	Accurate and timely submitted invoice
	Collections	Courteous and timely management of agency resources
	Cash Applications	Accurate posting
Information Systems	Info System Planning	Integration of strategic and action plans
	Training	Enhance staff computer literacy
	Maintenance	Support information system
	Reporting	Management & external reporting

continues

Table 9–14 continued

Process	Activities	Product
Human Resources	Resource Planning	Integration of strategic and action plans
	Training	Enhance staff competency
	Recruitment	Attract, interview, & hire new or replacement staff
	Benefits & Comp	Design, maintain, & evaluate benefit system
	Personnel	Implementation of action plans
General Mgmt & Finance	Plan & Develop Strategy	Strategic planning and subsequent action plan development
	Financial, Cost, & Tax Report	Internal and external reporting
	Coordinate & Deploy	Focus resources and mentor agency staff
	Accounting, AP, PR	Product and results dependent upon specific business function
	Process & Options	Implementation of action plans
	Supplier Management	Identification of input requirements and improvement plans
Plan, Develop, & Market	Market Analysis	Identification of opportunities, trends, and threats
	Customer Service & Reception	Communication link with stakeholders
	Coordinators/Liaison	Generate referrals
	Community Education	Community service
	Contract Development	Generate new business
Quality Improvement	QA/Inspect	Clean up and inspect for accuracy
	Training	Enhance staff competency
	Process Improvement	Enhance organizational processes and performance

organizational goals may provide a framework that will protect the integrity of the agency without damaging employee morale and customer satisfaction.

Another way to use the concepts of an ABCM system is to look at the cost drivers or root causes of an activity. A cost driver is an event or occurrence that causes an activity to take place. When the agency telephone rings with a referral, a chain of activities is triggered. Understanding the source of the trigger and the subsequent chain of activities facilitates the development of activity-oriented performance measures. Activity-oriented performance measures may be stand-alone indicators or they may be rolled into a composite indicator to reflect results at the process or agency levels.

Evaluation of the initial assessment visit process begins by understanding the flow of events as illustrated in Figure 9–5. In this simplified example, a referral

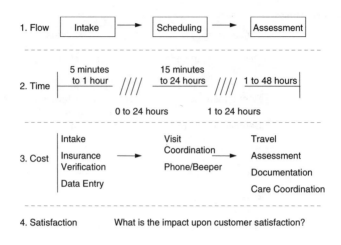

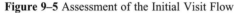

Figure 9–5 Assessment of the Initial Visit Flow

comes in, a visit is scheduled, an initial assessment visit is performed, and the subsequent paperwork is submitted to the office. The trigger or root cause is the phone call with the referral. It has triggered several activities that can be costed. The cycle time associated with this process also can be identified. In this example, the minimum time to complete the initial assessment visit is approximately three hours. Because of bottlenecks and delays, however, this process from referral to completed assessment could stretch out to five days.

Evaluating a process from the perspective of cost, time, and customer satisfaction enables managers to evaluate the impact of process changes. For instance, what happens if the cost of the initial admission visit is decreased? What impact does this have on customer satisfaction? Or, what happens if visit time is decreased? What happens if the total time from referral to the completion of the assessment visit is decreased? How does this impact cost and customer satisfaction?

A patient problem is a driver of cost. A patient who is admitted onto service with an uncomplicated postsurgical wound will require fewer services than a patient with a chronic condition who requires frequent nursing and aide visits. One of the goals of understanding how patient problems impact cost is to identify what resources particular classifications of patients consume, what outcomes the same group is able to achieve, and whether this customer group is satisfied. Regardless of whether the patient grouping follows the 18 HHUG categories that were developed as part of the prospective payment demonstration, or whether a different patient classification system is used, the goals remain the same.[12] The goals should be to increase the effectiveness of care delivered, improve customer satisfaction, and reduce cost. Understanding how specific patient problems impact cost, clinical outcomes, and patient satisfaction becomes the starting point for continuous improvement of services.

Furthermore, if the agency's ABCM system is set up using a relational database methodology, it will be able to retrieve data for a specific patient problem within any classification category the agency is using. These data will enable management to look at the nuances of patient problems to obtain a better understanding of the range of visits by discipline, the amount of supplies or antibiotics required for the healing process, the amount of telephone interaction and support activities, and any other activities that are being tracked by the agency. Understanding specific activities by patient problem and the range of resources consumed provides an agency-specific process for examining differences between teams of professionals, physicians, and referral sources. Understanding resource consumption by patient problem also provides a baseline for assessing and quantifying the use of alternate care methodologies such as tele-health or negotiating for additional visits to prevent rehospitalization of a patient.

Integrating the concepts of cost and quality provides a multidimensional way to assess agency operations. The goal is to make operations as efficient as possible while balancing the effectiveness of operations from a customer's perspective. From this perspective, ABCM becomes a tool that is operationally based by providing a metric; a cost that can be used to complement the metrics of time and customer satisfaction.

PROSPECTIVE PAYMENT

Prospective payment already exists in the home health community. Many states have paid on a per-visit basis for years, and managed care has introduced episodic and capitated payment methodologies. Eventually, the federal government will transition away from a system of cost reimbursement to one that allows home health providers the opportunity to make a profit in exchange for assuming risk. Currently, the IPS has shifted risk to providers but does not provide an opportunity for profit.

Figure 9–6 illustrates various payment types and the level of risk, rewards, and opportunities that are associated with each payment methodology. Figure 9–6 does not illustrate the IPS, which in a sense is a contradiction, because it increases provider risk without an opportunity for reward.[13]

Table 9–15 identifies specific risk, rewards, and opportunities with each payment system identified in Figure 9–6. As risk increases, providers need to be adopting an advanced costing system such as ABCM for many of the reasons discussed above. The adoption of these concepts will provide managers with a tool to evaluate cost per case and administrative overhead, and to develop process improvement strategies.

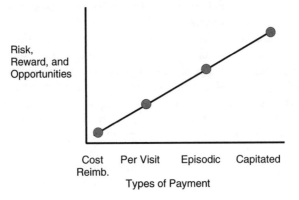

Figure 9–6 Relationship between Risk and Payment Methodology. *Source:* Adapted from T. McKeon, Efficient Operations: A Strategy that Crosses Clinical and Administrative Disciplines, *Home Healthcare Nurse*, Vol. 4, No. 5, © 1996, Lippincott-Raven.

The transition to a prospective payment system has been dragging on for years as the federal government attempts to gather sufficient data to make an informed decision regarding an episodic payment system. This time delay is providing a tremendous opportunity for home health providers to begin the implementation of an ABCM system. From a short-term perspective there is an opportunity to better understand agency cost structure. This information is valuable because it creates immediate competitive advantage for negotiation with MCOs today. It also identifies where changes will need to be made to survive under the new IPS and to position the agency for the eventual transition to a fully prospective payment system. From a long-term perspective, operational efficiency equates with profit under per-visit, episodic, and capitated payment systems. The more efficient an agency can become, the more profit potential it will have, and the more likely it will be to remain financially viable.

The concepts of ABCM have far-reaching ramifications and are critical in a prospective payment environment and the development of accurate costs. But ABCM's real power is in the management of processes to be discussed in the chapter on process management. Act now; develop your internal benchmarking system using an ABCM system. It will create strategic advantage.

CONCLUSION

This chapter has provided a brief overview of the concepts of ABCM. ABCM is a management tool that has broader applications than solely costing and pricing

Table 9–15 Relationship of Risk, Rewards, and Opportunities to Payment Methodology

Type of Payment	Risk	Reward	Opportunities
Cost Reimbursement	1. Denied cost. 2. Providers must follow rules (lower of cost, charges, or limits). 3. Utilization management risk remains with payer. 4. Cost risk remains with payer.	1. Relatively risk-free way of doing business. 2. Compensated for reasonable expenses. 3. Owner salary and related expenses could be greater than other sources of employment.	1. Cost reimbursement window is closing. Providers should be using this time to create efficient operating environments. 2. Opportunities to maximize reimbursement.
Interim Payment Systems (IPS)	1. Denied cost. 2. Providers must follow rules (lower of cost, limits, or per-beneficiary cap). 3. Utilization and cost management are providers' responsibility. 4. Readmissions, chronic cases, and volume issues.	1. Relatively risk-free way of doing business. 2. Compensated for reasonable expenses. 3. Owner salary and related expenses could be greater than other sources of employment. 4. Loss-leader for other profitable business.	1. Cost reimbursement window is closing. Providers should be using this time to create efficient operating environments, train and develop staff, and create customer-focused, values-driven, process-oriented organizations.
Per Visit	1. Opportunity for profit or loss. 2. Business is volume driven. 3. Utilization management risk remains with payer. 4. Cost risk is providers'.	1. Profits and losses are a function of pricing, cost, and volume. 2. Breakeven analysis is relatively straightforward.	1. Relatively risk-free business. Challenge is to maximize volume and control costs. 2. Channel profits into streamlining systems to increase profitability.
Episodic	1. Utilization management risk transferred to provider. 2. Provider determines whether to accept the referral.	1. Profit or loss is a function of pricing, cost, volume, and understanding service requirements. 2. Potential opportunity for	1. Development of prospective assessment tools linked to pricing and outcomes. 2. Increased importance of understanding

continues

Table 9–15 continued

Type of Payment	Risk	Reward	Opportunities
	3. Must be able to provide services within a prospectively determined amount.	creative pricing and bundling of services.	relationships between episodic case cost and administrative costs.
Capitated	1. Utilization management risk transferred to provider. 2. Provider accepts all referrals. 3. Must be able to provide services within rate based upon number of covered lives.	1. Profit or loss is a function of pricing, cost, volume, and understanding service requirements. 2. Contractual negotiations should consider organizational capabilities, high cost or utilization cases, and specific services to provide.	1. Development of prospective assessment tools linked to pricing and outcomes. 2. Increased importance of understanding relationships between case cost, administrative costs, and changing patterns of health care delivery system.

services. Surely, these are important uses; however, understanding the relationship of costs to outcomes, cost to time, and cost to customer satisfaction creates a strategic management advantage that provides a differentiating framework from all those providers who are not willing to invest in a management philosophy that will help to reshape their organizations.

The power of this philosophy does not come from its independence but rather its interdependence with all facets of agency operations. Interdependence is required to foster internal customer relationships. More important, if organizational processes are to become as efficient and effective as possible, it will require the collective efforts of all players within the organization. To be successful, an ABCM system requires that everyone contribute to the collection of data, to the refinement of cost drivers, and to take action once results are provided. This requires a joint ownership of the management system; otherwise, it will become another "we versus them" tool that has the potential to become as ineffective as traditional financial reporting.

Understanding the relationship between cost drivers, activities, and output measures enables managers to transition into an activity-based budgeting format. To then ask managers to explain variances, however, perpetuates the old paradigm of traditional financial reporting systems. Instead, if the concepts of ABCM were used to develop budgets and to evaluate systemic and process-oriented changes, then managers could invest their time in capacity analysis and focus on the maximization of human resources and customer satisfaction instead of spending their time on explaining variances.

Transitioning to a process-oriented management structure also requires not only aligning performance measures, but having the tools that will support a process orientation. ABCM meets that need. In fact, when linked to multiple indicators such as time, quality, and customer satisfaction, cost becomes a dimension that helps to explain processes in a fundamental language that every executive understands—the dollar. This creates a powerful position for home care managers. Understanding process cost and its relationship to clinical pathways and various programs that are offered by the agency enables astute managers to negotiate from a place of knowing, instead of by the seat of their pants. This position of power will enable managers to create win-win contracts with managed care organizations, enter into partnerships that are mutually rewarding, and generate enough surplus to invest in the agency's future.

NOTES

1. R.A. Fazzi and R.V. Agoglia, Managed Care's Expectations: Final Results from a National Study, *Caring* 15, no. 1 (1996): 10–16.
2. R. Fusco, Home Care—An Emerging Solution to the Healthcare Crisis, *Hospital Topics* 72, no. 4 (Fall 1994): 32–36.
3. R.A. Fazzi and R.V. Agoglia, What Home Care Executives Should Know about Managed Care Organizations: Preliminary Results from a National Study, *Caring* 14, no. 10 (1995): 78–85.
4. G. Cokins et al., *An ABC Manager's Primer* (Montvale, NJ: Institute of Management Accountants, 1993), iii.
5. D.T. Hicks, *Activity-Based Costing for Small and Mid-Sized Businesses* (New York: John Wiley & Sons, 1992), 56.
6. Hicks, *Activity-Based Costing.*
7. W.E. Deming, *Out of the Crisis* (Cambridge, MA: MIT Press, 1993), 88.
8. M.D. Shields and M.A. McEwen, Implementing Activity-Based Costing Systems Successfully, *Journal of Cost Management* 9, no. 4 (Winter 1996): 15–22.
9. C.R. Janis, The Role of the Home Health Nurse, *Healthcare Information Management* 11, no. 2 (Summer 1997): 15–22.
10. D.R. Baldwin, Implementation of Computerized Clinical Documentation, *Journal of Home Healthcare Practice and Management* 10, no. 2 (February 1998): 48–56.
11. H. Goldberg, Prospective Payment in Action: The National Home Health Demonstration, *Caring* 16, no. 2 (February 1997): 14–27.
12. Goldberg, Prospective Payment in Action, 14–27.
13. T. Mckeon, Efficient Operations: A Strategy that Crosses Clinical and Administrative Disciplines, *Home Healthcare Nurse* 14, no. 5 (May 1996): 358–361.

PART III

Integrating the Components and Succeeding

CHAPTER 10

Making Data Meaningful

Data are critical to managing processes, maximizing patient/community health, improving services, maximizing a financial return on investments, evaluating outcomes, demonstrating the value of services, evaluating service performance, and rendering care. Providers also use data as the foundation for benchmarking and provider scorecards. Data are the infrastructure for both information and knowledge. Data—summarized and displayed in meaningful ways—create information. Without data, decisions are based on the "best guess." With flawed data, decisions are made with incomplete or inaccurate facts.

The need for authentic data is growing. Fortunately, the capability of gathering data is also growing and improving, mostly through the enhanced availability and affordability of technology. Computer processing is faster, cheaper, and more sophisticated than ever before. Software has entered the world of clinical information systems; it has progressed from supporting clinician tasks to providing clinical information as a strategic resource for practice. Despite this increased need for data collection, aggregation, and analysis across numerous tracking systems, however, data integrity must be maintained. Data management principles to follow in generating useful data were outlined in Chapter 3. The six data characteristics that support these principles are

1. Relevancy: Data must support the clinical and business values and goals of the agency.
2. Currentness: Data need to be updated as providers reassess what information is critical to the achievement of strategic goals.
3. Consistency: Data must be captured using consistent terms, with consistent definitions, at a consistent level of use for all groups used in comparing the collected data.
4. Accuracy: Data definitions must be clear and precise.
5. Timeliness: Data need to be documented as they are obtained.

233

6. Comprehensiveness: To be useful, a data set must measure all the dimensions relevant to the issue at hand.[1]

Maintaining these six characteristics is essential for making data meaningful. The appropriate collection of data; their organization, aggregation, and befitting presentation; and comparisons are also instrumental to their meaningfulness.

This chapter will address

- data collection at the point of care
- the Outcome and Assessment Information Set (OASIS)
- electronic data gathering
- data collection from consumers
- an organizing framework for data
- aggregating data
- presentation of data
- benchmarking

DATA COLLECTION

The data to be collected are determined by the clinical and business values and goals of the agency and by the information needed to maintain and improve those values and goals. Feedback from those being served is a rich source of data for generating continuous quality improvement (CQI) and for survival. The logic behind this thinking is clearly articulated by Stephen Plume.

- Those served are the ultimate judges of the quality of the work.
- Given a choice, people will always choose value.
- People now have choices in health care.[2]

Success as a health care organization, therefore, depends on the ability to understand and meet the wants and needs of those served. Data can be collected from the patient at the point of care, from consumers (e.g., patients, payers, physicians, employees) through surveys and focus groups, and from the community at large. Each of these methods will be discussed further.

Point of Care Data Collection

Data are collected at point of care in order to determine the patient's needs as a starting point for care, to reassess patient needs during care, and to evaluate the value (efficiency and effectiveness) of care. Accurately collecting data at this point as part of the routine process of daily care is the least expensive method of obtaining data. These measurement data are also being aggregated to examine agencywide patient outcomes and overall patient services. (Figure 3–3 depicts this rolling up of data.) This aggregation, however, must meet all the characteristics mentioned above. Two ways to accomplish this measurement that have an immediate impact on home care are the inclusion of OASIS and the incorporation of electronic data collection at the point of care. Each of these will be addressed.

OASIS

The OASIS data have been determined as appropriate for all Medicare adult home care patients. They are not designed for maternity, pediatric, or hospice patients. The collection of these data will soon be mandated by the Health Care Financing Administration (HCFA). The challenge for agencies is to integrate these questions into their existing assessment process. Questions must be non-duplicative, which means that any question an agency currently has that is covered by an OASIS question must be removed from its assessment document and replaced by the similar OASIS question. OASIS questions must be incorporated intact (i.e., exactly as published in the OASIS data set). Some of the OASIS questions, however, do have "other" as a choice. For these questions, the agency can add its own choices in place of other as long as the given choices are left intact. The process of integrating the OASIS questions may be more difficult than it appears because the agency questions will probably not cover the exact area covered by the OASIS question; or in fact, they may overlap. For example, many of the items for the pain assessment for Agency One can be found on Table 10–1. The two OASIS questions on pain are shown in Table 10–2.

Combining the OASIS data set on pain with the agency's existing pain assessment could result in a pain assessment similar to that found in Table 10–3.

Integrating the OASIS data set into an existing assessment form is a process that may need to be undertaken by professionals who have the authority and expertise

---

Table 10–1 Examples of Pain Assessment for Agency One

Pain Assessment	Description
Pain	None; affects quality of life; itching
Pain intensity	0–10
Pain frequency	Continuous; every 1 to 3 hours; every 4 hours or more
Pain affects activity	Yes; No
Quality of pain	Ache; chronic; dull; sharp; stabbing; intractable
Pain duration	Less than 1 hour; 1 to 2 hours; 2 to 3 hours; 3 hours or more

Table 10–2 OASIS Questions on Pain

(MO420) Frequency of pain interfering with patient's activity or movement:
  0—Patient has no pain or pain does not interfere with activity or movement
  1—Less often than daily
  2—Daily, but not constantly
  3—All of the time

(MO430) Intractable pain: Is the patient experiencing pain that is not easily relieved, occurs at least daily, and affects the patient's sleep, appetite, physical or emotional energy, concentration, personal relationships, emotions, or ability or desire to perform physical activity?
  0—No
  1—Yes

Source: Courtesy of Center for Health Services and Policy Research, 1997, Denver, Colorado.

---

to make the required revisions. It could, in fact, be an opportunity to completely renovate all an agency's assessment (and reassessment) forms and formats. Because of the thoroughness of OASIS, many of the resulting assessment forms are longer than before. The added level of detail and consistency aids in the reliability of the data collected.

Unfortunately, requiring the assessment to be done in a predetermined format may appear to the clinician as changing the locus of control from the individual to the system. Whenever a clinician perceives his or her professional autonomy being threatened, he or she will rebel. This rebellion can take the form of negative attitudes and resistant behaviors that can jeopardize data integrity. Giving clinicians the opportunity to contribute to the process, as well as providing ongoing education and support, alleviates these negativities. Table 10–4 offers 13 tips for implementing OASIS.

Pencil to Pentium*

The need to collect more data at point of care is becoming obvious as the need for tracking more data items is required. The clinician must capture items not only to assess the care at that point in time, but also to compare data from one point in time with other points in time and/or with other patients. OASIS is an example of the additional data to be tracked. Another example is Joint Commission's ORYX initiative and the tracking of interventions and outcomes in clinical pathways and disease management. As the amount of data increases, it becomes more difficult to capture and track manually. In fact, at some point it will be impossible to track the data manually yet effectively enough to stay in business. Fortunately, comput-

---

*Source: Adapted with permission from D.A. Peters, Mobile Computing: Pencil to Pentium, *The Remington Report*, Vol. 5, No. 5, p. 34–38, © 1997.

Table 10–3 OASIS Pain Assessment for Agency One

Pain Assessment	Description
Pain	None; itching
Pain intensity	0–10
Pain duration	Less than 1 hour; 1 to 2 hours; 2 to 3 hours; 3 hours or more
Pain frequency	Continuous; every 1 to 3 hours; every 4 hours or more
(MO420) Frequency of pain interfering with patient's activity or movement:	0—Patient has no pain or pain does not interfere with activity or movement 1—Less often than daily 2—Daily, but not constantly 3—All of the time
Quality of pain	Ache; chronic; dull; sharp; stabbing
(MO430) Intractable pain: Is the patient experiencing pain that is not easily relieved, occurs at least daily, and affects the patient's sleep, appetite, physical or emotional energy, concentration, personal relationships, emotions, or ability or desire to perform physical activity?	0—No 1—Yes

erized mobile recording is available. Computerized mobile recording is the documentation of patient data and events on an electronic device (e.g., laptop, hand-held, or pen-based computers) from the field at the time care is rendered. These data are then communicated back to the central office at the same time the mobile computer receives updated information. Recent technological advancements are timely in making automation more feasible, affordable, and desirable than manual processes. The benefits of mobile computing include

- reduced turnaround time for paperwork
- neat and readable documents
- reduced errors and turnaround time for reimbursement
- quick access to improved management and quality improvement reports
- savings on administrative costs since clinicians don't have to go to the office to record information
- increased staff autonomy because of the ability to send data over the wire rather than returning to the office to hand it in
- improved interdisciplinary communication because the record can be accessed and updated quickly and easily by all authorized staff

Table 10–4 OASIS Implementation Tips

---

1. Ensure that key people understand the commitment in terms of time, money, and resources.
2. Allow three months to create new data collection forms.
3. Eliminate duplication in the data collection forms.
4. Retain the exact wording of the OASIS data set within the assessment form.
5. Design forms that are logical and practical to apply. This type of design will assist with staff buy-in.
6. Pilot new forms initially to identify any problems. When problems have been eliminated, use agencywide.
7. Check with staff periodically to make sure everyone interprets the wording and measurements in the same way. Offer support and instruction to those who have identified inconsistencies.
8. Advise staff to fully reassess health status at follow-up points, not just those areas where they suspect change.
9. Involve all major disciplines, not just nursing. OASIS is discipline-neutral so physical therapy, speech therapy, and occupational therapy are some of the other therapies that can help answer the questions.
10. Keep OASIS in front of staff. Mention OASIS at every meeting and in newsletters and memos.
11. Celebrate successes with staff when progress is made.
12. The agency medical director is a key player and needs to be involved throughout the implementation process.
13. Ensure that any software used to incorporate OASIS into the clinical record system is capable of updates. The current data set is OASIS-B, a refinement of the original set, OASIS-A. Updates can be expected periodically.

Source: Adapted from J. Marcus, One Agency's Experience in the HCFA Demonstration Project, *Home Health Management Institute,* p. 12, © 1997, Aspen Publishers, Inc.

Other benefits focus on the quality of documentation as:

- improved consistency of documentation, including the standardized use of terms and the implementation of agencywide standards of care
- more complete and accurate recording due to the availability of prompts to alert clinicians to missing data
- reduced redundancy since clinicians do not have to enter the same information on several different forms
- the ability to track and retrieve outcomes and interventions with associated variances and costs

Given all these benefits of computerization, it would seem appropriate for all agencies to convert to mobile documentation. At some time it may be necessary to do so for the sake of survival. Converting to mobile documentation, however, is not as easy as simply exchanging a pencil for a laptop. Such a conversion transforms the entire documentation process within an agency. It actually can be the catalyst for a transformation or reengineering of the entire agency. No thing or person goes untouched once an agency decides to convert to mobile computing. To be successful in this undertaking, there must be a plan and a team empowered to develop and execute the plan. The details of the plan and the composition of the team are agency specific, but there are six critical areas that need to be addressed.

1. *Start-Up and Ongoing Costs.* Obvious costs include the software product(s) and the hardware required to meet agency demands. Not so obvious are the costs of modems, additional dedicated phone lines, and printers. Replacement and/or extra mobile computers are also important for new staff and for use when an employee's computer is down for maintenance or repair. Vendors often provide periodic enhancements to their software at no charge, but these updates may require more disk space and possibly hardware upgrades, which do cost money. In addition, there is a learning curve (it takes time to learn) for staff when new software enhancements are released, resulting in a possible dip in productivity at the time of introduction. Having a means to test these new updates is important and could reduce any productivity dip, although it could also include some hardware costs. Another significant cost related to productivity is the cost of additional per diem staff and/or lower expected productivity during the initial learning curve.

2. *Procedures, Policies, and Forms.* Many existing agency procedures, policies, and forms will require a change. For example, old documentation procedures will need to be revised. The new procedure needs to include how to handle documentation for staff (such as aides, contract or part-time staff) that do not have their own mobile computer. Will they continue to document on paper? What is the procedure for entering that data onto the computer system (e.g., by whom and when)?

The agency's policy and procedure for handling disasters will need to be expanded to include mobile documentation. How is charting handled if/when the computer goes down, or electricity is off, or phone lines are down? What is the policy for servicing clients when chart information is not available, and what is the procedure for updating chart information from those visits once the disaster is over?

These questions lead to the issue of forms. When an agency introduces mobile computing, all form sets must be redesigned so they are aligned with the screens on the electronic system. This alignment provides for standardization between staff who use paper charts and those on the electronic system and facilitates any required data entry from paper charts. Printing these revised form sets is another cost consideration.

3. *Position and Competency Redefinitions.* One obvious change in staff position descriptions that involve documentation is a minimum level of computer

skills. All positions are affected by the change to electronic documentation even when the person is not directly responsible for electronic documentation; therefore, position descriptions and competencies need to be reevaluated. For example, with mobile computer documentation and the associated report writers that are available, quality improvement personnel may find their main role is one of data manager. This role may or may not require the same talents that they currently need. Viewing the activities associated with the positions from the perspective of activity-based cost management (ABCM) would facilitate the identification and matching of appropriate resource capabilities to job requirements.

Responsibilities also shift. For example, who updates the documentation system and the clinical system libraries? Who offers the general support for the use of the system and assists users in understanding the technology and the functionality? This assistance is especially important in facilitating the daily communication of data that occurs between the documentation input device and the main data repository at the agency.

4. *Structure and Process Redesign.* The business infrastructure, patient/caregiver interaction, and caregiver work habits are examples of the depth to which an agency is affected.

- Business infrastructure: One of the benefits of mobile documentation is that staff no longer need to come into the office on a daily basis to hand in paperwork. The agency, however, must decide how to support the staff in the field. For example, how will field staff be kept informed about changes and how will socialization be promoted when they may only see peers once a week? Processes, such as the flow of data, also will have to be reworked. Forms will now be generated by a computer that require a signature from someone off-site (e.g., verbal order forms). How can these forms be distributed and signed in a timely fashion?

- Patient/caregiver interaction: Many staff feel that introducing an electronic device or laptop into the home is a barrier to patient interaction. Experience seems to indicate, however, that this is a measure of staff discomfort rather than patient concern. Many patients actually show an interest in the computer and creative staff make use of the intrigue to get patients more involved in their own care.

- Work habits: Many staff are accustomed to finishing paperwork at the end of the day. Since mobile documentation works optimally in current time, documentation is best done during the visit. This change in work habits can be troublesome to many.

5. *Training and Overcoming Resistance.* It is common for staff to feel threatened by an automated documentation system that tracks everything including all staff activities. Many of the staff may not be computer literate, which makes it

even more threatening. The best way to deal with these feelings is through open communication that includes

- an explanation of what is happening, how things are changing, and timelines and milestones
- a users' group to discuss concerns
- quarterly updates on how to use the system, shortcuts that are available, and how to make the system work for you

All staff must meet the skill level needed to operate a computer prior to system training. A skills inventory test on the computer including typing, mouse and other elementary computer skills followed by remedial training, one-on-one support, and a validation test are helpful.

System training is usually done with the train-the-trainer approach. There should be an educational plan that includes a course description, curriculum, and schedule. Helpful training tools include training manuals, reference materials, and flowcharts that outline the data entry process for laptop entry and entry from paper copy. The effectiveness of the training should be measured with some type of post-test and an ongoing review of computer-generated material to ensure the accuracy of data. After the initial system training is completed, remedial training will need to be offered to those who just can't master it, and ongoing training will be required for all staff when vendor enhancements are released.

6. *System Preparation.* Equally important to preparing staff is preparing the system. The amount of preparation depends on the product. One important task is reviewing the clinical libraries that come with the product for consistency with agency terms and guidelines for care. Another major preparation step is getting patient data loaded into the system from paper. If an agency is using other products from different vendors, or if an agency wants to transfer data from a hospital system, the two products may not be compatible. Common problems between systems can include different data formatting, different patient identifiers, or different field lengths. In these cases, interfaces are required in order to avoid rekeying data. It is important to explore this need early in the conversion process and allow time and money to develop and test the required interfaces.

The last big decisions are when and how to go "live." Will it be full agency implementation after a pilot, or team by team? Will all cases be converted and previous data entered or will only new cases be put on the system? Entering all the data can be onerous, but having staff chart some cases on paper and some on a laptop can be confusing and frustrating. There are also billing ramifications. If all the patient data is not on the system, some bills will have to be generated manually and some electronically. Will it be necessary to run two systems (the old and new) concurrently for a couple of months to be sure the financial calculations in the new system are accurate? There is no one answer for any of these questions; it depends on the agency's unique situation. Other agencies, consultants, and the vendor itself all may be good resources regarding the best way to handle an individual situation.

When to go live is also an agency-specific decision; some of the considerations in making the decision include financial factors such as the start of the month or fiscal year, staff training completion, hardware and infrastructure installation, testing, backup or "disaster" plans, extra support staff availability, and vendor support coordination.

The remaining question is, How do you choose a vendor? There are now well over 200 national and regional vendors offering home care information products and services.[3] Before beginning the search, develop a plan that incorporates the priorities and outcomes that are to be accomplished by the acquisition of a system. Once you know what you want then answer the following questions: Do you want to work with one of the large national vendors, or will a regional or specialized company be a better choice? Do you want to acquire the hardware and software or work with a service company? Do you want a comprehensive solution that offers clinical documentation and tracking, general ledger, billing, human resources, scheduling, and more? Or do you want a specialized program just to track outcomes or OASIS, or to document care planning? The following are some steps to take to maximize chances of finding a system that meets your needs:

- Define system requirements: Prepare a list of system specifications that reflect what you want.
- Send out a request for proposals based on your specifications to vendors that fit your agency requirements as determined by your plan.
- Evaluate the vendor proposals. Watch out for "futures" (e.g., what is planned but not clearly delineated for the future). Look for phrases such as "in testing" or "in development" which may identify vaporware (e.g., proposed software presented as current, but not really completed).
- Determine semifinalists and schedule demonstrations and site visits. Ask for a copy of the vendor customer list and select customers at random for phone references.
- Identify finalists and investigate further. Check the vendor's track record for delivering working enhancements and updates in a timely manner. Check its reputation for supporting the product after it is purchased and installed (e.g., problem solving and hand holding). Remember, you are doing more than buying a product; you are establishing a partnership. Negotiate a contract that includes performance criteria for implementation and training, system testing and acceptance, and ongoing support and maintenance.[4]

Data Collection from Consumers

Consumers of home care are numerous. There are the patients and their families, payers, physicians, suppliers, and internal consumers—employees and contract staff. Knowing the wants and needs of each of these groups is imperative for understanding how to interact and communicate with them. Consumer data also are collected to achieve the following goals.[5]

- Identify and prevent problems
- Evaluate agency performance
- Plan staff education
- Improve public image and reputation
- Identify and plan new services
- Give feedback to payers, accreditors, and others

Two common methods for collecting these data are surveys and focus groups. A third method that has not been fully embraced is complaint solicitation. The following is a detailed discussion of each of these methods.

Surveys

The most frequently surveyed group of consumers is patients. Surveys can take the form of written questionnaires, telephone calls, or personal interviews. In home care, a patient satisfaction survey is normally used to determine if a patient's expectations were met. Patient satisfaction is essentially a subjective judgment reflecting the degree to which an individual's actual experience matches his or her preferences regarding the experience.[6] In 20,000 questionnaires sent out in 114 home care agencies, the key drivers of satisfaction have been found to be the following:[7]

- how well family informed regarding treatment
- how well emergencies were handled
- how technically skilled nurses were
- how well initial plan met needs
- how problems/complaints were handled
- how friendly nurses were
- how involved families were in planning
- how sensitive aides were to the inconveniences that health problems cause

Unfortunately, agencies are often not getting valid or useful results from their surveys. One reason is that the results can be difficult to interpret. Survey findings often mix the views of the patient's guardian (whose views may represent a different set of interests) with those of the patient rather than provide a separate survey. Another reason is that the population using home care services is methodologically difficult to survey because they are dependent on the services they receive to remain at home. They may fear that giving negative feedback will jeopardize their ability to continue to receive services now or in the future.[8]

Getting valid results begins with understanding what it is that you want evaluated, and what information you need to obtain from whom. Focused surveys that examine one diagnosis or service are more revealing than those looking for overall satisfaction. Satisfaction is not the only information that can be obtained through surveys. In fact, some believe satisfaction to be too subjective to be useful and are turning to quality of life or level of health as more objective measures. Quality of life can be seen as physical, psychosocial, and spiritual well-being that incorporates both a subjective opinion about well-being and an objective assessment about functional status.[9] Other content in surveys could deal with interpersonal relationships, teaching and preparation for discharge, and safety. Furthermore, surveys are not limited to current and former patients and families, but can include all agency customers such as referral sources, physicians, suppliers, and payers.

After determining the what and who, the next step is to design or adopt a survey questionnaire, pretest it, and administer it. The following are some tips for designing a survey questionnaire:

1. Design the questionnaire for maximum readability, clarity, and visual appeal. Adapt it to the population being surveyed (e.g., for the older population use large, bold print; for the pediatric population write the questions for the parent to answer). Ask questions the respondents can answer such as, Did you have enough information to . . .? rather than putting them in the position of judging another's performance.
2. List questions down the page or in booklet format, if there is more than one page. The maximum length is 75 questions.
3. Use a simple and consistent rating scale (e.g., very poor, poor, fair, good, very good) that goes across the page. If a quantified measure is added to this scale such as very poor = 1, poor = 2, and so on, then an agency can track improvement in the responses over time.
4. Sequence questions from the general to the specific. The specific questions should appear in the order in which care occurred.
5. Use everyday language and avoid medical jargon and complex terms. Wording should be at the sixth-grade level. Avoid vague questions like, Was care consistent?
6. Each question should contain only one issue or characteristic. Avoid double-component questions like, Did you feel that the nurse was caring and courteous?

Recommendations for administering surveys include the following:

- Use mail surveys as the primary method. Mail surveys save considerable time and money and yield the best data. Personal interviews and telephone surveys yield a bias toward more positive results.
- Include an optional name field and also code the survey with a unique identifier. There does not seem to be any difference in response rates when the form is coded.
- Survey both current and discharged patients, but identify which is which. Survey discharged patients within two weeks of discharge. For patients with a length of stay longer than three months, survey every three months and at discharge.
- To boost response rates, tell patients at discharge that they will be surveyed, include a signed letter from the CEO with the survey, and provide return postage.[10]

Another survey approach to gathering data from consumers and potential consumers is a market service survey. The answers to market survey questions will indicate what matters to clients and potential clients (e.g., what they want and/ or need) within a given market (e.g., geographical area, managed care organization). This type of survey is valuable for an agency's internal market (employees) as well. Internal measures can then be set up to track how well the agency provides services that matter to customers. Types of data an agency may want to gather in this manner include

- what programs are important
- what service characteristics are important
- what is the relative importance of each consumer want
- what level of performance within each program will meet consumer expectations
- what level of performance on each service characteristic will meet consumer expectations[11]

Focus Groups*

Focus group interviews use a qualitative research technique that is useful in obtaining data about the feelings, ideas, and opinions of a small group concerning a given service, experience, or other phenomenon that are applicable to the larger universe. They are relatively easy to conduct and have been primarily used in the business world for market research to help businesses learn about their customers.

Source: Adapted from D.A. Peters, Improving Quality Requires Consumer Input: Using Focus Groups, *Journal of Nursing Care Quality*, Vol. 7, No. 2, pp. 34–38, © 1997.

Now focus groups are being utilized increasingly in health care. Focus groups provide other benefits to the consumer and home care agency.

- They serve as a teaching and learning tool at several levels. For example, participants have the opportunity to ask questions about funding and other agency services. One agency, making calls to discharged consumers to find potential focus group participants, discovered a group of clients who needed care again. These consumers' cases were reopened to care and the agency began planning for more routine follow-up on this type of client.
- They are a marketing tool. Agency strengths identified in the groups can be used in marketing to others in the community.
- They are a social experience. People have a reason to get out and be with other people with similar experiences in an enjoyable, informal setting. Sometimes it is a starting place for friendships and the exchange of phone numbers.
- They can serve as a support group session for some persons. Sharing of stories can serve as a reminder to each that he or she is not the only one that has gone through these experiences.

Focus groups gather people together for an easy exchange of information. The synergism of the group dynamics allows for the potential of serendipitously uncovering important understandings about consumers and their care. To be successful, however, focus groups require a trusting, secure, and comfortable environment. Participants need to feel secure in speaking freely about their needs and care. Several items need to be considered before convening a focus group. A listing of 10 of them follow. These were obtained from focus groups organized at eight different agencies across the country as part of the *In Search of Excellence* project, a $1.2 million grant from the W.K. Kellogg Foundation to the National League for Nursing to develop outcomes for examining the quality of home care services, utilizing consumers as the primary source of data.[12]

1. *Purpose.* The reason for convening the group should be well articulated.

2. *Size and Composition of Groups.* Groups can be any size, although 10 to 12 participants is considered ideal. In the *In Search of Excellence* project, more needed to be invited to compensate for no-shows. In addition, the type of person to be invited needs to be identified and based on the information to be gained. For example, focus groups could target Medicare patients, managed care patients, or patients who have received services from a specific discipline, such as social work or physical therapy. If there are concerns in these categories or changes in the numbers of cases being served, discussions might elicit possible problems and/or solutions.

3. *Setting.* The setting needs to be nonthreatening, comfortable, and accessible for persons with disabilities. Off-site locations may be less threatening, although on-site locations are more convenient and less expensive. It is also valuable to provide some type of food as an incentive for people to participate.

4. *Time.* The time the session(s) are held needs to be convenient for the participants. The maximum time allotted should be about two hours, which allows time for the participants to eat and socialize, in addition to participating in the discussion.

5. *Invitations.* How the consumers are invited influences their willingness to participate. With the *In Search of Excellence* project, the most successful way was for their nurse to personally invite them and then have the agency follow up with a telephone call or confirmation letter.

6. *Transportation.* Providing transportation is probably necessary for at least some of the participants, especially those with limited mobility (e.g., persons who are wheelchair-bound) or with limited funds. Ways that were used in the *In Search of Excellence* project included having the nurse bring the participant in, reimbursing for use of public transportation, and hiring taxicabs.

7. *Group Leader.* One way to ensure a nonthreatening environment is to not have agency staff present; the group leader should be from outside the agency. The leader should, however, be familiar with the topic being explored, skilled in group process, and knowledgeable about working with the elderly (or whatever age group is participating). The role of the group leader is to create a supportive climate that encourages participants to contribute openly and honestly. The leader should articulate the purpose of the meeting, cover the predetermined topics and questions, and facilitate the group interaction. Facilitation can take the form of encouraging participation, injecting probing comments, presenting questions in an unbiased way, asking transitional questions, determining how group members feel about ideas expressed by others, and summarizing the answers given.

8. *Recording.* In order to get the most information from these gatherings, documentation of the proceedings should be retained. This retention can be handled by having a nonparticipant be a recorder or by using a mechanical tape recorder at the session. If a tape recorder is used, participants should be told that the session is being recorded, and perhaps even sign a consent form. The *In Search of Excellence* project groups signed consent forms, and there was no evidence that it affected anyone's participation.

9. *Budget.* Focus groups can be held at a reasonable cost. The amount allowed in the *In Search of Excellence* project was $250/site (which was one meeting per site), although many agencies required less. Items that might require funds

include the facilitator, food, transportation for the participants, and room rental if held off-site.

10. *Interview Outline*. Using the purpose of the meeting as a guide, an interview outline should be prepared so that all salient points are covered and all groups are asked for the same information. In some of the focus groups in the *In Search of Excellence* project, it was easy to follow the prepared interview outline. In other groups, the group took off on its own after the first question and stories of home care experiences did not end until the facilitator called the session to a close. In still other groups, some participants came with prepared speeches while others simply responded to the questions.

The experience of the *In Search of Excellence* project was that consumers were delighted to be able to participate. Some of the elements that characterize the care they desire are

- support to gain independence, including being given the opportunity to make choices
- caring and compassion demonstrated by touch, eye contact, and use of their name
- honest feedback regarding their status
- competency in caregivers who will admit to not knowing an answer and then find the answers they don't have
- consistency in caregivers and/or only informed changes in caregivers (e.g., patient was told there would be a different caregiver)
- caregivers who respect their time
- a sense of humor, a smile, and a lift for their spirits on difficult days

Complaint Solicitation

No one likes complainers. Agencies solicit consumer satisfaction with the expectation that everyone is satisfied, and that is appropriate. Not everyone will be satisfied, however, and the greatest learning on how to improve services comes from the consumers who are not satisfied. Complainers are an agency's friend, much like pain is a person's friend; it is letting you know that something is wrong. If the pain is in your back, maybe you are lifting too much and should lift less; if the pain is a headache, maybe you are under too much stress. The message is that something is wrong and you have the opportunity to change it. So it is with customers who complain. They are telling you something is wrong. Maybe they had inappropriate expectations about services; maybe they were admitted to the wrong program (do they really belong in home care?). Their complaint is an opportunity for the home care agency to learn something about the way it is doing business. Therefore, the agency needs a way to make it relatively easy and safe for a consumer to make a complaint. It could be in the form of an 800 number to call that is separate from the agency's main number, or a stamped envelope given to new patient admissions in which they can send in a complaint to an address different from the agency's main address. In any event, complainers offer an often untapped resource for agency improvement.

Data Collection from the Community

It is important for an agency to gather community data for several reasons. First, with the movement to managed care, it is ultimately the level of health of the community that measures the effectiveness of the health care providers. Second, understanding the community composition, demographics, resident wants and needs, social and cultural norms, social and physical environment, health care services and resources, beliefs, values, and attitudes allows for the individualization of planning health programs and activities. Obviously, before collecting any community data, an agency must decide what it wants to assess.

Community can be defined in several ways. It can be geographic: a defined location and the people living there. It can be sociocultural: a perceived community of interests and/or common experience. The latter would include the community formed by all persons enlisted in the same managed care group. Third, it can be political: defined by a boundary such as a state, county, region, or agency service area.

In addition to collecting data from agency consumers and/or community residents (or enrollees) as described above, supplemental data can be collected from a defined community using some or all of the techniques discussed below.

Use of an Assessment Tool

A community assessment tool is one way to systematically obtain information about community dynamics and health status. It organizes data in a meaningful manner; identifies community strengths, potential needs, and problems; and identifies needed interventions.[13] The key areas to be assessed include demographics, health status, social and cultural status of people in the community; the community environment, including physical and social elements; and the health care delivery system, including resources and services. Assessment tools may be available from state and local health departments.

Analyzing Available Statistics

It is important to analyze a range of available community health or health-related data such as demographics, mortality, utilization, and disease rates and data about health-related phenomena. Depending on the definition of community being used, these data can be obtained from health departments, city planner's offices, hospital records, or payer's claim forms. Comparing statistics with other communities and examining statistical trends over time can be very revealing and serve as benchmarking data to determine progress in improving the level of health. These data can also assist with

- predicting health needs
- identifying aggregates at risk
- determining priorities
- evaluating outcomes
- documenting accountability
- supporting the need for reimbursement/funding[14]

Interviewing Community Leaders

The values, attitudes, and interests of community leaders often influence and/ or reflect the values, attitudes, and interests of the community. Therefore, these individuals can provide knowledge about community values and attitudes, power relationships, and factors that may enhance or detract from a community's state of health. This information is important when attempting to improve the level of health in the community and/or wanting to establish new programs. Depending on the definition of community being used, persons that might be helpful include professionals in other health care agencies, local politicians, clergy, business owners, local librarians, managed care coordinators and administrators, and physicians.

DATA ORGANIZATION*

It is one thing to collect the clinical data that an agency needs to do business, and quite another thing to be able to extract these data as information. In fact, it has been said that the home care industry is data rich but information poor. This saying means there is much data but no way to extract them to provide information. Roadblocks to extracting information include nonrelational electronic databases, reliance on manual data collection that is not coded or filed by variables, and lack of standard language or terms. An additional key element to accurate extraction of clinical data is understanding the concepts that incorporate the data elements and how they relate to each other. Much of this book has been devoted to defining these concepts, which include outcomes, guidelines, clinical paths, flowcharts, protocols, standards, and policies. The purpose of this section is to organize them

---

*Source: Adapted from D.A. Peters, Outcomes: The Mainstay of a Framework for Quality Care, *Journal of Nursing Care Quality*, Vol. 10, No. 1, pp. 61–69, © 1995, Aspen Publishing, Inc.

into a relevant picture or conceptual framework and to depict how they relate to each other in creating a higher level of quality care.

A conceptual framework enhances the definition and understanding of patient care. Using a common framework allows for the universal understanding and sharing of terminology and concepts, organizes data, facilitates the investigation and evaluation of the elements of care through quality management, assists in understanding the process of change, and promotes the effectiveness of generating information with quality management tools. Conceptual frameworks can also be valuable for educating staff. The conceptual framework for organizing data for quality care is depicted in Figure 10–1. The components of the framework include

- the outcomes that are used to reflect quality
- the external environment that surrounds the organization and influences client care
- the mission/vision/values of the organization
- professional standards operationalized as policies, flowcharts, position descriptions, and performance skills and qualities that define clinician behaviors
- care guidelines operationalized as procedures, protocols, critical pathways, and care plans that define care management
- unifying tools that provide the opportunity to bring together professional and patient/consumer viewpoints

Costs are part of outcomes and results. They are also associated with each of the activities that are incorporated into the concepts identified.

The external environment provides the context in which outcomes are met and patient-focused care processes occur. Under systems thinking, the environment (including consumer expectations, clinician expectations, regulatory and professional directives, legal mandates, and health care scorecards) is crucial in explaining what outcomes need to be measured and to what degree they are being met. Internally, there must be a clear and well-defined shared vision to get people to work together. The agency mission defines the unique contribution that the organization strives to make. The internal values answer the question of how individuals in the organization want to act, consistent with the mission and along the path to achieve the vision.

The professional side of care (professional standards) and the client's side of care (care guidelines) are integrated by using certain identified tools. These critical tools include feedback (from surveys, questionnaires, complaints, and personal contact), an information system that incorporates and builds on a data set, and a system for CQI and/or research. The purpose of these tools (all of which have been discussed elsewhere in this book) is twofold: (1) to unify and improve

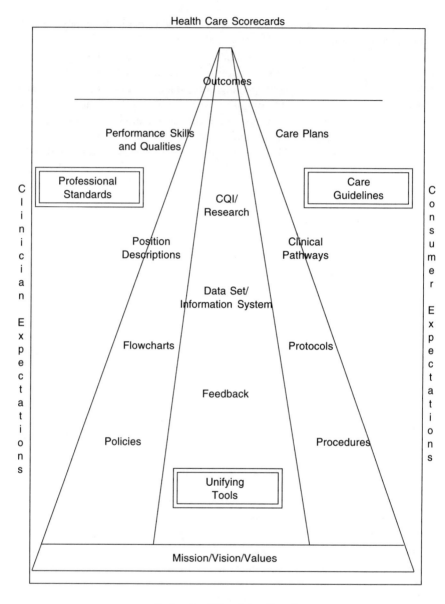

Figure 10–1 Organizing Framework. *Source:* Adapted from D.A. Peters, Outcomes: The Mainstay of a Framework for Quality Care, *Journal of Nursing Care Quality*, Vol. 10, No. 1, pp. 61–69, © 1995, Aspen Publishers, Inc.

on the professional standards and care guidelines, and (2) to optimize the attainment of the agreed-upon client outcomes.

The need for an information system with a consistent data set that allows for the tracking and synthesis of care planned, care rendered, and variations that occurred during the process is obvious. Ultimately the information system provides the capacity to understand which care alternative—using various procedures and protocols—achieves the best outcome at what cost using what clinician.

The information system, manual or electronic, is the data repository for information about the performance skills and qualities of the clinician and the care requirements of the client so that the two partners in care can be better matched. Ultimately, the abilities and experiences of the clinician need to match the unique requirements in the patient pathway or care plan. The better the match, the more conducive the environment is for meeting the agreed-upon outcomes in the shortest period of time.

Furthermore, the more comprehensive and detailed the data set, the more factual information the clinician will have to make knowledgeable decisions rather than blind selections or best guesses. The more the information system is understood and kept current, the more quality will be defined by the actual caregiving process rather than by the demands or regulations from the external environment. For example, imagine that an MCO authorizes only three visits for a particular patient. The agency, however, has historical information that shows that a minimum of three visits for this type of patient results in a hospital readmission. Furthermore, agency information demonstrates that six visits will provide for optimal outcomes and no hospital readmissions. With this data set, the agency can strongly negotiate for the additional three visits.

DATA AGGREGATION/TRANSFORMATION

The next step to making data meaningful, after its collection and organization, is to aggregate the data and use the resulting information. Because of the expanding scope of data that need to be collected and tracked, it is necessary to use an electronic system for aggregation of essential data elements. In an electronic environment, it is important that all the data about the agency's patients (demographics, utilization, outcomes, and survey results) reside on a single database. Furthermore, the database should be relational, meaning that all data elements are related to each other so one can specify which data elements are to be reviewed and analyzed in relation to others.

It should be noted, however, that the data may be integrated from several sources via highly sophisticated database interfaces. The standard interface for health care is the Health Language 7 (HL7). The interfacing of health care data provides an integrated hospital, ambulatory, home care, and consumer health information infrastructure as the basis for a seamless integrated delivery model managing both resources and care. Administrative, financial, clinical, patient, and demographic data from numerous providers will be integrated and analyzed to produce disease and health state management spanning a lifetime. Home care has much to offer on this continuum, but if data collection remains paper based, the home care contribution will remain invisible as the electronic data is aggregated and analyzed.

As more data become available from a variety of sources and are utilized to examine and improve care, there are certain stipulations to consider. First, the data must meet all the characteristics defined at the beginning of the chapter. Be especially sensitive to data accuracy and consistency when using outside data sets. Second, when two or more patient samples are being compared (e.g., different managed care providers, different agencies) on performance measures, such as outcomes, then risk factors must be taken into consideration. Risk factors include age, race, diagnosis, comorbidities, and functional limitations that influence the ability of a person to achieve a maximum outcome. Controlling for patient risk factors helps to isolate quality differences by determining what portion of observed differences is due to patient factors under the control of the agency versus those not under agency control.[15]

There are two basic means to adjust for risk factors: stratification and statistical. The most obvious way is stratification, or grouping of similar types of patients. Here, a patient group is divided into subgroups or strata based on the risk factors for the outcome being evaluated. If done precisely, the two resulting groups will be homogeneous—comprised of exactly the same type of patients and, therefore, comparable. Some of the characteristics that can be used to stratify patients include

- age
- sex
- medical diagnoses
- nursing diagnoses
- functional disabilities
- psychological, cognitive, and psychosocial functioning
- health status
- home environmental characteristics

The most common approach to statistical risk adjustment involves multivariate modeling. Basically, this approach employs a variety of techniques to produce a model that predicts an outcome measure using multiple risk factors. The predictive formula can then be used to obtain an expected agency outcome rate that can be compared to the actual agency outcome rate. The exact specifications of the model vary among patient groupings and across outcomes of interest.

Regardless of the risk adjustment method or combination of methods that are used, risk adjustment will never be perfect. Reasons for imperfection include[16]

- It is impossible to adjust for everything
- Collecting data is expensive and logistically complicated
- Collecting highly sensitive data is difficult (highly sensitive data includes income or personal factors such as ethical matters)

How much risk adjustment is necessary depends on how the information is going to be used. Furthermore, a single risk-adjusted performance measure should never be the sole basis of judgments about quality; it should be only one factor of many that are considered.[17] Home care is still in the infancy stage of comparing data. What is important to remember when comparing data is that there may be differences due to intrinsic factors (risk factors) that are outside of the agency's control. One starting point for considering risk factors is a case mix report as used in OASIS (see Exhibit 6–2 for an example) that compares patients' characteristics in an agency's sample with the sample from another agency or from another time period in the same agency. If in "eyeballing" the report, one finds no major differences, then risk adjustment is probably not an issue. Even if there are differences, quality improvement activities, especially more data gathering, may be helpful in improving outcomes.

Another consideration when aggregating and comparing data is patient classification by complexity or intensity of care. Intensity of care refers to the amount of resources consumed by a patient during an episode of care. It is also important information for clinical practice improvement, along with the other clinical and financial data. Unfortunately, very few reliable and valid classification methods have been developed in the home care industry, although many subjective classifications for intensity are done at an individual agency level. There are several reasons for the lack of patient intensity classifications, including the heterogeneity of the nature of home care activities and services, the diverse home care population, and the lack of available patient-specific workload data. Data about clinician workload (resources consumed) are very rarely kept as part of the patient record or even tagged to an individual patient, making it difficult to measure. Now, however, more data collection is being done electronically, and management information systems are being combined with clinical information systems. These improvements should aid greatly in tagging individual patient data with clinicians' workloads.

One tool that has been developed is the Community Health Intensity Rating Scale (CHIRS).[18] CHIRS is a patient classification system designed to predict resource consumption by quantifying the intensity of a community health client's need for agency services. The CHIRS concept of need includes the physiological aspects of care as well as incorporating the client in the context of his or her support system (e.g., family, home environment, and community resources). CHIRS scores, therefore, incorporate both the physiological and nonphysiological patient needs. Including both of these areas is especially important as home care enters the arena of managed care, where the goal of care is to educate and empower clients toward long-term independent management of their own health status and health problems. CHIRS has been found to significantly explain variation in resource consumption in several different studies.[19-21] It has also been applied to different patient populations including general home care, maternal and child health, frail elderly, HIV/AIDS patients, patients using high technologies, and substance-abusing homeless families, and it is currently being adapted for school use—as the School Health Intensity Rating Scale (SHIRS).

CHIRS was originally a prototype classification tool that used the nursing process format. Fifteen parameters represented the home health domains of environment, psychosocial, physiological, and health behaviors. For each of the 15 parameters, the tool included a patient profile to illustrate the extent of nursing input required for patient care within each of the four levels. The categorical ratings were minimum nursing care requirements (Level 1), moderate (Level 2), major (Level 3), and extreme (Level 4). Unfortunately, this format was challenging to use in the workplace, so it has been revised into a comprehensive patient assessment format divided into the original 15 parameters. The responses for each of the assessment questions are weighted, offer a score for each parameter, and produce a final intensity score between 15 and 60.

PRESENTATION OF DATA

Once data are collected, aggregated, and analyzed, the final step is presentation. Most data presentation depicts outcome measures in order to evaluate performance of services, value of services, opportunities for improvement, or other areas. Exact presentation is important for accurate evaluation. There are a few key principles to follow.

1. Keep the presentation format simple, whether it be graph, table, chart, or other.
2. On each graph, table, or chart, include only the data necessary for the indicator or measure being evaluated. Put other variables and supporting data on separate tables, graphs, or charts.
3. Format the presentation of data to the audience. (For example, the same data may have a different focus for a third-party payer than it will for a clinical

management team because these groups are looking for different information. The third-party payer wants to see a demonstration of the value of the services for which it is paying; the clinical management team is interested in evaluating the performance of the personnel. The former may take the shape of a scorecard; the latter may take the shape of an information system report.)

4. Include in the report the purpose, the definition of statistical comparison methods used (if any), and the results.

BENCHMARKING

Another way to evaluate services is through data comparisons of similar processes/activities/outcomes within an agency or across agencies. These comparisons can be useful in maintaining and improving agency processes and activities and thereby add value to agency operations. This type of data comparison is known as *benchmarking*. There are four different types of benchmarking.[22]

1. *internal benchmarking*: comparing similar internal processes/activities/outcomes to discover the best practices within an organization for replication elsewhere
2. *competitive benchmarking*: comparing an agency process/activity/outcome with the industry's best competitor in order to provide a performance level to surpass
3. *functional benchmarking*: comparing an agency process/activity/outcome with an organization that excels but is not in the same industry
4. *generic benchmarking*: comparing a vital agency process with the best practices of this process across industries

The key steps to benchmarking are as follows:[23]

1. *Define the Internal Process To Be Benchmarked.* Some of the processes that have been benchmarked in home care include continuity of care, rehospitalization, nosocomial infections,[24] and efficiency of infusion shipments.[25] Aspen Publishers' *Home Health Data Quarterly* looks at home care benchmark statistics by agency type, product line, geographic location, community type and population, and average visits per month.

2. *Develop a Database That Describes the Performance of the Process.* Sources of data are numerous; however, they are also diverse and sometimes difficult to locate. Some reliable sources include research literature; other home care agencies; product/service vendors; third-party payers; local, state, and federal governments; local community; and professional associations.

3. *Identify the Extraordinary Performers.* This identification can be done by evaluating the data.

4. *Identify the Factors That Drive the Superior Performance.* What is the extraordinary performer doing that the others are not that makes a difference in the performance of the process?

5. *Adopt Those Superior Performance Activities/Factors into the Agency Doing the Benchmarking.* Although benchmarking can be helpful in assessing agency processes, it should not be the sole means of evaluation because limitations exist in a pooled or reference data set. Limitations to these types of data that currently exist include representativeness of the sample, reliability, adequacy of risk adjustments to render the data comparable, adequate control of variables, adequacy of the statistical analysis of the data, the degree of the validity of the data for the intended use, and electronic issues such as lack of standards for coding, incompatible information system platforms, and inability to integrate across data sources. In other words, when comparing benchmark data always be certain that the comparison is apples to apples. Furthermore, be sure that the benchmark data is really "elite" data—data of excellence. Grabbing statistics from a report or from another agency may provide a means for comparison, but the comparison may be one of mediocrity rather than excellence. With the intense interest in data and data comparisons, and the resulting proliferation of evolving data sets, benchmarker beware and be discriminating!

CONCLUSION

One of the keys to success in the new paradigm is data. It is not sufficient, however, just to have data. The data must have meaning, maintain integrity, and be retrievable. With the amount of data that must be tracked and analyzed, an electronic means to capture it as part of a clinician's daily routine becomes essential. It is more efficient and accurate, and it provides the ability to track and sort large sets of data. This chapter discussed the implications and challenges of implementing an electronic system. The longer agencies wait to implement such a system the longer it will be before they will have timely and essential data, the more expensive it will be to collect and analyze the data they do have, and the more hidden the value of the home care industry will remain to the rest of the health care continuum.

Collecting data at the point of care is only one of the crucial elements for making data meaningful. Data must also be collected from other consumers of the agency's services to determine their expectations and how well those expectations are being met. The concepts within which data reside (such as standards, guidelines, outcomes, and clinical paths) must be understood to see how they interface and interact. A framework depicting these concepts and their relationship has been presented.

Finally, data must be aggregated, analyzed, and presented for evaluation. Tips on how to do these steps were offered as well as the limitations currently surrounding these processes. Some of these items will be revisited in the following chapters because data are instrumental in all agency operations and services. Without data there is no means of managing processes, making care meaningful, or reporting to stakeholders.

NOTES

1. D.A. Peters, The Details Are in the Data, *Computertalk for Homecare Providers* 5, no. 2 (1997): 43–45.

2. S.K. Plume, Effective Strategies for Tracking Patient Information (Paper presented at the Disease Management Congress, Phoenix, AZ, March 6, 1997).

3. *The Corridor Connection*, Successful Home Care Automation, *The Corridor Connection* (September/October 1997): 3.

4. *The Corridor Connection,* Successful Home Care Automation, 3.

5. S. Young and S.A. Kaiden, Measuring Patient Satisfaction in Home Care (Paper presented at the National Association for Home Care Annual Meeting, Boston, MA, October 20, 1997).

6. P.F. Brennan, Patient Satisfaction and Normative Decision Theory, *Informatics: The Infrastructure for Quality Assessment and Improvement in Nursing* (San Francisco: UC Nursing Press, 1994).

7. M.F. Hall, But All My Patients Love Me! (Paper presented at the National Association for Home Care Annual Meeting, Boston, MA, October 20, 1997).

8. U.S. General Accounting Office, *Long-Term Care: Status of Quality Assurance and Measurement in Home and Community-Based Services*, GAO Report, GAO/PEMD-94–19, Washington, DC: March 1994.

9. P. Petryshen et al., Outcomes Monitoring: Adjusting for Risk Factors, Severity of Illness, and Complexity of Care, *Journal of American Informatics Association* 2, (1995): 169–182.

10. Young and Kaiden, Measuring Patient Satisfaction.

11. R.C. Whiteley, *The Customer Driven Company* (Reading, MA: Addison-Wesley Publishing Co., 1991).

12. D.A. Peters, Improving Quality Requires Consumer Input: Using Focus Groups, *Journal of Nursing Care Quality* 7, no. 2 (1993): 34–41.

13. S. Clemen-Stone et al., *Comprehensive Community Health Nursing*, 4th ed. (St. Louis, MO: Mosby, 1995).

14. Clemen-Stone, *Comprehensive Community Health Nursing.*

15. L.I. Iezzoni, *Risk Adjustment for Measuring Healthcare Outcomes* (Chicago: Health Administration Press, 1997).

16. Iezzoni, *Risk Adjustment.*

17. Iezzoni, *Risk Adjustment.*

18. D.A. Peters, Development of a Community Health Intensity Rating Scale, *Nursing Research* 37, no. 4 (1988): 202–207.

19. Peters, Development of a Community Health Intensity Rating Scale, 202–207.

20. B.J. Hays, Nursing Care Requirements and Resource Consumption in Home Health Care, *Nursing Research* 41, no. 3 (1992): 138–143.

21. Hays, Nursing Intensity as a Predictor of Resource Consumption in Public Health Nursing, *Nursing Research* 44, no. 2 (1995): 106–110.

22. R.C. Camp and A. Sweet, Benchmarking Applied to Health Care, *Journal of Quality Improvement* 20, no. 5 (1994): 229–238. As reported in P. Howard, Benchmarking Home Health Care Data, *Home Health Care Management and Practice* 9, no. 4 (1997): 52–63.

23. B.A. Campbell, Benchmarking: A Performance Tool, *Journal of Quality Improvement* 20, no. 5 (1994).

24. K.L. Hudock et al., Benchmarking in Home Care, *Caring* 15, no. 2 (1997): 72–77.

25. P. Howard, Benchmarking Home Health Care Data, *Home Health Care Management and Practice* 9, no. 2 (1997): 52–63.

CHAPTER 11

Steps to Managing a Process

Administrators have been taught to manage operations using profit and loss (P&L) statements. Consequently, managers are often recruited based upon whether they have had previous P&L responsibility. There is an inherent assumption that managers who have P&L responsibility will be fiscally sensitive to the financial requirements of a health care organization. This fiscal sensitivity is usually a valid assumption because the managers who have P&L responsibility are often involved in the budgeting process, make decisions that have financial consequences, and are on the distribution list for monthly financial statements. Often managers receive monthly financial statements in a predetermined format that report results by department, branch, division, or company. These predetermined formats have often been designed to parallel the organizational chart or informal reporting hierarchies, or to meet the needs of the IRS or the fiscal intermediary.

Financial reporting presents a challenge for many managers because traditional financial statements are being used to meet two goals. The primary goal of most financial reporting systems is to convey results to stockholders, creditors, and regulatory agencies. A secondary goal is to provide managers with information to run their respective operations. When a manager is handed a monthly financial statement he or she can quickly identify whether the organization made money and, if the financial statement is in a comparative format, he or she can determine whether results were under budget, over budget, or better than those of a previous reporting period. The problem is that managers are unable to identify from the financial statements whether their staff were productive, whether they satisfied customers, whether there were improvements in delivery time, and how their operations contributed to the organization as a whole.

A shift in approach, or perspective, is to think about agency operations in the context of processes. The agency as a "whole" is comprised of a group of interrelated processes. Each process consumes resources in the form of labor, materials, supplies, technology, and capital. Resources are consumed by individuals performing specific activities such as data entry, direct care, and travel. Each activity produces an output that either goes directly to an external customer (direct care) or goes to an internal customer (data entry).

The shift to a process orientation enables managers to focus on the chain of events that occurs in a process from a starting point to an end point. In a sense, a shift to a process orientation requires viewing the organization in a horizontal fashion. This viewpoint is a departure from the traditional approach that sees an organization in a vertical departmental or functional format. Processes also have a cross-functional orientation that has the potential to move beyond departmental boundaries. This distinction is relevant because within a departmental system the employees of a department become good at their specific tasks and pass their completed tasks (output) on to the next department. This process is illustrated in Figure 11–1. Often this handoff does not consider the needs and requirements of the next group of processors.

Figure 11–1 illustrates three different subprocesses that occur within three different departments in a departmental structure. Each process is made up of inputs (I), activities (A), and outputs (O) and is sequential in nature. Stated differently, Department B cannot begin its activities until Department A finishes, and Department C cannot begin until Department B has completed its activities and produced an output in a format that is usable by Department C. Figure 11–1 also illustrates that Department B's and C's costs and subsequent results will be dictated by the effectiveness of the sequence of activities that started in Department A.

Figure 11–1 also illustrates the difficulty managers have in making effective decisions based upon a traditional financial reporting structure that charges or allocates payroll dollars, benefits, and departmental expenses to specific departments. The reporting process identifies total dollars spent but does not provide indicators of how effective each department was in meeting the needs of its internal customers (Department B is Department A's internal customer), how efficient the process is from the perspective of cycle time and cost, or whether the

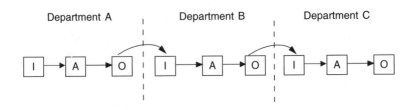

Figure 11–1 An Illustration of How Processes Comprising of Inputs, Activities, and Outputs Cross Departments

process as a whole (Departments A, B, and C) is providing value to the external customers (patients) it is serving.

Managing the process requires viewing organizations in a horizontal perspective rather than a vertical one. If one of management's goals is to pursue strategic objectives, then resources need to be aligned with the pursuit of these objectives. An approach to optimizing resources is to understand the relationship between customers and suppliers, resource consumption and output, and results and strategic priorities. It is a process of continuously questioning the status quo, seeking feedback, assessing results, and taking action.

This chapter describes

- managing the process
- developing a process-driven organization
- improving organizational performance

Many of these issues and concepts have been addressed previously in the book, but they have been brought together here for the purpose of reviewing all the steps to process management and improvement. These steps are illustrated in Figure 11–2, which identifies the 10 key concepts critical for process management and will be used as a guide to identify tools that can be used for the management of processes while creating a process improvement model.

DEFINE THE PROCESS

The first key concept for process management is to define the process. A basic process model for an agency differentiates between two types of processes: primary and secondary (see Figure 9–3). The primary process is referred to as the patient-focused care process. This process is the organization's reason for being. It is also the process that creates external value and revenue for the organization. The secondary processes are considered support processes. They support the organization's reason for being from beginning (upstream process) to end (downstream process).

A tool useful in understanding existing processes is a flowchart. A flowchart is a visual representation of a sequence of events and activities that make up a process. Flowcharts have beginning and ending points, identify various events (such as manual processes, decision points, the production of reports, filing or storage activities, and meetings), and illustrate the flow of activities or sequence of events. Once constructed, a flowchart will provide a visual representation of all activities that would occur in a given process. Examples of flowcharts were presented in Chapter 7.

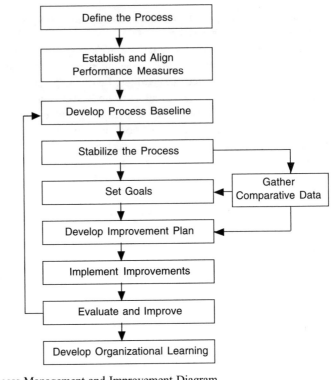

Figure 11–2 Process Management and Improvement Diagram

Defining the process does not stop with developing a flowchart. The flowchart provides a visual representation of a flow of activities that can then be used for determining customer/supplier relationships among a series of activities or throughout an extended process. The concepts of customer and supplier applies to both internal customers and customers outside of the organization. For instance, Figure 11–1 illustrates that a customer/supplier relationship exists among Departments A, B, and C. Department C also needs to consider an end user or external customer. In this example the external customer could be a patient, referral source, physician, payer, or regulatory body.

Customer/supplier relationships can also be identified by looking at the sequence of activities that occurs within a specific process. Activities are an aggregation of common steps, tasks, and actions. Another element of defining the process is to identify each of the activities that occurs within a specific process. Common activities associated with each process and the potential customers and products associated with each activity were illustrated in Tables 9–11 and 9–12.

An approach to foster accountability in the managing of processes is to create a process improvement team that consists of representatives of the process illustrated by the flowchart. Once the team has been assembled and a charter or mission has been developed, the team can be used to "step through" the process. The stepping-through process can be one of using the flowchart as a control sheet to verify the sequence of activities, identify customer requirements, develop internal customer satisfaction assessment instruments, and identify areas where bottlenecks or errors could occur. Eliminating bottlenecks and errors usually contributes significantly to process improvements. Another reason to step through the process is to identify the amount of time it takes to complete the process. In fact, by repeatedly stepping through the process, it is possible to develop a time-line with supporting time measurements, such as a minimum, maximum, and mode, for process completion.

ESTABLISH AND ALIGN PERFORMANCE METRICS

The second key step in managing the process is to develop a sound performance measurement system. Figure 3–3 illustrated a performance measurement hierar-chy that cascades from strategic measures at an organizational level down to process indicators, which cascade down to the work unit or team level. Con-versely, these measures should also have the ability to be aggregated or rolled up from the work unit or team level to support process and strategic measures. The utilization of a cascading performance measurement system enables the align-ment of strategic goals across processes.

An approach to performance measurement development is to determine how value is provided from the perspective of the customer. Value is said to be in the eye of the beholder. Therefore, a natural starting point is the identification of strategic priorities since these are what is of value to the organization and its stakeholders. For illustration purposes, let's say an organization has four strategic priorities. They are

1. to become as cost-effective as possible
2. to demonstrate high-quality outcomes
3. to demonstrate organizational learning and continuous quality improvement
4. to satisfy stakeholders

These are generic strategic priorities that could be used by any home care agency. Each of these strategic priorities has an internal and external customer element. Cost-effectiveness and organizational learning are intrinsic: These pri-orities benefit the internal organization, its owners, and the staff by striving for improved processes and long-term viability. Demonstrable quality and stake-holder satisfaction are extrinsic: They provide value to the patients, payers, and physicians who are being served by the organization. Therefore, a performance measurement based upon strategic priorities needs to consider what provides value from the customer's perspective and the organization's perspective. The following formula shows that value has two components—efficiency and effectiveness. Utilizing the two elements of this formula provides an approach to balancing the diverse and often polar requirements of developing a performance measurement system.

$$Value = Efficiency + Effectiveness$$

Value is the sum of efficiency and effectiveness indicators. Measures of efficiency would include cost and time reductions. Measures of effectiveness would include improvements in satisfaction and clinical outcomes. To have effectiveness without efficiency, or vice versa, would lead to the possibility of developing a dysfunctional organization. Stated differently, reliance upon efficiency measures could create short-term opportunities from a financial perspective but impair long-term viability by not paying attention to the needs of customers. Conversely, relying solely upon indicators of effectiveness might allow an organization to demonstrate impressive clinical outcomes and high customer satisfaction ratings, but its cost structure might be prohibitive in a cost-sensitive marketplace. The measuring and monitoring of indicators of both efficiency and effectiveness provide a format for demonstrating the provision of value. Measures of value could be used to support the balanced scorecard concept introduced in Chapter 4. Examples of measures that could be used at each of the three levels (system dimensions) can be found in Figure 11–3.

Figure 11–3 identifies six categories of performance measures (three for efficiency and three for effectiveness) at the strategic or agencywide level. Cascading down to the process level, it is necessary to create process-oriented performance measures that support the objectives at a strategic (agency) level. Therefore, the development of performance measures needs to support these objectives and also have the ability to be aggregated to assess whether strategic goals were being met. Table 9–10 illustrated this concept with cost per visit. The illustration identified baseline process cost by category and identified two-year

	System Dimension	Efficiency	Effectiveness
Cascade Down	Agencywide (Strategic Level)	Reduced Cost Reduced Time Enhanced Capacity	Increased Customer Satisfaction Contract Loyalty (Retention) Clinical Outcome Improvement
	Processes	Process Simplification	Service Line Segmentation Customer Focus
	Individual, Work Unit, or Team	Improved Time Management Activity Analysis	Contribution to Team, Process, and Agency Goals Skill Improvement

Figure 11–3 Cascading Indicators of Value

goals. Both the baseline and stretch target goals (e.g., goals that will stretch the accomplishments) are aggregated to support the organization's strategic measurement system for the first strategic priority—to become as cost-effective as possible.

Table 9–10 is an example of how the strategic priority—cost-effectiveness—may be measured and monitored at the process level. This example relies solely on measures of efficiency (e.g., cost per visit). Therefore, there needs to be comparable measures of effectiveness, such as was demonstrated in Table 9–12, that evaluate customer satisfaction by process; otherwise the agency would run the risk of skewing its perception of value creation. These measures support the fourth strategic priority—to satisfy stakeholders.

Table 11–1 uses a matrix to identify additional examples of performance measures or indicators that could be used to support the organization's strategic objectives at the process level. One of the issues with any performance measurement system is to collect data that will make a difference and answer the "so what" question. Therefore, managers need to take a step back and ask hard questions of themselves, their customers, suppliers, and staff before deciding what is to be measured. Measurement prioritization is important not only because there is a need to limit the amount of indicators to those indices that are truly meaningful,

Table 11–1 Performance Measure Matrix

| Process | | Value Indicators | |
	Efficiency	Effectiveness
Patient-Focused Care Processes	Upstream	Reduce time to complete an admission visit.	Increase patient and MCO satisfaction.
	Core Processes Downstream	Increase productivity. Reduce A/R days.	Improve ADLs. Increase patient satisfaction with discharge and follow-up.
Support Processes	Information Systems	Reduce response time.	Improve staff access to data.
	Human Resources	Reduce recruitment cost.	Enhance training retention.
	General and Financial Management	Reduce time devoted to the budgeting process.	Reduce the number of reporting errors.
	Plan, Develop, and Market	Reduce cost per new contract.	Reduce contract development time.
	Quality Improvement	Dollar savings from process improvements.	Percent of staff trained in CQI strategies.

but also because measurement also creates an odd paradox: The measurement system will determine how people act. In other words, you get what you measure. It is for this reason that outcomes should always have a positive focus rather than a negative one. It also demonstrates how process level objectives need to be supported by individual, or work unit, measures. Then, measures can be rolled up from the individual level through to the agency level.

Although the value indicators listed in Table 11–1 are written as goals, these measures of value also can be written and quantified as outcomes. Furthermore, value indicators can be broken down into more specific pieces. For example, the core process effectiveness indicator "Improve ADLs" could be diagnosis-specific to address high-volume, high-risk, or high-cost diagnoses.

DEVELOP PROCESS BASELINE

Developing a baseline is the third essential element to managing the process. Developing a baseline requires collecting data about each process. For instance, if data are to be collected to demonstrate stakeholder satisfaction with respect to each process, then the organization needs to identify what service elements contribute to stakeholder satisfaction. Elements need to be identified by process and their relationship to the stakeholder. How to collect these data was addressed in Chapter 10. Suggestions for what data to collect are depicted in Table 11–2.

Table 11–2 illustrates how to start developing this approach using a process orientation. Understanding and evaluating customer requirements will require some research. This research can be accomplished through searches of previously published materials, face-to-face conversations, or focus groups. The challenge is to identify sets of primary requirements and secondary requirements that differentiate between basic service expectations and elements of service that go beyond traditional expectations.[1] There also may be a need to identify what elements of

Table 11–2 Stakeholder Satisfaction Matrix

| | | External Customers | | | Internal Customers | |
	Process	Patient	MCO	Physician	Staff	Owner(s)
PFC	Upstream	1.				
	Core Processes	2.	3.	4.		
	Downstream				5.	6.
Support	Information Systems	7.				
	Human Resources			8.		
	General and Financial Management				9.	
	Plan, Develop, and Market					10.
	Quality Improvement	11.				

the process are seen by the customer and what elements of the process are blind to the customer.[2] For instance, one of the traditional indicators of patient satisfaction may be to assess whether staff arrive at the patient's home within 15 minutes of the anticipated arrival time. An indicator that demonstrates attempts to go beyond this basic service expectation is that the staff be present at the home when the patient is discharged from the hospital. These are all elements of the process that can be seen by the patient. An element of the process not seen by the customer is the call(s) made by the scheduler to assign an appropriate staff member to the visit.

The following numbers correspond to the numbers on the grid in Table 11–2. The following suggestions are merely possibilities, not an all-inclusive listing of opportunities to demonstrate customer satisfaction.

1. Upstream process from the perspective of the patient
   - Was there a smooth transition from the hospital to the home?
   - Was the patient involved in the development of an initial plan of treatment?
   - Was the patient's family involved in the development of an initial plan of treatment?
2. Core process from the perspective of the patient
   - Were all disciplines responsive to the needs of the patient? If not, which ones were not?
   - Was the patient kept informed of the treatment process?
3. Core process from the perspective of the managed care organization (MCO)
   - Were outcomes met on time, early, late, never met, or changed?
   - Was there consistent communication between the team leader and the MCO case manager?
4. Core process from the perspective of the physician
   - Was the physician kept up to date on patient progress?
   - Was the care team supportive of physician wishes?
5. Downstream process from the perspective of the staff
   - Is intake information gathered completely during the upstream process to meet the goals and objectives of the downstream process?
   - Is the intake information accurate?
   - Is documentation submitted on time during the core processes so that the goals and objectives of the downstream process can be realized?
6. Downstream process from the perspective of the owner(s)
   - Are receivables being collected on time?
   - Are data retrievable to meet the needs of third-party inquiries?
7. Information system process from the perspective of the MCO
   - Are reports provided on a timely basis (e.g., the third day of every month)?

- Do reports meet the needs of MCO case managers and analysts?
8. Human resource process from the perspective of the physician
   - Do clinical staff have the technical competence to meet my evolving needs?
   - Are administrative staff responsive to my needs?
9. General and financial management process from the perspective of the staff
   - How does management recognize the contributions of all staff?
   - Does management demonstrate its commitment to the organization's values on a daily basis?
10. Planning, development, and marketing process from the perspective of the owner(s)
    - Does the community assessment process identify new business opportunities?
    - Are all other processes satisfied with the efforts and contributions of this process?
11. Quality improvement process from the perspective of the MCO
    - Does this organization's improvement efforts in cost effectiveness match the MCO's expected level?
    - Does this organization's improvement efforts in clinical outcomes match the MCO's expected level?

Keep in mind that the category labeled "owner(s)" could identify agency-specific objectives and goals as illustrated in Table 11–3 rather than just satisfaction from the perspective of the stakeholder.

In developing a process baseline, step one is identifying what data are critical to managing the organization's processes. The development of a cross-disciplin-

---

Table 11–3 Process-Oriented Objectives from an Owner or Agency Perspective

Process	Process Objective from an Owner or Agency Perspective
Upstream	Identify what percentage of patients completed the admission process within 24 hours.
Core Process	Identify what percentage of patients achieved expected outcomes on time.
Downstream	Identify the effectiveness of the record retrieval process.
Information Systems	Identify the percentage of activities that are dependent upon manual intervention.
Human Resources	Identify staff satisfaction by discipline and job category.
General & Financial Management	Identify whether the management reporting system is meeting the needs of internal customers.
Plan, Develop, & Market	Identify growth opportunities by service line.
Quality Improvement	Quantify the dollar value of quality improvement initiatives.

ary team, the use of focus groups consisting of customers and/or suppliers, and strategic planning sessions provide some of the opportunities for the identification of data needed to assess whether the organization is on target in the pursuit of its vision, mission, and strategic objectives. The preceding examples are not intended to be an all-encompassing list of performance measures but merely a list of possibilities.

Once performance measures have been identified, then the second step is determining additional or supporting measures that will provide balance in the analysis of processes. Figure 11–4 illustrates the interrelatedness of processes to other elements of the larger system. The dark circles at the four points of the diamond (cost, organizational growth, stakeholder satisfaction, and quality) represent the four strategic priorities that were earlier mentioned.

All processes are made up of activities. Activities are an accumulation of steps, tasks, and actions. Within each process is an abundance of data. For instance, the patient-focused care processes have a wealth of data related to the patient and payer that can form a baseline for process management and improvement activities. Support processes have business-related data that are specific to the various service lines that the organization supports. All processes can gather data about the staff that work within each process grouping, the agency, or business unit.

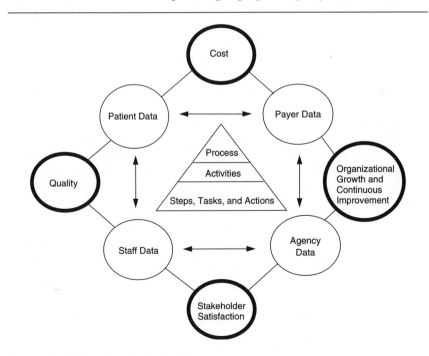

Figure 11–4 The Interrelatedness of Data

It is the relationship among activities, customers, staff, business policies, and requirements that will dictate how successful an organization will be in pursuing its strategic goals. When combined and viewed in a multidimensional format (e.g., from the perspectives of cost, quality, and time), data can provide a baseline to guide all process management activities. These data are accumulated in the pursuit of strategic priorities such as cost-effectiveness, stakeholder satisfaction, organizational learning and continuous improvement, and demonstrable quality. Ideally, the collection, storage, and retrieval of data should use a secure and automated system that will facilitate the relational analysis of all service dimensions.

Developing a baseline for improvement-oriented activities can also be very specific. For instance, members of the downstream process may decide that they want to identify billing errors that were contributing to their collection problems. They decide to collect data about the number of claim rejections. To accomplish this objective they created a basic checksheet as shown in Table 11–4.

In this example, it was decided that in order to specifically analyze rejected claims, one column would identify the type of errors and another column would identify the quantity of errors. A third column was added to summarize the errors. Once rejected claims were summarized, the members of the downstream process constructed a Pareto Chart to share their findings with other members of the patient-focused care process.

A Pareto Chart is named for the creator of the Pareto Principle, Vilfredo Pareto (1843–1923). The Pareto Principle basically states that a few categories (20 percent or less) will provide approximately 80 percent of the opportunities for improvement. The Pareto Chart combines a bar chart with an aggregate accumulation line to create a visual tool for explaining results. A Pareto Chart based on the data in Table 11–4 is illustrated in Figure 11–5.

The Pareto Chart can be used to illustrate results or to determine a baseline or starting point for process improvement activities. To complete the above example, the downstream process used collected data to identify areas where staff

---

Table 11–4 Billing Error Checklist

Billing Errors—July 1996		
Type of Error	Number of Errors	Total Errors by Type
Incomplete UB-92	JHT JHT JHT JHT JHT JHT JHT JHT JHT II	47
Missing Insurance Data	JHT JHT JHT JHT IIII	24
Wrong Codes	JHT JHT JHT II	17
Secondary Payer	JHT II	7
Wrong Name	JHT	5
		100

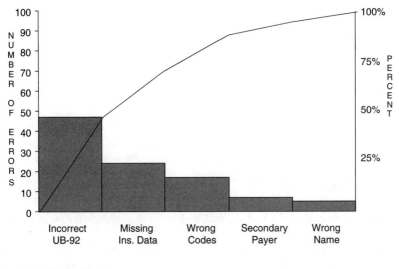

Figure 11–5 Pareto Chart

needed to be trained or retrained and policies and procedures needed to be revised to prevent the continuation of collection problems.

STABILIZE THE PROCESS

A stable process is one that will produce predictable results. For example, in a perfect world this means that all documentation is completed accurately, entered into the information system correctly, and filed properly, and meets customer requirements. Reality, however, is that humans make mistakes. Presuming that everyone attempts to do his or her best on every job, then mistakes occur because of poor training, forgetfulness, or being rushed. Sometimes errors occur because of equipment failure, interruptions by a third party, or a change of shift or personnel.

W. Edwards Deming referred to this phenomenon as *variation*.[3] Variation can easily be seen when looking at a run chart. A run chart is another visual tool that plots results sequentially across a range of time. Figure 11–6 illustrates a run chart for medical record errors that is based upon a monthly sample of 50 records per month.

Over the course of a 12-month period there was a range of errors that were as low as 4 in October and as high as 23 in July. This is an example of variation. Deming refined this concept and identified two types of variation: common and special cause. His premise was that *common cause variation* was a result of the

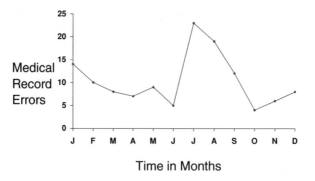

Time in Months

Figure 11–6 Run Chart Depicting Medical Record Errors

---

process that management had created and *special cause variation* was due to extenuating circumstances.

Deming demonstrated the phenomenon of variation with what has since been referred to as the funnel experiment.[4] During the experiment, the funnel is held stationary above a table or sheet of paper, beads are dropped through the funnel, and an "x" is placed on the table where each bead hits. After 50 beads are dropped through the funnel there will be many "x's" on the paper within a tight range. When the funnel is fixed in place, its output (the beads) will exhibit common variation, hence multiple "x's" close together on the paper. If someone accidentally hits the table while a bead is going through the funnel and the bead hits the table farther away from the norm, this is an example of special cause variation.

A process that is stable rarely exhibits special cause variation and, therefore, can be used for forecasting.[5] This concept is an important premise in process management. First, the goal of every process is to serve customers by producing some form of output. If the output is error-prone or unsatisfactory from the customer's perspective, then the customer may become dissatisfied and complain. If the customer is not satisfied with the organization's response, he or she may seek another supplier. The goal of process management is not only to satisfy customers, but to identify how the process can efficiently meet a customer's needs.

To determine whether a process is stable requires converting a run chart (Figure 11–6) into a control chart. This conversion is accomplished by statistically determining upper control limit (UCL) and lower control limit (LCL) lines drawn on either side of the process average. The statistical methodology (which type of control chart and how the limits are calculated) will depend upon whether data are count (discrete or attribute data) or measurement (continuous or variables data) data and whether the sample size is constant or variable. A total of seven different types of control charts are listed below.

For measurement or continuous data:

1. $\overline{X}$&R chart—Average and range chart for fewer than 10 items in a subgroup of data
2. $\overline{X}$&S chart—Average and standard deviation for more than 10 items in a subgroup of data
3. individual's chart (XMR)—Individual value and moving range (moving range because can't have a range of one) for one observation in a subgroup of data

For count or discrete data:

1. c chart—Number of nonconformities with a constant sample size (plots number of defects)
2. u chart—Number of nonconformities with varying sample size (unequal subgroups, therefore plots ratio)
3. p chart—Proportion defective (plots a percentage to account for different size subgroups)
4. np chart—Number defective (plots exact number of items on chart for equal size subgroups)

The most frequently used chart is the individual's chart. Table 11–5 outlines the type of question and data structure addressed by each type of control chart.

The control chart is constructed using data that has been collected and plotted on a run chart. The run chart is then modified to include three horizontal lines. The two outer lines are referred to as UCL and LCL and the center line is the central

Table 11–5 Data Structure/Question for Each Type of Control Chart

Type of Control Chart	Question/Data Structure
$\overline{X}$&R chart	What is the turnaround time for submitting a sample of 8 claims daily?
$\overline{X}$&S chart	What is the turnaround time for submitting a sample of 20 claims daily?
Individual's chart	How many claims are submitted each week?
c chart	Out of a sample of 50 claim submissions each week, how many defects (errors) are found?
u chart	Out of all the claim submissions each week, how many defects (errors) are found?
p chart	Out of all the claim submissions each week, what percent have one or more defects (errors)?
np chart	Out of a sample of 50 claim submissions each week, how many have one or more defects (errors)?

tendency line, or average. Points that are outside of the control limits, either upper or lower, identify a process that is unstable. In addition, eight successive points that are on one side of the center line (either above or below) are also considered to represent an unstable process. Unstable processes are also known as being out of control. Figure 11–7 illustrates the concept of a control chart using the medical record errors examples presented in the preceding run chart (Figure 11–6). Count data were used for a constant sample size. This data structure requires an np chart.

Table 11–6 illustrates the data for the calculation of UCLs and LCLs. The limits are derived by calculating the number of errors found in each batch of 50 medical records. Results are tracked for each month in a 12-month period. Using the results from the past 12 months it is possible to calculate the average number of errors that occurred over the course of 12 months.

The average proportion of errors per record or $\bar{p}$ (pronounced p bar) is calculated by summarizing the error proportion column and dividing by 12 (or K), for each month in the data sample.

$$\text{Calculate}\,\bar{p} = \frac{\sum p}{K} = \frac{2.5}{12} = .208333$$

The central tendency line, or average errors found in the medical records, is calculated by summarizing the amount of errors for the 12 months and then dividing by 12.

$$\text{Calculate CL} = \bar{np} = \frac{\sum np}{K} = \frac{125}{12} = 10.41667$$

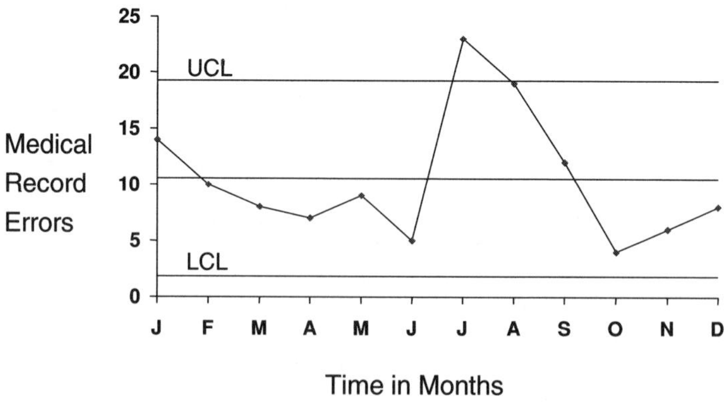

Figure 11–7 "np" Control Chart Depicting Medical Record Errors

Table 11–6 Data for Calculation of UCL and LCL

	Medical Record Errors (np)	Total Records Reviewed (n)	Proportion (p)
Jan	14	50	0.28
Feb	10	50	0.2
Mar	8	50	0.16
Apr	7	50	0.14
May	9	50	0.18
Jun	5	50	0.1
Jul	23	50	0.46
Aug	19	50	0.38
Sep	12	50	0.24
Oct	4	50	0.08
Nov	6	50	0.12
Dec	8	50	0.16
Total	125	600	2.5

The UCL is calculated by adding the sum of the errors (10.41667) and three times the square root of the sum of the errors multiplied by one less $\bar{p}$ (1 − .20833 = .7917). The resultant calculation produces a UCL of 19.0317.

$$Calculate = \bar{np} + 3\sqrt{\bar{np}(1-\bar{p})}$$
$$= 10.41667 + 3\sqrt{10.41667(1-.20833)}$$
$$= 19.0317$$

The LCL is calculated by subtracting from the sum of the errors (10.41667) three times the square root of the sum of the errors (10.41667) multiplied by one less $\bar{p}$ (.7917). The resultant calculation produces an LCL of 1.8016.

$$Calculate = \bar{np} - 3\sqrt{\bar{np}(1-\bar{p})}$$
$$= 10.41667 - 3\sqrt{10.41667(1-.20833)}$$
$$= 1.801636$$

Based upon the results illustrated in Figure 11–7 it is easy to identify that one point is out of control. In this example, the out of control situation was investigated and found to have occurred because of new field staff that were hired and sent into the field without properly completing the training program. This action resulted in rework and wasted resources.

The goal is to achieve stability in all processes because once a process has stabilized, it is possible to begin the improvement process.[6] Some of the factors to consider when looking at individual processes are the design of the process, management interventions, bottlenecks, manual systems, the impact of suppliers, part-time staff, contracted staff, and the impact of training.

An example of investigation for stabilization is the assessment of the initial visit flow (process), which includes intake through the actual assessment (see Figure 9–5). The illustration indicates that the minimum time to complete an assessment visit from the time of intake is several hours, and the maximum time is five days. The illustration also indicates five areas (intake, the time between intake and scheduling, scheduling, the time between scheduling and the assessment, and the actual assessment) where variation can occur. Charting each area of variation and the aggregate will provide an opportunity to begin to stabilize this process. Emphasis also could be placed on limiting the variation caused by the bottlenecks (represented by diagonal lines in the figure).

A Clinical Application

Tracking variances for clinical pathways was introduced in Chapter 8. A control chart has been developed (based on the clinical pathway for pneumonia found in Exhibit 8–2) as another means to determine whether actual utilization results are stable. The appropriate control chart for the data format in this example is an Individual's chart. The individual's or X chart tracks data for each occurrence. Actual utilization is reflected in the upper portion of Figure 11–8 as evidenced by the X measure. The lower portion of the chart is the moving range. The moving range is the difference between visits per case recalculated for each subsequent case. If results for either the X measure or moving range are outside of the control limits, then the process is unstable. Figure 11–8 indicates that both the X measure and the moving range charts are in control. Stated differently, there are no results that are outside the statistically calculated control limits.

Table 11–7 illustrates the data for how the X chart or individual's chart and moving range charts were calculated.

Calculating the control limits for the pneumonia clinical pathway requires two calculations (moving range and X measure). The first calculation determines the moving range. The average variability ($\overline{R}$m) was calculated using the values generated that reflect the difference between the number of visits for one case compared to the subsequent case. Summarizing the variation and then dividing it by one minus the total number of cases (K–1) provided an average variability of 1.913. Calculation for the moving range chart:[7]

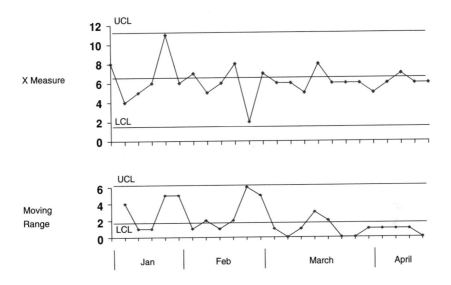

Figure 11–8 Clinical Pathway Control Chart for Pneumonia

$$\overline{R}_m = \frac{\sum R_m}{K-1} = \frac{44}{23} = 1.913$$

The UCL was calculated by multiplying $\overline{R}_m$ by D_4. A value for D_4 is based upon the number of observations or samples (pathways) and in this situation two samples are used to calculate the range, therefore, D_4 has a value of 3.267. This r results in a value of 6.250 for the UCL. The LCL has a value of zero because D_3 is equal to zero. D_3 and D_4 are obtained from a supplied chart of factors. See Table 11–8.

$$UCL_8 = D_4(\overline{R}_m) = (3.267)(1.913) = 6.250$$
$$LCL_8 = D_3(\overline{R}_m) = (0)(1.913) = 0$$

The calculation of the X measure for the individual's chart begins with calculating the average number of visits across all episodes of care that pertain to this clinical pathway. In this example, 24 cases resulted in 148 total visits for an average of 6.167. Calculation for the individual's chart:[8]

$$\overline{X} = \frac{\sum X}{K} = \frac{148}{24} = 6.167$$

Table 11–7 Data for Calculation of Clinical Pathway Control Chart Limits

Month of Service	Utilization of Pn Pathway (pt. number)	Actual Visits	Moving Range ($\overline{Rm}$)
January	1	8	
	2	4	4
	3	5	1
	4	6	1
	5	11	5
February	6	6	5
	7	7	1
	8	5	2
	9	6	1
	10	8	2
	11	2	6
March	12	7	5
	13	6	1
	14	6	0
	15	5	1
	16	8	3
	17	6	2
	18	6	0
April	19	6	0
	20	5	1
	21	6	1
	22	7	1
	23	6	1
	24	6	0

To arrive at the UCL, the average is then added to the result of multiplying E_2 by the previously calculated range ($\overline{Rm}$). The same calculation is used to determine the LCL except that the result is subtracted instead of added.

$$UCL_x = \overline{X} + E_2(\overline{R}_m) = 6.167 + (2.66)(1.913) = 11.256$$
$$LCL_x = \overline{X} - E_2(\overline{R}_m) = 6.167 - (2.66)(1.913) = 1.078$$

(Note: E_2 is a factor, similar to pi,   ; E_2 equals 2.66.)

As stated, in this example the pneumonia (Pn) pathway was utilized 24 times over a four-month period. Actual utilization ranged from a high of 11 visits to a low of 2 visits. The majority of the visits were consistent with the clinical pathway, which calls for six visits. There are several interesting points to note. First, there appears to be a higher degree of variation in the earlier cases of pneumonia than in the later cases. This variation could be attributable to patients' having a higher intensity of care requirements or staff's unfamiliarity with the care interventions. Another point to note is that one patient had only two visits. It appears that this

Table 11–8 Table of Factors for X and R Charts

	R Chart Factors		X Chart Factors
Number of Observations in Subgroup (n)	*Lower D_3*	*Upper D_4*	*A_2*
2	0	3.267	1.880
3	0	2.575	1.023
4	0	2.282	.729
5	0	2.115	.577

Source: Reprinted with permission from M.D. Sloan, *How to Lower Health Care Costs by Improving Health Care Quality*, p. 111, © 1994, American Society for Quality Control.

patient was discharged prior to the completion of his or her course of treatment. This discharge could have been due to rehospitalization or death.

Another chart to complement the control chart would be the identification of whether outcomes were being met. Eight expected outcomes were associated with the clinical pathway of pneumonia (see Exhibit 8–2). Figure 11–9 represents the tracking of the percentage of these outcomes that have been met on a monthly basis.

Figure 11–9 identifies the percent of monthly pneumonia episodes whose patients achieved all eight outcomes. For example, 0.6, or 60 percent, of the patients in January achieved all expected outcomes associated with the pneumonia pathway. By April the number was up to 80 percent. A trend line has been drawn to illustrate the continuous improvement with this pathway and the results

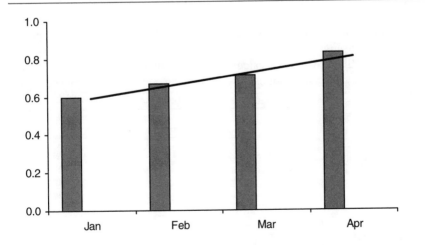

Figure 11–9 Outcomes Met for the Clinical Pathway of Pneumonia (Percentage Achieving All Eight Outcomes by Monthly Episodes of Pneumonia)

that are being achieved. One might infer from this improvement in outcomes and from the decrease in utilization variability (see moving range for March and April in Figure 11–8) that there has been stabilization in this clinical pathway. This initial inference will require additional monitoring, however, since once a process has stabilized there are still additional opportunities for improving the quality of care and investigating the use of alternative resources. For instance, substituting a LPN for a RN may decrease the cost of the clinical pathway. This substitution, however, may also increase the cost of the clinical pathway if additional visits are required for instruction or if there is a decrease in completed outcomes.

GATHER COMPARATIVE DATA

Comparative data can come from the budget, an interim forecast, or a previous month or year. Comparative data can also be the result of a strategic planning session, data gathered from published research, or based upon some other goal-oriented process. As discussed in Chapter 10, comparative data for the management of processes is typically referred to as *benchmark data*. Benchmark data are found within and outside of the organization. Internal benchmark data can be developed as part of process improvement initiatives. They represent improvement goals for the upcoming year. For instance, by using a traditional financial statement format, the concept of benchmarking can be illustrated. If an organization currently has a 2 percent bottom line (revenue less expenses) and an improvement objective to reach 5 percent by the end of next year, the 2 percent is the baseline, the 5 percent is the internal benchmark or goal, and the difference— 3 percent—is the gap or hurdle. Internal benchmarks can also be developed using the concepts of activity-based cost management (ABCM), discussed in Chapter 9 and illustrated in Figure 11–10.

Figure 11–10 illustrates the calculation of an internal benchmark using an ABCM system. The calculation is developed using activity cost associated with

	Formula	Application	Result
Example A	$\dfrac{\text{Activity Cost}}{\text{FTE}}$ =	$\dfrac{\$20,000}{50}$ =	$400 per FTE
Example B	$\dfrac{\text{Activity Cost}}{\text{Total Activity Cost}}$ =	$\dfrac{\$20,000}{\$4,000,000}$ =	.005

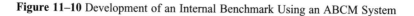

Figure 11–10 Development of an Internal Benchmark Using an ABCM System

training. In this example, the activity of training consumed $20,000 in labor, benefits, supplies, and external seminar costs for 50 full-time equivalents (FTEs). Example A illustrates how an internal benchmark could be calculated on a FTE basis. Example B illustrates how the activity cost of training can be compared against total activity cost for the organization. In this example there was activity cost of $20,000 compared to $4,000,000 of total activity cost. The result of this calculation indicates that 0.5 percent of the activity cost incurred by this organization has been utilized for the purposes of training.

Once calculated, internal benchmarks can be compared and contrasted against improvement goals. For instance, it may be this organization's objective to increase its training costs from $400 to $800 per FTE for 1 percent of total activity cost.

Another way to use the concept of benchmarking is to compare cost or productivity measures against benchmarks from within the home health industry. For instance, nursing productivity is an indicator of the efficiency of field nurses. When using benchmarks from outside of the organization, however, one needs to make sure that the benchmarks are calculated in the same way by all involved in the benchmarking process. An example of outside benchmarking can be seen in Table 11–9, which examines nursing productivity as an indicator of the efficiency of field nurses in three different scenarios.

Table 11–9 illustrates one method of calculating the average nursing visits per day. The average visit-per-day calculation is based upon an eight-hour day less a half-hour break, or 450 minutes, to be consistent with the National Association of Home Care's (NAHC's) approach to productivity as defined by its Uniform Data Set for Home Care and Hospice. Total visit time is then divided into 450 minutes to arrive at an estimate for nursing productivity. Using the model in Table 11–9 one can see that a 10-minute reduction in visit time (scenario A vs. B) will have a rather significant increase in productivity (from 5.0 visits per day in scenario A to 5.6 average visits per day in scenario B).

Table 11–9 Nursing Productivity Benchmarks

| | Scenario | | |
Activities	A	B	C
Direct Care	35	30	30
Documentation	23	20	18
Travel	22	20	17
Coordination	10	10	10
Average Visit Time (minutes)	90	80	75
8-Hour Day (minus 30-minute break)	450	450	450
Average Visits/Day	5.0	5.6	6.0

Benchmarking does not have to stop at the gathering of statistics for comparison with internal results, however. The process of benchmarking can become even more involved and expensive. The more elaborate process of benchmarking (as outlined in Chapter 10) involves studying another organization's system, learning why it is able to produce better results, and then returning to your organization to implement findings. Hopefully, the same positive results will be recreated.

Benchmark data can also be gathered from outside of the home health industry but within the health care industry. For instance, a home health agency may be interested in comparing data on staff retention with a long-term-care facility. In addition to evaluating the calculation of performance measures, it is important to understand the underlying process. There may be differences in rules and regulations, work and staffing requirements, support systems, equipment, or pay scales that could influence results. Benchmark data can also be gathered from outside of the health care industry. Information gathered from an airline about its scheduling process, however, may have little applicability to the home health industry.

Benchmarking results from outside the home health industry should not necessarily be ruled out. Figure 11–11 utilizes benchmarks that compare the results of the cost of payroll processing using an ABCM system with the best results from Fortune 100 companies and the best results on a worldwide basis.[9] In this example, it costs an agency $9.50 to produce a payroll check in contrast to $5.00 for the best of the Fortune 100 companies and $1.72 for a world-class organization.

Ultimately, the goal of acquiring comparative data is to develop an external yardstick to gauge the management and improvements of internal operations.

SET GOALS

Once performance measures have been identified, a baseline developed, and the process stabilized, improvement-oriented goals are set. Goals can be set in relation to comparative data or based upon an internal, growth-oriented goal. The achievement of goals cannot be accomplished from within a vacuum. Stated differently, achieving a strategic goal (e.g., enhancing the organization's cost-

Formula	Application	Agency Results	Fortune 100	World-Class
$\dfrac{\text{Payroll Processing}}{\text{Number of Payroll Checks}}$ =	$\dfrac{\$42,000}{4,420}$ =	$9.50	$5.00	$1.72

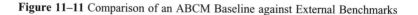

Figure 11–11 Comparison of an ABCM Baseline against External Benchmarks

effectiveness) will require everyone's assistance. Goals can be specific to one process or cross multiple processes.

An example of a goal that would be specific to the core process would be enhancing the capacity of the nursing staff to see more patients. The performance measure associated with this objective would be an indicator of nursing productivity, such as the average number of visits per day. The goal might be to increase productivity from 5.0 to 6.0 visits per day.

A goal that would cross all processes would be to enhance organizational cost-effectiveness by reducing the average cost per visit. For instance, Table 9–10 illustrated a goal of decreasing the average cost per visit from $70.35 to $61.00, for a 13.3 percent reduction in average visit cost. In this illustration, goals have been established for each process as coparticipants in the achievement of the organization's strategic goals. All process owners need to work toward the achievement of organizational goals; otherwise, the possibility of resorting to a departmental mentality that ignores membership in the larger system exists.

Another example utilizes data provided by the organization's ABCM system and is based upon Figure 11–11. An improvement goal associated with Figure 11–11 may be to reduce payroll processing cost from $9.50 to $7.00 per payroll check. Accomplishing this goal requires evaluating organizational payroll policies and enlisting the support of other process owners. For instance, a large portion of the activity cost associated with payroll processing may be attributable to the payment of myriad visit rates based upon when field staff worked, what day they worked, whether they qualified for a bonus, whether they were in an overtime situation, the type of visit, and other factors. A strategy to accomplish this goal may be to convert everyone to salary. This conversion would reduce the cost of processing per payroll check but would create other issues within the system (agency).

Again, goals cannot be created in a vacuum. Goals and subsequent improvement plans need to consider all aspects of the organization that could be influenced by changes. If goals are to be achievable, they must have finite time frames associated with them, accountability must be established for their accomplishment, resource requirements must be established, and systemic implications must be assessed.

DEVELOP IMPROVEMENT PLAN

Once goals have been developed, an improvement plan is created. Generally, managers are ideal for developing an approach to solving problems, developing performance measures, and gathering baseline data. Sometimes there is hesitancy to put plans into action because of the risk of failure, a fear of uncharted waters, or perhaps an unwillingness to make unpopular decisions. These concerns need to be dealt with by creating a safe, supportive environment within the agency that encourages risks and creativity.

The action plan grid (Table 11–10) is a tool to foster ownership and account-ability. Using the grid also assists with team ownership and removes some of the individual risks and concerns.

The action plan grid creates a visual tool that paints a picture for all to see, and identifies who, what, where, when, and how. Creation of an action plan provides a starting point or foundation that identifies the action owner or accountable person, the agreed-upon approach, actions to support the agreed-upon plan, and barriers and aids required for its successful implementation. The grid also provides an opportu-nity to identify resource requirements and performance measures for the evaluation of interim and final targets. Additional columns can be added to the grid to cross-reference events that need to be completed sequentially or concurrently.

For instance, one example of an organizational goal is to increase productivity from 5.0 to 6.0 visits per day. Based upon the data in Table 11–9 this would require a reduction of 15 minutes in average visit time. If one were to ignore the importance of activities that add value, then a goal of reducing activity time could be accomplished by targeting any of the activities associated with the visit. Reducing the amount of direct care time or care coordination, however, would decrease the provision of value from the perspective of the customers (patients) being served and the nurses who provide care. Rather, the activities of travel and documentation do not add value to either customer group. Therefore, to target a reduction in non-value-adding activities would not be harmful from either group's perspective. In fact, it is unlikely that any home health nurse became involved in home health nursing because of the documentation.

Because Table 11–9 identifies visit time by activity category, it is possible to quantify the financial impact of a decision to increase nursing productivity from 5.0 to 6.0 visits per day. This quantification is illustrated in Table 11–11.

Table 11–10 Action Plan Grid

Action Owner	Approach	Actions	Completion Date	Resource Requirements	Performance Measures

Table 11–11 Valuation of an Improvement in Nursing Productivity

Average Visits/Day	5.0	6.0
Productive Days	230	230
Annual Visits	1,150	1,380
Annual Cost	$42,000	$42,000
Cost per Visit	$36.52	$30.43
Value of Improvement (per Visit)		$6.09

Table 11–11 calculated the average cost per visit using average visits per day and multiplying the average visit assumptions by the number of productive days to arrive at an annual visit estimate.[10] Annual visits were divided into an annual cost of $42,000 ($35,000 salary inflated by a 20 percent benefit factor) to arrive at a cost per visit. Table 11–11 indicates a savings of $6.09 per visit. Assuming that this improvement will benefit 80 percent of the 60,000 nursing visits that are performed, this improvement in productivity would yield a savings of $292,320 (48,000 x $6.09). Furthermore, this approach is consistent with the agency's value system because the agency is decreasing non-value-adding activities while supporting its strategic priorities of stakeholder satisfaction, organizational growth, and increased cost-effectiveness.

The preceding calculation could provide the incentive to invest in a new information system that utilizes laptop computers because the new information infrastructure would yield an average savings of several minutes per visit. Concurrently, it might be decided to transition the care delivery structure into a team model based upon geographic area. The underlying strategy for this approach is that there would be better care coordination, improved scheduling, and less travel for field staff.

Once the improvement plan is identified, an action plan would be developed that would identify who is responsible for investigating the purchase of a new information system, evaluating training requirements, and setting implementation timelines. Concurrently, the action plan would be updated to identify who is responsible for developing a geographic team structure, evaluating potential changes in scheduling methodology, and determining whether changes were required for weekend and evening coverage.

The quantification of improvement plans also helps to gain senior management support. In this example, it would be necessary to quantify the cost of hardware, software, training, and the duplication of activities in running a parallel system. Monitoring implementation progress would also be critical to keep duplicate costs for parallel processing to a minimum. Once support and approval have been provided, the hard work begins. The purpose of the action plan grid is to lay out each sequential step, attach time frames, and assign accountability. See Table 11–12 for an example of a completed action plan grid.

Table 11–12 Action Plan for Productivity Enhancement Project

Action Owner	Approach	Actions	Completion Date	Resource Requirements	Performance Measures
Director of Professional Services	Perform literature research to identify technological innovations and their application to clinical documentation.	1. Gather data from the Internet. 2. Utilize university library. 3. Contact national and state home care associations.	12/1/96	Internet access	None
Director of MIS	Work with clinical team to identify field staff activities.	1. Develop data collection tool. 2. Design tables to collect data from field staff and store in database.	12/31/96	Database program	None
Team Members	Develop RFP for industry software vendors.	1. Identify wish list. 2. Prioritize requirements for enhancing field staff productivity.	1/15/97	Word processing software	None
Director of MIS	Review RFPs and schedule on-site demonstrations.	1. Review RFPs. 2. Identify vendors who meet agency requirements and schedule demonstrations. 3. Coordinate team schedules with on-site demonstrations.	3/15/97	Team time	Response rate
Field Staff	Record time spent on designated activities.	Forward to MIS for entry into database.	2/28/97	Revised day sheets	All paperwork to be submitted within 24 hours of completed visit

Table 11–12 continued

Action Owner	Approach	Actions	Completion Date	Resource Requirements	Performance Measures
Analyst	Compile and summarize activities.	Produce report and forward to CFO.	3/15/97	None	None
CFO	Work with clinical team and DOPS to identify the potential for reducing the amount of time associated with documentation.	1. Review documentation requirements for admission visit, routine visit, visits requiring IVs, and discharges. 2. Agree upon assumptions. 3. Calculate savings and potential return on investment. 4. Review software proposals for cost of hardware, software, and training requirements.	3/31/97	Team time	Agency thresholds for return on investment Impact to agency cost structure
CEO	Present proposal to board for approval.	1. Make presentation. 2. Field questions. 3. Obtain approval.	4/15/97	None	None
Director of MIS	Place order and coordinate training.		4/30/97	None	None
CFO	Coordinate financing.	Meet with bankers.	4/30/97	None	None
Analyst	Review post-implementation results.	Discuss results with project team. Take action to ensure results will be achieved.	7/31/97	None	Increased productivity

An agency does not want to take on a project that results in a negative return on its expenditure of time and resources. One of the tools that can be used to substantiate the need for an improvement project is a cost-benefit analysis. Cost-benefit analysis looks at the relationship of cash inflows and outflows to determine net present value (NPV) or return on investment (ROI).[11] These financial tools need to balance financial ramifications with impacts to internal and external customer satisfaction, quality-oriented services, and the organization's vision and values. Sometimes, however, tradeoffs will need to be made, such as excepting a lower ROI in exchange for maintaining a high level of stakeholder satisfaction.

IMPLEMENT IMPROVEMENTS

This step is the first one in process management and improvement that moves outside of the planning function. Implementing improvements requires taking action. It requires working toward a future-oriented goal and, more often than not, juggling multiple priorities at the same time. Implementing improvements could include installing new equipment, training on a new information system, or training in new protocols. It is generally a time of change, and its achievement will depend upon how successful the team or organizational culture has been with prior implementation efforts.

Implementing improvements is also about change. Change can cause concern for the staff that they may lose their jobs, that there is no substantive reason to change or work harder, or that the new system will not work as well as the old system. Change can cause resistance and be met with sabotage.

Change, however, is a fact of life. One way to deal with resistance is to enlist the support of those affected by the change; explain what is in it for them. The preceding example addressed nursing productivity. How many nurses would react favorably to the agency's administrator telling them that they have to work harder and do more visits without additional compensation? Not many. If the agency's administration, however, illustrated that by reducing the amount of non-value-adding time (e.g., repetitive data entry) one could enhance productivity without affecting existing work schedules, there would be a better reaction. Furthermore, by building upon "what is in it for us," it is possible to illustrate that through the reduction of non-value-adding activities, patient interaction time would not be affected and documentation and travel time should decrease. These notions should create a favorable reaction. After all, the majority of nurses chose home care because of the patient interaction, not to travel or do paperwork.

As discussed in Chapter 5, values are the glue that creates a shared vision in an organization. In the preceding example, a process and organizational improvement objective was established that affected one group of individuals. Instead of focusing solely on a metric of 5.0 or 6.0 visits per day, however, the underlying processes/activities (e.g., documentation, travel, patient interaction) were as-sessed to identify where there was an opportunity to create a win-win situation for the staff, the customers, and the agency. Through the concept of value, a strategy was developed that honored the needs of both the staff and the agency without affecting the customer. If, however, the emphasis was placed solely on the metric of 5.0 or 6.0 visits per day, a we-they situation could occur. This kind of situation has negative implications for customer and staff satisfaction.

Process management and subsequent improvement objectives require the assistance of the agency's staff. Without a willingness to support the process and accomplish the agency's goals, staff will always have the ability to thwart progress. Communication with staff, answering the "what is in it for us" question, the alignment of incentive systems, and providing continual support and feedback are several of the tools that can be used to enlist everyone's support in accomplish-ing improvement objectives.

EVALUATE AND IMPROVE

Review results. Is the project on track from a time and cost perspective? Is the process producing the results that were initially projected? The review process is critical for course correction. Management has a responsibility to review results and to take corrective action. Corrective action requires refocusing resources, contacting consultants, or identifying new improvement objectives. Its specific nature depends on the situation.

Process evaluation depends on the agency's information infrastructure. For instance, the development of an ABCM system will provide the ability to assess process cost on a monthly basis. Process time may be available on a monthly basis as well. Customer satisfaction surveys may only occur on a quarterly, semiannual, or annual basis; therefore, the agency should consider intermediate indicators of customer satisfaction to supplement process management goals. For instance, senior management may visit payers, physicians, and referral sources on a staggered basis to gather information about the agency. Field staff may provide informal feedback that was based upon conversations with the physician's office manager.

Informal sources of information should be taken "informally," but they can provide clues to impending problems. Once information is gathered, it should be aggregated and assessed. All potential sources of information should be evaluated for relevance, and also for inclusion into the management of processes (which is outlined in Figure 11–2). This evaluation is represented by the feedback line that runs from the Evaluate and Improve step in the management process (Figure 11–2) back to the step Develop Process Baseline. This feedback provides the opportunity to develop a new, improved, process baseline and to manage the new, improved version of the process. Process management techniques will evolve, data will become better, and, as the organization evolves, the management of processes will become second nature.

ORGANIZATIONAL LEARNING

Organizational learning is an oxymoron because organizations do not learn, people do. What organizational learning refers to, however, is getting everyone working toward common goals. It is learning from past successes and mistakes; it is breaking recurring patterns that do not contribute to agency goals; it is commitment to excellence; and it is the development of a corporate culture that supports personal growth, participation, and experimentation. Organizational learning occurs when everyone is involved in the development of strategic direction, the management of processes, and the ownership of results. It is a shift from a superior-subordinate relationship to one of partners or co-owners.

Staff represent a huge untapped resource that, if cultivated through effective leadership, provide every organization with an opportunity to transcend the status quo. Leadership's challenge is to provide an environment that is characterized by trust, opportunities to learn and grow, and an incentive system that aligns personal and professional values and goals. Leadership must be willing to hold itself accountable on a daily basis for adhering to the organization's value system. Leadership needs to become a role model in the shift from functional, or departmentally driven, organizations to organizations that are process oriented. It needs to work with staff as mentor in this metamorphosis and to be held as accountable as staff.

The reality is that developing a process orientation may be threatening to leadership, if it views itself as a white knight, hero, or the sole beacon of inspiration for the organization. A shift to a process orientation and organizational learning will occur through the promotion of teamwork and a willingness to foster commitment and shared vision, instead of depending upon control and fear to manage relationships. Commitment will occur when management moves from blaming staff for problems to examining the underlying processes that management has developed and perpetuated. This transition will not happen overnight, but the tools and technologies are already available to support the development of organizations that are customer focused and process oriented.

Organizational learning is more important than ever to agencies in the process of transitioning from a relatively safe structure, such as cost reimbursement, to an environment dominated by managed care and prospective payment. Organizational learning is not dependent upon external seminars; it is an internal philosophy. It focuses on growing the entire organization by cultivating personnel.

Growth can take many forms: It can occur by giving staff opportunities to be team leaders, to champion projects, and to assist the organization to accomplish its goals. Growth can also occur by giving staff the tools and opportunities to improve their interpersonal skills, critical thinking abilities, and negotiation skills. Growth inspires a willingness to experiment, to achieve higher goals, and to make a meaningful contribution. Harnessing this energy toward common goals will benefit not only the individual, but the organization as a whole.

CONCLUSION

The development of a process-oriented management structure shifts the perspective of agency management from a vertical (hierarchical) orientation to a horizontal (collaborative) orientation. This chapter examined the concepts of ABCM, cycle time, customer satisfaction, performance measurement, benchmarking, and statistical process control to illustrate how multiple tools can be used effectively in the management of processes. Moreover, the chapter illustrated how the tools of process management can be used for improvement of processes.

These tools are community oriented; they provide information that can be used by staff to improve their daily work life. Results will depend on leadership's willingness to share successes and rewards and move away from management of symptoms to the management of root causes. Long-term success requires digging deep into the roots of organizational processes and eliminating core problems. Without a willingness to dig deep and take action, there is the likelihood of perpetuating problems and treating symptoms instead of correcting root causes.

Processes have multiple components, different levels of customers, and the potential to span an organization. A commitment to a common value system and vision will provide a basis to encourage the human element (staff) to use the tools mentioned in this chapter to accomplish organizational goals.

NOTES

1. J.R. Hauser, How Puritan-Bennett Used the House of Quality, *Sloan Management Review* 34, no. 3 (Spring 1993): 61–70.
2. R. Anthony, Note on Service Mapping, Harvard Business School, #9–693–065, November 30, 1992.
3. W.E. Deming, *Out of the Crisis* (Cambridge, MA: MIT Press, 1982), 310.
4. Deming, *Out of the Crisis*, 327.
5. Deming, *Out of the Crisis*, 340.
6. Deming, *Out of the Crisis*, 354.

7. S. Coburn et al., *Management Accounting* (January 1995): 56–60.
8. Coburn et al., *Management Accounting*, 56–60.
9. Coburn et al., *Management Accounting*.
10. T. McKeon, *Home Health Financial Management* (Gaithersburg, MD: Aspen Publishers, 1996), 176.
11. T. McKeon, *Home Health Financial Management*, 411–419.

CHAPTER 12

Making Care Meaningful

There are two important elements in making care meaningful: the technical element (correctness) and the human element (creativity). Care is meaningful when it is technically correct—when it is appropriate, relevant, effective, efficient, and timely. This book has dealt with many of these issues in the form of outcomes, standards, costs, and process management. This chapter will look further at continuous quality improvement (CQI), the umbrella for these issues. Specifically, how does CQI compare to research and quality assurance (QA)? How is CQI different for service organizations than for industries that manufacture products? Why is there staff resistance to CQI? What is outcome-based quality improvement (OBQI)? The chapter will also address the issue of the cost of rendering technically meaningful care.

The other element of meaningful care relates to creativity. This element puts people into the equation of care; people are, after all, the most important ingredient. People are what health care is all about, although it seems sometimes that the people ingredient gets displaced because of the pressure for "correctness" (e.g., productivity and reduced costs). What is meant by creativity is that care is different for each person to whom it is rendered and by each person rendering it. The provider of care must be creative with his or her clinical knowledge to be sure that care maintains its value by being matched with the wants and needs of the recipient. This customization of care is becoming more challenging and exciting as the recipients become more knowledgeable in the area of health and thus more empowered to care for themselves. The customization is further enhanced with patient/provider synergy that can be strengthened with good interpersonal skills. Along with the above-mentioned examination of quality improvement, this chapter will discuss

- the empowered consumer
- the notion of a customer-centered agency

- the process of learning from both the perspective of the care provider and a learning environment

RESEARCH, QUALITY ASSURANCE, AND CONTINUOUS QUALITY IMPROVEMENT

Ways of maintaining the correctness of care include research and CQI. These are data-driven processes that seek data to analyze practice systematically and to improve agency effectiveness and efficiency. The manipulation and presentation of data results in information. Understanding the information results in knowledge. With information and knowledge, intelligent decisions can be made to make care meaningful.

The beginning for measuring correct care is good data, or data with integrity. Data have been discussed extensively throughout the book. What is important to remember is that not all data are useful for the purposes of meaningful care. Some data are collected because they are easy to collect. Other data are collected because they have been collected for years and are thought to serve a purpose. Data that do not translate into information that provides knowledge and support for organizational strategies, patient outcomes, quality initiatives, and an indication of progress toward goals do not support meaningful care.

Definitions

Research

Research is a method of systematic inquiry based upon scientific theory to discover and interpret facts for the purpose of improving care. It is a tool that is used to contribute to the body of knowledge for giving care.[1] Data are used in research activities in specific statistical analyses that are then discussed and communicated through the professional and, with increasing frequency, the lay literature. This statistical use of data in research is reflected in quality improvement methods such as CQI, which is becoming more sophisticated in its use of statistics. The intent of research, however, differs from that of quality improvement. The intent of research is to look beyond the immediate problem and to generalize to other situations, while the intent of quality improvement is to investigate a current problem in a particular situation or institution and to remedy it.

Research, however, does contribute to the meaningfulness of care as it unveils new knowledge on how to care for certain diseases and conditions. It enriches everyone's understanding of diseases as it probes etiologies and increases everyone's comprehension of the delivery of health care as it examines regional variances and investigates differences in care processes and protocols for different diseases and different locations. For example, the upper Midwest is known as the mastectomy capital of the country, showing higher rates of mastectomies (vs. lumpectomies) than the East and West coasts, or even the South. This variance is true despite the fact that studies show that the chance of surviving early-stage breast cancer is the same no matter which treatment is used.[2]

QA

QA is seen as an outdated, old paradigm, term. It perpetuates the image of inspectors searching for samples of poor quality. QA can be defined as systematic inquiry to evaluate patient care and identify, study, and correct deficiencies in the patient care process.[3] It is still utilized particularly in the area of risk management. Here, QA specialists continually gather data on defined deficiency or risk (e.g., falls, infections). The data are summarized and then used as feedback to determine whether or not the agency is "assured" of quality or if deficiencies or risks are present. This feedback provides the agency an opportunity to respond to the deficiency (e.g., if quality is not assured) in a problem-solving manner. Although new knowledge may be gained, it is specific to the particular agency where the data were generated, and not necessarily generalizable to the industry at large.

QA contributes to the "correct" element of meaningful care, since deficiencies must be eliminated for "correct" care to occur. Defining correct as the absence of deficiencies, however, is old paradigm thinking. As discussed in Chapter 1, quality in the new paradigm has a more positive focus (e.g., looking always for ways to improve the rendering of care, making this care more meaningful each time it is offered).

CQI

CQI deals with problems also, but from a broader perspective. CQI collects and analyzes data in order to search for the underlying (root) causes of poor performance within a process (including the patient-focused care process). Once the underlying cause is identified, then changes that eliminate, reduce, or neutralize the cause are developed and implemented. Finally, the revised operating process is monitored in order to maintain the new performance.

CQI contributes to the meaningfulness of care by constantly improving the process of rendering care. CQI techniques for data analysis are very similar to those of research. The difference, however, is that the results may not be as generalizable depending on the scope of the CQI project. Furthermore, CQI requires an action plan, implementation of the plan, and an evaluation of the effectiveness of the change to remedy the cause of poor performance. Research, on the other hand, focuses on the discovery and not the performance improvement.

Attaining performance improvement is no small accomplishment. Paul Plsek describes five subordinate and significant breakthroughs that are required before the improvement in performance is achieved. They are

1. Breakthrough in *attitude*. The historical performance level must be challenged and the need to do better instilled.
2. Breakthrough in *organization*. Processes cross organizational lines so process improvement must do the same.
3. Breakthrough in *knowledge*. New levels of understanding of how the process operates and what causes poor performance are required.
4. Breakthrough in *cultural patterns*. Staff are accustomed to the old ways of doing things so training must be provided and resistance to change dealt with.
5. Breakthrough in *results*. The change must be evaluated to verify improved results and then monitored in order to sustain the results.[4]

Selecting the process or problem to address can be determined by

- Listening to external customers to determine what expectations are not being met
- Asking the internal customers who actually work on/with the processes for problems they consider important
- Reviewing internal management reports to discover those places where standards are not being met
- Reviewing external benchmark reports for comparisons that are unfavorable
- Reviewing reports and/or processes for areas of complexity
- Reviewing reports and/or processes for bottlenecks

The means to improve or maintain the process was described in Chapter 11.

CQI IN SERVICE ORGANIZATIONS

As health care and home care continue to embrace the philosophy of CQI, it is important to note the differences that are apparent between using CQI in service organizations and using CQI for the manufacturing of products. To omit the presence of these differences would limit the effectiveness of CQI and potentially diminish the meaningfulness of care. Being aware of the differences can also foster a smoother transition into the process of evolving quality. The following is a brief discussion about some of the differences.

Different Level of Personnel[5]

Personnel in service organizations, particularly health care, are more likely to be professionals. This difference affects the approach used in framing the process of quality improvement. Professionals can take offense at programs geared to "improve the quality of their work" since they often pride themselves in giving "quality care." Furthermore, clinicians want to believe that their work leads to good outcomes because bad outcomes can hurt people; only bad practitioners have bad outcomes. A more service-oriented approach would be to emphasize improvement in client/customer satisfaction as part of a balanced approach that includes practictioner satisfaction and cost-effectiveness, rather than only improvement in outcomes.

Different Nature of Work

In a service organization, the volume and flow of work cannot be planned as it can in manufacturing a product. Because of this unpredictable ebb and flow, service companies need to base their work on a philosophy where service capacity focuses on peak volume rather than average volume. In other words, agencies must have sufficient staff to service their highest demand times rather than their average demand. This preparedness could include the availability of experienced home care per-diem staff. The contrast in manufacturing is the "just-in-time" operation where all the necessary ingredients for a product converge at the point of delivery exactly when needed.[6] Unfortunately, if a home health organization operates on the just-in-time philosophy and demand increases, the agency has to compensate for the increased demand by delaying the first visit to a client, reducing the amount of time spent with other patients to increase productivity, or stretching staff by sending out persons who are less prepared. All of these behaviors can affect quality.

A consequence of working with an unpredictable ebb and flow of service demand is more fluid schedules, making it difficult to plan lunches and breaks, let alone meetings to discuss quality improvement.[7] Ways to address this difference include starting CQI activities with supportive (as opposed to clinical) agency processes (e.g., information systems, human resources, management, or marketing); holding frequent but short (15 minutes) CQI meetings; supplementing committee meetings with e-mail communication; and linking CQI activities to an individual's performance objectives.

More Difficult To Measure Services Than Products

An obvious difference between service and manufacturing is that products are tangible and services are not. One can't touch or feel a service, nor is a service easy to inspect once it is completed. Quality is determined by the numerous patient or customer encounters with field staff or other front-line personnel. At the time of the encounter, all that is needed to provide that service must converge. Home health care has been perceived as a service, and it has been difficult to measure. It has been difficult to capture both the processes that get everything in place to perform the service (patient visit) as well as the content of the encounter. Sound approaches are being made, however, to remedy this situation, such as calculating costs of the clinical activities, conducting employee attitude surveys, and evaluating the support processes. It is interesting to note that in an industry that relies so heavily on encounters with field staff and front-line personnel to measure quality, so little investment is made in the development of these individuals.

Different Cultural Perspective[8]

The cultural perspective in manufacturing is more impersonal than the cultural perspective in service organizations. In general, no one in manufacturing takes offense to counting, categorizing, or analyzing processes. Efficiency, "zero deficits," and statistical process controls are all acceptable terms and concepts. Health care, as a service organization, is more personal. The main process is patient-focused, competent, loving care. It is difficult to think of this process in terms of defects or being statistically controlled. Even terms connoting efficiency are hard fought. The more acceptable way of dealing with this difference is to balance efficiency with effectiveness, patient satisfaction, and community health when evaluating services related to direct patient care.

These contrasts also dictate a difference in maintaining performance excellence in a service organization. In manufacturing, all that is required is to run the production line as smoothly as possible. The product is already designed. Variances in production can be charted and controlled. In a service setting and in home care, the design of the service is not complete until the field staff interact with the patient. Patients (or other customers) can introduce variances that cannot be controlled in advance (e.g., a patient is not capable of following the pathway as established and wants to modify it, such as delaying learning to do a dressing change). Therefore, to maintain performance excellence, an agency must define its working quality standard or goal, understand what the customer needs or wants even though this changes, and understand its processes to determine if the service capacity is sufficient to meet the quality goal. When the service capacity is insufficient (e.g., the number of patients or types of needs exceed the capacity of the staff and skill mix), one of two things can happen: (1) work is assigned to staff with less experience or skill than required by the job at hand, or (2) less time is spent with each patient. Regardless, quality suffers.[9]

RESISTANCE TO CQI BY CLINICIANS

There is always resistance to change. The better the etiology of the defensiveness is understood, the easier it is to address. There are some specific clinician issues related to implementing CQI to consider. The resistance to attending meetings, gathering data, analyzing problems, making use of the results, and changing the processes is all rationalized by practitioners who believe that each agency in home care is unique or serves a unique (sicker) caseload. "Each patient is different" is a common cry; there is no average home care patient on whom to apply these quality management principles. Similarly, the resistance to providing patient data is rationalized by the concern for patient confidentiality. It is common for clinicians to resist handing in paperwork with the data that are needed for analysis and then to say that the data are unreliable when the analysis is presented.

As discussed previously, it is true that CQI in home care is different from CQI in manufacturing, but the differences can be managed. The root of the defensiveness is more likely a psychological mechanism that clinicians use to protect themselves from vulnerability and guilt when things go wrong with their patients. The mechanism used is believing that they are in control of what is going on.[10] Therefore, another way to look at what is happening is to see it as a shift in the locus of control, actually the locus of accountability, from the clinician or professional to managed care systems, government agencies, and payers.

Traditionally, clinicians have relied on their own skill and independence to make their clinical decisions. The autonomy of home care is often an attraction for clinicians. To feel confident to make these decisions, however, clinicians must feel in control of what is going on (i.e., they know what the result of their action will be). Failing to believe they are in control would force them to acknowledge that they can't do right by their patients, or make their patients better. The only way to acknowledge adverse outcomes, then, is to believe that bad outcomes are a result of faulty decision making. This thinking further leads to fear of blame by others (e.g., if they have bad outcomes they must be bad practitioners since bad outcomes only happen to people who are incompetent). Unfortunately, this thinking was reinforced by QA activities that always looked for the "bad apple" to blame. Now CQI wants to standardize clinical activities (e.g., clinical pathways, protocols), which removes the control (e.g., the clinician cannot make his or her own decision but must follow the standard guideline) and clinicians feel threatened. Thus, the bemoaning of "cookbook health care."

Overcoming this type of resistance requires a change in thinking from the old "control" paradigm to a new paradigm that acknowledges the complexity of care. The new paradigm asserts that the clinician functions within a situational context and recognizes that better outcomes of care can be achieved with better information and agency support. A move toward acceptance of the new paradigm is to hold regular meetings, even if they are short, to define processes and outcomes that constitute quality care. Holding routine meetings that discuss adverse outcomes such as infections, falls, or medication errors can also be helpful as long as the focus is on improving practice, not investigations to find blame. The regular nature of these meetings will replace the fear with support and, thereby, reduce resistance.

More significant is the long-term establishment of a corporate culture that supports creativity and critical thinking within the system structure. The goal is to provide a culture that offers security and safety in order to promote clinician experimentation with standardized guidelines to meet individual patient needs. Without experimentation, practice can rapidly become impersonal, stale, and outdated. In a CQI environment, however, the clinician is held accountable for both the successes and failures for these "experiments." Thus the need for a safe supportive culture.

OUTCOME-BASED QUALITY IMPROVEMENT (OBQI)

One form of CQI that is gaining popularity, due to the forthcoming OASIS mandate, is OBQI. OBQI was discussed briefly in Chapter 6. It is the use of the OASIS data as the basis for an outcome-based quality improvement program. Sometime after the mandate for the collection of OASIS data is finalized, the next expected mandate will be to submit the data to the Health Care Financing Administration (HCFA), or its selected contractor, in order that national benchmarks can be determined. The question is, however, if an agency is collecting all of these data, how can the agency use them prior to receiving reports from HCFA? The purpose of this section is to describe how to establish an OBQI program using OASIS data. Alternatives for how to utilize these data before the HCFA-generated reports are available also will be presented.

Collect OASIS Data

The first step in establishing any successful OBQI program is to collect the OASIS data. This step may seem self-evident, but the key is that a process is established within the agency that collects data and maintains the integrity of that data. This data collection is not an easy task, and setting up the system and collecting the data as a baseline for future comparisons may be as much as an agency wants to do.

One aspect of maintaining integrity is to be sure that data collection follows the rules in the mandate (e.g., the questions must be incorporated in their entirety with no changes). How to incorporate OASIS into the assessment was discussed in Chapter 10. In addition, the agency must determine how the clinician will be prompted to collect the follow-up data every 60 days and at discharge, who will monitor the follow-up process, who will enter the data into the computer for analysis (or who will analyze the data), what the reports will look like, and who is responsible for reviewing the reports.

Reports can be presented in whatever format provides the desired agency information. Examples of reports similar to the ones expected to be generated by the OASIS project were presented in Chapter 6 (Exhibits 6–1 and 6–2 and Table 6–2). Another example of how data could be reported is shown in Table 12–1.

These data are collected from the OASIS questions dealing with integumentary status. The report indicates by patient and by aggregate for each company (or program line, business unit, or team) the number of patients with a wound at admission to home care and the number with a wound at discharge. It then indicates how many of those with a wound at admission had a wound at discharge; and how many of those who were admitted with no wound had a wound at discharge. At the patient level it indicates the type of wound, the start of care and discharge dates, and the number of comorbidities present.

A similar example for resource utilization of emergent care is found in Table 12–2. These data are collected from the OASIS questions dealing with emergent care and from some of the demographic questions.

This report indicates by patient and in the aggregate, the number of patients who used emergent care for each company, program, business unit, or team. By patient it also indicates the start of care date, the discharge date, the type of facility where emergent care was rendered, the reason for the emergent care, the number of disciplines involved in the case, the total number of home care visits, the length of stay, and the number of comorbidities. The reasons for emergent care are also presented in the aggregate. The reasons OASIS (question MO840) uses for emergent care are[11]

1. improper medication administration, medication side effects, toxicity, anaphylaxis
2. nausea, dehydration, malnutrition, constipation, impaction
3. injury caused by fall or accident at home
4. respiratory problems (e.g., shortness of breath, respiratory function, tracheobronchial obstruction)
5. wound infection, deteriorating wound status, new lesion/ulcer

Table 12–1 Wounds Outcomes Report

Patient Name	MR #	SOC	DC Date	Presence of Wound at ADM	Type Wound at ADM	Presence of Wound at DC	Type Wound at DC	Number of Comorbidities
Karen Jones	24332	9/1/96	5/19/97	Y	PU	N	NA	4
Samuel Smith	52245	8/12/97	10/11/97	Y	SW	Y	SW	2
Timothy Walker	87523	1/12/97	9/26/97	Y	PU	N	NA	1
Harriet Thomas	67755	6/12/96	2/22/97	N	NA	N	NA	7
Andrea Benet	33675	5/30/97	10/29/97	Y	SW	N	NA	1
Ann White	62345	2/16/97	5/5/97	N	NA	N	NA	3
William Green	72261	4/8/96	12/28/96	N	NA	N	NA	4

Total for Company A	Total Wound at ADM	Total Wound at DC	ADM-Yes DC-Yes	ADM-Yes DC-No	ADM-No DC-No	ADM-No DC-Yes
7	4/57%	1/14%	1/14%	3/43%	3/43%	0/0%

Patient Name	MR #	SOC	DC Date	Presence of Wound at ADM	Type Wound at ADM	Presence of Wound at DC	Type Wound at DC	Number of Comorbidities
Tony Small	78784	1/12/97	10/10/97	N	NA	N	NA	1
Sam Brendan	47477	3/18/97	9/26/97	Y	SW	Y	SW	3
Brett Green	80075	11/27/96	8/30/97	Y	PU	Y	PU	5

continues

Table 12–1 continued

Patient Name	MR #	SOC	DC Date	Presence of Wound at ADM	Type Wound at ADM	Presence of Wound at DC	Type Wound at DC	Number of Comorbidities
Robert Ford	42274	6/19/97	9/9/97	N	NA	Y	SU	3
Janet Kerr	36626	4/23/97	8/17/97	Y	PU	N	NA	4
	Total Wound at ADM	Total Wound at DC	ADM-Yes DC-Yes	ADM-Yes DC-No	ADM-No DC-No	ADM-No DC-Yes		
Total for Company B	3/60%	3/60%	2/40%	1/20%	1/20%	1/20%		
5								
	Total Wound at ADM	Total Wound at DC	ADM-Yes DC-Yes	ADM-Yes DC-No	ADM-No DC-No	ADM-No DC-Yes		
Total for All	7/58%	4/33%	3/25%	4/33%	4/33%	1/8%		
12								

Note: PU = pressure ulcer, SU = stasis ulcer, SW = surgical wound, NA = no observable wound

Source: Reprinted with permission from Delta Health Systems, Altoona, Pennsylvania.

Table 12–2 Resource Utilization of Emergent Care Outcomes Report

Patient Name	MR #	SOC	DC Date	Emer. Care Used	Fac. Type	Reas. Emer. Care	Num. DSCP Types	Num. Vsts. All DSCP	LOS	Number of Comorbidities
Jane White	23332	9/1/96	5/19/97	Y	ER	1	4	86	169	4
Jore Green	45245	8/12/97	10/11/97	Y	ER	6	3	52	60	2
Tony Limb	65523	1/12/97	3/11/97	Y	UK	9	5	42	60	1
Brendan Gray	88755	6/12/96	10/10/96	Y	DR	4	2	30	120	7
Kim Bennet	98675	5/30/97	10/29/97	Y	OP	2	3	8	152	1
George Ford	23345	2/16/97	5/5/97	Y	DR	5	2	60	78	3
Bill Weaver	77261	4/8/96	7/7/96	Y	OP	UK	3	60	90	4

Total for Company A	Emer. Care	Rea. One	Rea. Two	Rea. Three	Rea. Four	Rea. Five	Rea. Six	Rea. Seven	Rea. Eight	Rea. Nine	Rea. Ten
7	7/100%	1/14%	1/14%		1/14%	1/14%	1/14%			1/14%	1/14%

Patient Name	MR #	SOC	DC Date	Emer. Care Used	Fac. Type	Reas. Emer. Care	Num. DSCP Types	Num. Vsts. All DSCP	LOS	Number of Comorbidities
Glenn Jones	76784	1/12/97	4/17/97	Y	ER	6	3	34	95	1
Sam Smith	33477	3/18/97	7/14/97	Y	UK	1	4	32	118	3
Brett Morrow	98075	11/27/96	5/26/96	Y	ER	8	4	43	180	5
Bob Kerr	48274	6/19/97	9/9/97	Y	OP	3	4	20	82	3
Ken Sherry	73626	4/23/97	8/17/97	Y	DR	4	2	18	116	4

continues

Table 12–2 continued

	Emer. Care	Rea. One	Rea. Two	Rea. Three	Rea. Four	Rea. Five	Rea. Six	Rea. Seven	Rea. Eight	Rea. Nine	Rea. Ten
Total for Company B											
5	5/100%	1/20%		1/20%	1/20%		1/20%		1/20%		
Total for All											
12	12/100%	2/17%	1/8%	1/8%	2/17%	1/8%	2/17%		1/8%	1/8%	1/8%

Note: EMER = emergent, NUM = number, DSCP = discipline, REA. = reason, ER = emergency room, DR = doctor's office, OP = outpatient, UK = unknown

Source: Reprinted with permission from Delta Health Systems, Altoona, Pennsylvania.

6. cardiac problems (e.g., fluid overload, exacerbation of congestive heart failure [CHF], chest pain)
7. hypo-/hyperglycemia, diabetes out of control
8. gastrointestinal (GI) bleeding, obstruction
9. other than the above reasons
10. reason unknown

These reports can be generated for a specific medical diagnosis, employee, time span, payer, or primary physician. They can also be monitored for active patients only, discharged patients only, or both.

Select Outcomes

The next step in establishing an OBQI project using OASIS data is to determine which outcomes are to be addressed. Selecting the outcomes can be accomplished in two ways: examining outcome reports and examining processes of care that may need improvement.

Option One

Examine outcome reports. One can look at agency-generated reports, electronic system–generated reports (as above), or reports generated by other sources. For example, many states have begun their own OASIS initiatives. The OASIS reports in Chapter 6 were generated by Outcomes USA, a benchmarking project by the Indiana Association for Home Care using the OASIS minimum data set. Over 120 home health agencies are participating in this program to date. If such a program is not available, agency reports can be compared over time, or among teams (business units or branches). Look for differences in variables that may indicate a need for risk adjustment. Taking any risk adjustment into consideration, look for results that indicate subpar performance, or a possible problem. For example, using the data in Table 12–1, it can be seen that of the five patients in Company B with wounds, three were admitted with wounds and they all still had their wounds at discharge. In Company A, however, seven patients had wounds during the same time frame, four were admitted with wounds, and only one still had a wound at discharge. Why was Company A able to get the wounds healed prior to discharge, and Company B unable to do so?

Option Two

Examine processes of care for various defined populations that may need improvement. An example of this is a diagnosis or condition that is expensive or resource intense. Here the OASIS outcome measures can be used as a baseline and as a means to determine improvement in the process. This alternative for using OASIS data is very similar to the process management described in Chapter 11 and depicted in Figure 11–2. The outcomes measures become the performance metrics. In actuality, however, it is not a process that is being examined, but a subprocess of the core process (patient-focused care process). If the area being examined deals with a diagnosis, the subprocess may take the form of a clinical pathway; if what is being examined is a condition (e.g., wound care), it may be a protocol rather than a subprocess.

Regardless of the method used, there are some key points to remember. First, the outcomes or processes chosen should have a sample size of at least 60 or more patients to make the data more generalizable and to limit the skewing of data with an unusual case. If there is an extreme outlier case, it can be removed to again limit the skewing of data. Second, the outcomes or processes selected should be relevant to agency goals. Finally, agency staff need to be able to influence the outcome, or process, selected by changing their behaviors. It is recommended that only one or two outcomes or one process (e.g., a clinical pathway) be chosen at the start.

Analyze the Process

After selecting the process, the next step is to analyze the process (i.e., investigate the activities that produce the outcomes) for areas that could be improved. If an outcome(s) was selected (option one above) then the process that leads to that outcome must first be determined. For example, referring to Table 12–1, Wounds Outcomes Reports, the subprocess (or in this case protocol) to examine why Company A did better than Company B is wound care.

At this point resistance, or defensiveness, may appear. It is important to anticipate it and then move beyond it. Dealing with it may take a while, but the analysis should continue during this time. One form of defensiveness is that clinicians think of their patients as "sicker." A way to determine if that is true is to adjust for case mix as discussed in Chapter 10. The simplest case mix is an "eyeballing" of demographic variables to see if there are large differences. For example, information available on Table 12–1 that may be pertinent includes length of stay, type of wound, and number of comorbidities. Demographics that might be valuable would be age, sex (could be determined by name), level of functional impairment, prognosis, and whether other caregivers were available in the home. Even if case mix data are not available, it is rare that "sicker" patients would be the only reason for subpar measurements/performance.

Another way to deal with defensiveness is to get people involved. Forming a multidisciplinary CQI team to handle the project is a good beginning. From here, suggestions and help can also be solicited from other staff members. The team should include clinicians who are interested in the chosen topic and whose practice could be affected by any changes in the subprocess, pathway, or protocol. The need is to determine the activities that are associated with this subprocess, pathway, or protocol. (Refer to Figure 8–4 to see the relationship of these items.)

A CQI technique that may be useful here and has not been previously discussed, is the cause and effect diagram. This technique is used to identify and display possible causes for a poor outcome or condition. It is sometimes called a fishbone diagram because it takes on the shape of fishbones. See Figure 12–1 for a sample diagram.

The effect (or problem) is stated on the righthand side of the diagram and all the possible causes are listed on the left side. For every effect (problem) there are likely to be several major categories of causes. The categories used in Figure 12–1 are patients, family/caregivers, clinicians, and methods. These are only suggestions. The major categories to select are the ones that assist team members to think creatively. The causes can be generated in two ways: (1) brainstorming, or (2) having team members investigate possible causes by examining the process prior to the meeting and bringing their ideas with them.

Determine Changes or Reinforcements

Once the current process is analyzed, required changes are then determined. There are numerous ways to determine these changes using various CQI tech-

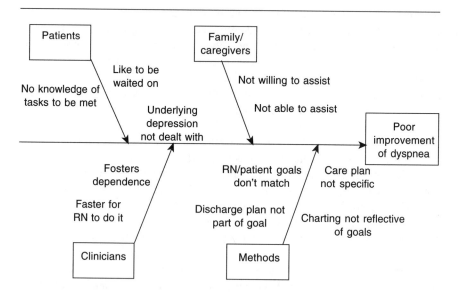

Figure 12–1 Fishbone Diagram

niques such as flowcharts and control charts, which have been discussed previously. Some of these techniques have been used as part of analyzing the process. Perhaps the simplest method is to start with brainstorming optimal care behaviors for this particular subprocess or protocol. Using the wound example, what would be the best practices associated with wound care? Of course, experts in the form of clinical specialists, journal articles, and medical Web sites could also be consulted.

Another approach is to compare the agency subprocess with a benchmark agency, or another team within the same agency that is getting better results, to see where the differences are in the subprocess. Again using the wound example, Company B could consult Company A to see what it is doing, and Company B could then incorporate the differences that represent improvements. The ultimate task is to determine the best practices (or better practices) and then compare those with current activities to see where the differences exist and make changes accordingly.

A third good option is to do a focused review of agency charts to see how often the optimal care behaviors are actually used (or how often they are missed). Suggested steps for performing the review are the following:[12]

1. Determine the most important behaviors list or critical path to utilize in the chart review.
2. Identify patients in the target population (e.g., patients who demonstrate the potential to achieve the outcome being studied at admission; patients who had not achieved the outcome being studied by discharge).
3. Select the time intervals to study to capture the required data (e.g., selected times such as the first 60 days, or the entire episode of care).
4. Select the reviewers.
5. Develop or adapt a review form that includes the criteria (behaviors being utilized), a scoring column, and an area for the totals.
6. Pilot the criteria and review form; revise as necessary.
7. Choose a record review sample (15–20 cases) selected at random from the target population.
8. Conduct the chart review.
9. Interpret the results in one of two ways: (1) the percentage of care behaviors present for each patient, or (2) the percentage of each behavior documented across all patients.
10. Clearly state the problem (e.g., the inadequate care behaviors) or the strength (e.g., the exemplary care behaviors—example: 82 percent of the wound care patients that were discharged with a healed wound received instruction on how to change a dressing; only 25 percent of patients who still had a wound at discharge received that instruction).

Develop a Plan of Action

A plan of action is simply a listing of suggestions or options for improving the outcome. It should be written out as a formal plan. One suggested form is the action grid presented in Chapter 11 (see Table 11–10).

Some generic approaches and actions for improving performance are listed in Table 12–3. Holding an inservice is the most popular approach, but it is limited in its usefulness. The persons requiring the inservice the most are the least likely to be present, those present that don't need it get bored, and it is expensive to pull everyone out of the field.

The goal of the plan is to improve the use of the defined optimum behaviors and thereby improve the outcomes. The performance measures for the plan would be the same OASIS-based outcomes that were originally used to assess the problem.

Implement the Plan

Once the problem is clearly stated, the findings summarized and reported, and a written action plan developed, it is time to communicate the plan to all involved. The actual implementation of the plan should coincide with the data collection for the outcome report. In other words, in order to see the results of the actions, the actions need to coincide with the data that are going to appear on the next report. If reports are generated every six months (January and July) from data that are collected from June to December and January to June, one would not want to implement a change in March because only half of the data on the report in July would represent the change. It would be best to implement the change in June or January.

Once the plan is implemented, charts of all clinicians affected by the change should be monitored on a monthly basis to ascertain whether the changes have been incorporated into their practice. Positive behaviors should be reinforced, even celebrated, and problems/questions should be addressed. Staff must be

---

Table 12–3 Action Plan Approaches and Actions

Approaches	Actions
Education	Inservice
	Mentoring/peer support
Clinical competencies	Demo/return demo of required techniques
	Incorporate into evaluation/orientation
New documentation tools	Implement clinical path
	Implement new protocol
	Disseminate new procedures

supported long enough for old habits to be forgotten and new behaviors to be well established. Actions and behaviors should be monitored for at least six months, perhaps longer, depending on the extent of the change.

Evaluate Changes

Examine the group of outcome reports that reflect the implemented change to determine the degree of success and whether further changes need to be made. If the results are still not at an acceptable level, go back to reanalyzing the process, determining changes, establishing an action plan, and so on. Regardless of the results, communicate the outcomes (and a discussion of what they mean) to the staff and all those involved. Even if the outcomes are good, they should continue to be monitored to be sure that the new behaviors are maintained. One way to do this is to add them to the agency quality plan.

This OBQI process makes good use of the OASIS outcome data in whatever format an agency chooses to use it, whether it be in the form of state-generated reports, vendor-generated reports, or agency-tabulated reports. Keys to success in using this process include the following:

- Obtaining OASIS outcome reports on a regular basis even if they only represent agency data. The data can be divided by team, branch, physician, clinician, diagnosis, or other.
- Having someone accountable for reviewing and reacting to the OASIS outcome reports.
- Using an iterative combination of data analysis and clinical judgment to achieve the best results.
- Developing a *written* plan of action.
- Having someone accountable for implementing and monitoring the change.
- Willingly revising the process again if indicated.

THE VALUE OF CARE

Another factor in the meaningfulness of care has to do with the value received—in other words, is the cost of care appropriate for the value received? Activity-based cost management (ABCM) is a tool to quantify the consumption of organizational resources. The quantification can be used to determine cost per episode of care and organizational profitability, or to determine the provision of value from the customer's perspective. The combination of the concepts of cost and quality will provide a framework for maximizing activities that provide value to the customer, minimizing activities that support business pursuits, and eliminating activities that add cost, but not value. Working within payer guidelines provides a methodology for determining what activities are valued by the payer and, consequently, should be maximized. Conversely, those activities that are not valued should be minimized. Understanding payer guidelines will provide a framework for organizations to identify services that provide value and activities that are critical for the provision of value from the payer's perspective.

The question that agencies need to have answered is whether the payer expects the home health care agency to operate on a medical or health model. A medical model focuses on returning the patient to independence, or their pre-episodic condition, using the most efficient route possible. It is a symptom-management process. A health model goes further, looks at the root cause of the episode, and attempts to reeducate the individual to correct his or her behaviors (or patterns) that may have caused the underlying problem and resultant symptom. The goal of a health model is either to prevent the illness or disease from occurring or, once it has occurred, to teach the individual to manage his or her own symptoms and care. The concept of health can even expand into the community by evaluating additional external (environmental) factors that may have negatively influenced the individual's problems. Outside, or community, factors that contributed to patient problems are addressed and improved where possible.

The challenge for providers is to identify which model supports their mission statement and which model is expected by their pay sources. For instance, imagine that a patient is discharged to a home health care provider who has contracted with the patient's managed care organization (MCO). Prior to discharge from the hospital, six home care visits were approved by the MCO for wound care. In this example, the MCO is operating under a medical model paradigm. It is interested in the patient's wound healing and the patient returning to work or no longer requiring health care services. From the perspective of the agency, it will need to provide the medical interventions necessary to accomplish this goal. Family and environmental assessments, nutritional teaching, and emotional support are not considered. The method of payment then has an impact on the type of activities that are provided. The agency may be able to accomplish the MCO's objective by substituting an LPN for a RN. The reimbursement received by the agency from the MCO for each visit would remain the same, but the agency cost could be less for the LPN. Or, the agency may perform the six visits and only do wound care. Again, the reimbursement from the MCO would remain the same, but reducing the number of interventions could reduce the cost per visit to the agency if the clinician is able to increase his or her productivity (number of visits per day).

The presumption of a lower cost per visit is dependent upon an agency's payment methodology. If the agency compensates field staff using a per-visit payment methodology, then there will be no change in the cost per visit. On the other hand, if the agency has transitioned field staff to salaried positions and additional visits can be performed as a result of a shorter visit (fewer interventions), then an opportunity exists for a lower cost per visit.

In the above example, the home health provider would only perform the necessary interventions, protocols, and procedures to heal the wound outlined in the MCO's medical model (e.g., return the individual to his or her pre-episode health status). If the MCO negotiated a wellness or health model with the home health care provider, however, then it might expand its interventions, protocols, and procedures to include assessing the patient's approach to nutrition and general well-being. It would then build education and related interventions into the remaining visits. These added interventions may increase the amount of direct care time associated with the remaining visits but may prevent later readmissions and/or hospitalizations.

Historically, the foundation of home care supported wellness and health models. Medicare brought in a medical model, and home care struggled for years to put a round peg in a square hole, so that home care services could be reimbursed. This process took several forms including much creative charting. Now in the era of MCOs, an agency needs to reevaluate its mission, vision, and values once again and then seek out payers that support them. This process may be an iterative one (e.g., an agency may need to provide data to the MCO to show the long-term savings of a wellness model rather than the short-term cost efficiency of a medical model).

Milliman and Robertson offer two principles for home health care providers to keep in mind with respect to the efficient delivery of health care services.[13]

1. The services provided must not include any service that is not medically necessary or that is more intense than is medically necessary, to produce improvement in health status that the patient has a right to expect.
2. The care should not be provided by a clinician with a greater level of expertise than is medically necessary to provide the medically appropriate care, unless the provider is willing to provide care at a cost that is equivalent to the cost for a provider having the appropriate level of expertise.

Table 12–4 illustrates the impact that different levels (Level A = medical, B = mixed, and C = wellness, health) of direct care have on nursing productivity. The longer the direct care, the fewer the number of visits. Albeit, in reality there would be a mix of visit type and duration on any given day or over the course of a month; however, the illustration offers an example for the pricing of services.

Table 12–5 illustrates how differences in the length of direct care (visits/day), composed of interventions and protocols, will affect cost per visit.

One point that is not recognized in these examples is that care also needs to be meaningful. Besides being efficient, the provision of care needs to be effective and accomplish stated goals and objectives. The question is, how broad are these

Table 12–4 Assessment of Nursing Productivity

Activities	A	B	C
Direct Care	30	60	90
Documentation	20	20	20
Travel	30	30	30
Coordination	10	10	10
Average Visit Time	90	120	150
8-Hour Day with 30-Minute Break	450	450	450
Average Visits/Day	5.0	3.75	3.0

goals and objectives—are they medically or health oriented? And do the rates paid by the MCO support the defined goals?

Table 12–5 illustrates the initial question which was, Is the cost appropriate for the value received? Table 12–5 illustrates cost per visit for three types of visits: A = medical model, B = mixed, and C = health model. Several assumptions were made in Tables 12–4 and 12–5. First, all activities were static with respect to the amount of time they consumed, except direct care. Second, a nurse would not have a mix of visits (e.g., some type A, some B, and/or some C), thereby mixing the costs per visit. The third assumption is that all wellness activities would be done during a home visit. Fourth, each group of activities builds on the preceding (e.g., B is more inclusive than A and C is more inclusive than B). Therefore, the additional value added is from the preceding group of activities (B from A and C from B). The additional value from A to C is $24.35. The point of the illustration is to exemplify that home care agencies are in a position to provide additional value to the MCO patient; however, they cannot continue to operate under a cost reimbursement paradigm. Home care agencies must negotiate the amount of additional value created through interventions targeted at wellness, nutrition, and general well-being into contract pricing. Otherwise, they need to revise their approach to the provision of care to be consistent with the MCO's philosophy.

It will be unfortunate, however, if MCOs do not recognize the value provided through interventions targeted toward patient wellness, nutrition, and general

Table 12–5 Identification of Additional Value Added to Each Nursing Visit

	A	B	C
Average Visits/Day	5.0	3.75	3.0
Productive Days	230	230	230
Annual Visits	1,150	863	690
Annual Cost	$42,000	$42,000	$42,000
Cost per Visit	$36.52	$48.67	$60.87
Additional Value Added		$12.15	$12.20

well-being. The field nurse has an opportunity to provide incremental value to the patient throughout the provision of additional interventions while she or he is in the home. Currently, a tool does not exist to quantify the long-term value of providing additional interventions. If one did exist, however, it would be interesting to know how many readmissions were prevented and how much patient quality of life was enhanced.

Adopting a time-based methodology for costing the activity of direct care identifies the total cost for that activity. Further refinement using the number of interventions associated with instruction, assessment, and direct care will assist agencies in developing finite approaches for the costing of clinical pathways. Once in place, this methodology will identify the type of interventions, protocols, and procedures to offer once a care model (medical or health) and payer and staff payment methodologies have been determined.

In addition to direct care, agencies need to negotiate additional activities, such as the transportation of laboratory samples, community education, free screening, flu shots, and a predischarge home assessment, into their contractual negotiations. Other considerations are telephone visits and telehealth technology. All of these activities represent a cost to an agency. If it does not provide value from the MCO's perspective and the MCO is not willing to compensate the agency for these activities, then a decision must be made. Either the agency will continue to provide these activities at its own cost as a service to the community, or the activities will be refocused to medical necessity if it reflects the agency mission, or the MCO contract will be dropped.

The new paradigm, however, offers a broader view of health care. The old paradigm is compliance-driven health care. This autocratic, medical model care is of questionable benefit to those in home care with chronic diseases. The new paradigm is a risk-driven, or evidence-based, care to prevent avoidable illness and focuses on self-management. In this paradigm, the agency invests in the community to help reduce risk. Already there are examples of hospitals or health systems buying traffic lights for accident-prone intersections with the resultant reduction of emergency room trauma cases. Home care agencies can follow this example.

This notion of risk-based care is further exemplified in capitation payment and the capitating of larger hospitals and health systems. When a hospital or health system is capitated, it shares the cost risk of care with the payer. Thus, it has a vested interest in keeping its catchment population as healthy as possible. Home care has a place in this scenario, and agencies need to consider how they can be of service, or give back to, the community (e.g., geographical community or covered lives in an MCO contract). Being of service is to enhance wellness while at the same time rendering care to individuals in need. The underlying need is for data on demographics and evidence of risk/need. One way to gather these data is through the community assessments discussed in Chapter 10. In addition, the more experience an agency has with gathering data about the care effectiveness and its cost (efficiency), the more solid its position for negotiating viable capitated contracts that will provide meaningful care.

THE EMPOWERED CONSUMER/PARTNERING

One of the cornerstones of the health management paradigm is consumer empowerment. Although everyone knows that people (individuals, families, or communities) have the diseases or conditions, it is easy for providers to get caught up with treating the condition and not the person. This focus on disease slides in unnoticed as practitioners are pushed to be more efficient, or payers base reimbursement on a physical situation and not what concerns the customer. As the health care system evolves from a sickness-based system to a system incorporating prevention and education, the recipient of care will have a more active role and be considered more a customer than a patient.

There are several factors merging that are generating an increase in demands from patients to actively understand, participate in, and influence their health status—in other words, to be empowered. These factors include[14]

1. increasing trend of consumers at all levels to demand more say and more information in all of their relationships with organizations—government, schools, hotel chains, airlines, and health care
2. increasing occurrence and treatment of chronic disease over acute disease
3. increasing economic involvement (and risk exposure) of patients as they pay for larger portions of their health insurance
4. increasing availability of health information in print media, television, and on the Internet (it is estimated that 38 percent of people use the Internet to acquire health and medical information)[15]
5. rapid growth of capitated contracts under managed care, which creates financial incentives to promote patient involvement and education

An additional factor is the growth of telehealth. Telehealth, a derivative of telemedicine, focuses on prevention through the use of patient education, early recognition of alterations in vital signs, awareness of changes in health status, and improved compliance in medication and treatment regimens. The current telehealth systems utilize a combination of audio, video, and data sent between patients and home health agencies. Systems use a number of telecommunications links including two-way cable, local area networks (LANs), wide-band pipes, or ordinary telephone systems. Recent developments in data compression have allowed for the transmission of more data over telephone lines, thus increasing the access of patients to telehealth systems since the majority of households have phones.[16] The increased ability to send data over phone lines allows for greater patient education through the use of videos. It also provides for a stronger provider/patient partnership in monitoring symptom measurements and accurate treatment/medication regimens.

As electronic communication of patient information becomes increasingly available, informed patients are likely to ask for copies. This request is especially true for communication via e-mail; in fact, patients may actively participate by sending their own e-mail. As patients join the communication stream, many of the barriers that prevented their involvement disappear. Given the ability and extra time to check additional resources, look up vocabulary, post questions on the Internet, and ask questions of other family members, motivated patients will compose well-thought-out questions and responses.[17]

An example of the overwhelming desire of patients to become informed customers occurred in Massachusetts in November 1996. At that time, Massachusetts became the first state in the country to make information on file at the State Board of Registration in Medicine available to the public. Customers could call a toll-free number (or log onto the Internet) to request physician profiles that included

- education, experience, and credentials
- any disciplinary action from the state medical board or hospitals
- number and size of any malpractice payments
- average number of malpractice claims for a specific specialty

There were more than 6,000 calls the first day, and the State Board of Registration has had to double the number of phone lines and operators in order to handle the volume.[18]

As consumers become more informed and empowered, several things will occur:[19]

- Consumers will be able to select agencies that perform well (e.g., meet their expectations) and avoid those that perform poorly.
- Gaps that are troubling within the system will become apparent, providing the opportunity for improvement.
- The opportunity for consumers to become better partners with the provider is enhanced.
- More public discussions about consumer expectations will appear.

It is obvious that agency success will be determined by how well an agency meets customer expectations. Thus, before any involvement with the consumer occurs, one must check to be sure that everyone involved in the relationship has the same expectations. This principle is important at the clinician level as well as at the agency level. The reason is that if the consumers' expectations exceed what the provider can offer, there will be dissatisfaction and disaster. Ultimately, the best way to deal with establishing equal expectations is through data, information, and communication. Mutual expectations can be established at the individual level at the start of care by jointly setting up expected outcomes and then reviewing and revising them as care progresses. At the agency level, setting up information accessibility for the agency's customers becomes paramount. The types of data that need to be formatted for customer information are depicted in Figure 12–2 and discussed below.

This figure depicts three concentric circles, the middle of which is broken into four segments. The innermost circle is the center, or beginning, of information—data. Much has already been discussed about data. Two pionts need to be reinforced here. First, data always need to be collected from the perspective of the customer in support of agency strategy and vision. Data that do not support agency strategies, patient outcomes, and quality initiatives, or indicate progress toward goals lose their meaningfulness. Second, data must provide the basis for taking action. Empowerment requires the accessibility of data in order for appropriate action to be taken. Information provides the ability for a customer to make an informed decision. If customers have access to information, they can take respon-

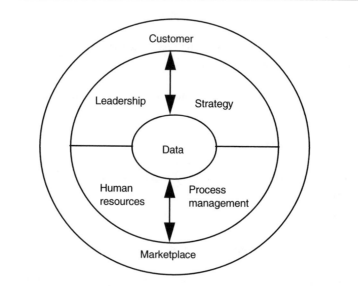

Figure 12–2 Information Accessibility for Customers

sibility for resolving problems, making appropriate decisions, and participating in the pursuit of their individual and group vision.

The outer circle in Figure 12–2 represents those to whom the data must be accessible—to and from the customer and marketplace. Who are the customers? Everyone whose decisions determine whether the organization or agency will succeed.[20] This group may be complex and multilayered, but it is important to know and serve it. There are three basic groups of customers that all organizations serve.

1. End users—The final customer outside the organization or the customer that uses the service (e.g., patients). Agencies must provide more information accessibility to this group of customers, but the other groups also need information.
2. Intermediate customers—People who assist in making services available to patients (e.g., payers, suppliers, surveyors, accreditors, physicians, referral sources).
3. Internal customers—Employees. People within the organization who use the service/product of a process and carry out the next function (e.g., nurses use the product [referral] of the intake process to provide the next function [care]) in order to serve the end user.

The middle circle in Figure 12–2 represents the four domains of data that must be formatted into information for the customers: strategy, process management, human resources, and leadership. The strategy and process management domains represent deployment of actions of the agency—what they are and how well they are done. The human resources and leadership domains represent the persons who are doing the deploying, including their philosophies and their abilities. The following discusses each of these areas in detail.

Strategy

Information accessibility for strategies includes the agency's strategic priorities and how they are being pursued or changed. As mentioned previously, health care reformation will require a more customer-centered approach by agencies, and the commitment to the overall health care needs of the community. The seven basics for developing a customer-centered agency are the following:[21]

1. *Create a Customer-Keeping Vision.* This vision is in concert with what was discussed in Chapter 5; however, be sure it depicts a state that is connected to the customer.

2. *Saturate the Organization with the Voice of the Customer.* Create a real intimacy with current, potential (especially members of an MCO), and prior

customers. Listen to those who are happy and those who are not. Use all the information to provide a better experience to current customers. Home care has been weak in this area. Unfortunately, if a patient complains, the usual response is that he or she is being unrealistic, or the payer won't pay for that. As home care becomes more competitive, agencies will benefit from listening and seeing what can be done. On the other hand, if an agency's action isn't adding value for customers, eliminate it.

3. *Sanction Customer Advocates.* This basic fundamental involves setting the unswerving goal of putting customer satisfaction first and remembering that employees are also customers and should be treated as such. The job of management becomes one of creating an environment that supports employees' pursuit of customer satisfaction. Employees really do want to serve their patients well.

4. *Smash the Barriers to Customer-Winning Performance.* This fundamental means that the barriers (physical, emotional, mental) that prevent employees from serving customers efficiently and effectively are eliminated. Make sure that staff have the physical resources (e.g., equipment) and the information and training to do their job. Eliminating these types of barriers results in both customer satisfaction and lower costs.

5. *Learn from the Winners.* Use benchmarking both in terms of measurement and in visiting companies that do it best. Depending on the process being investigated, health care may not always be the best place to look. Other service industries, such as the airlines, may provide valuable information.

6. *Measure, Measure, Measure.* Measurement has been discussed previously, but there are five important principles to keep in mind when measuring: (1) know why you are measuring, (2) let customers tell you which end results to measure, (3) continually ask how well you are doing (customer satisfaction), (4) track the processes as well as the end results, and (5) tell employees everything you learn.

7. *Talk the Talk and Walk the Walk.* Leaders at every level, including the clinician that makes the home visit, must embody the agency's purpose and vision. Leaders act upon customer feedback to design today's activities and tomorrow's services. Leaders continue to keep their fingers on the customer pulse to anticipate their needs, creating the "ah-ha" level of quality.

Process Management

This is the aggregated data presented as information on the quality of everyone's activities. Unfortunately, little is known about the type of health quality information end users want and about how to best present the information so it is meaningful and useful. Without this perspective, data about health care quality run the risk of being irrelevant. On the national level, there is some feedback that indicates that customers are not pleased with the Health Plan Employer Data and Information Set (HEDIS) report cards; they want indicators more relevant to their needs. They find the current measures irrelevant and not understandable.[22]

The Foundation for Accountability (FACCT), a nonprofit organization established in 1995 to ensure that consumers have reliable information to make health care decisions, is working with consumers to determine what measures would be more meaningful. FACCT seeks to assemble and endorse portfolios of existing measures that shed meaningful light on the quality of care. Its goal is to have its measures used by government agencies, consumer groups, regulators, and accreditors. In 1996, FACCT produced measures for breast cancer, diabetes, major depressive disorders, health risks, and customer satisfaction with a health plan. In development are proposed measures for asthma, arthritis, heart disease, alcohol use, health status, and pediatric care.[23]

The reality is that consumers are becoming more knowledgeable and involved across the country. Individual agencies need to be aware of this movement and engage the consumer more in determining end results that are meaningful.

Human Resources

The data required in human resources relates to the information that clinicians, employees, and intermediate customers and patients need to make decisions. This information includes both customer priorities and the impact that customer decisions have on the larger agency process. It answers questions such as, Who is able to do what on this health care team? How are the accountabilities shared in reaching desired outcomes? For example, are patients given copies of their plan of care or pathway? If not, how does the patient get this information? Does the patient have defined interventions to carry out (for which he or she is accountable)? How does he or she know what they are? How does the patient learn how to do them? If someone on the team was supposed to teach him or her and didn't, what was the impact and how does the patient then get the information? Who else on the team is qualified to teach it? How does that person get the assignment? The questions go on. All of these data aid the patient in self-management of disease symptoms and health status.

The other type of data needed is on the staff themselves. Data are needed to evaluate staff competencies for meeting current and future needs. Data are also valuable for enabling "niching." Niching allows people to specialize their work activities according to their own preferences. Niching allows staff to complement one another and do what they like and do best. For example, if one nurse is good at assessments but not teaching, she or he could do the assessments on patients and someone else who enjoys teaching could do the patient education. Having such data available allows for staff with different specialties to be placed on the same team.

Leadership

The data on leadership includes the measurement of leadership effectiveness. These data include the concept of a 360–degree review process (by all those surrounding the leader), as described in the next chapter. Successful leaders carry out the customer-centered basics listed above under Strategy. Additional leadership behaviors include the following:

- Personally put the customer first.
- Promote the agency vision.
- Constantly seek new ways to learn—"student for life."
- Facilitate/teach.
- Believe in and invest in employees.
- Build customer-focused teams.
- Celebrate successes.
- Encourage collaboration—"partnering."
- Lead by example.
- Accept feedback from stakeholders, customers, and employees.

The key to all this information accessibility is listening, listening to what is said by each and every customer. Listening is the cornerstone for communicating and sharing. Listening with C.A.R.E. (Compassion/commitment: Attention: Respect: Empathy) fosters rapport, trust, team spirit, and effectiveness. It also encourages empowerment by building confidence. It is important to focus totally on the person speaking, encourage the person speaking to be clear about what he or she is saying, listen to what is being said with a clear mind, rather than thinking about a reply, and be open to alternative outcomes.

PROCESS OF LEARNING—LEARNING ENVIRONMENT

As customers become empowered, the health care system will continue to change in more dynamically complex ways. It has already been stated that to maintain the meaningfulness of care, agencies and individuals must capture this opportunity and redesign services in concert with customer expectations and needs. This change is an evolution, not an event; the way to deal with the change is to establish a systems approach to learning as well as managing. This approach creates an environment where all become "perpetual students." Perpetual students accept each event as it unfolds and then use the experience as an opportunity for creating a better day, or better event. This continual learning is the foundation of CQI. In order to establish such an environment, three tools are required: (1) systems design/thinking, (2) a cultural system for the learning journey, and (3) group tools for team building. Each of these will be discussed further.

Systems Design/Thinking

Much has been discussed about processes and systems and their importance in this book. The question remains, however, How does one think in terms of system design? The following steps will move one from events thinking to systems thinking:

- Start thinking about a given problem or situation before acting on it. One way to begin is to have each person involved in the situation tell the story of the problem or events from his or her point of view. This describes the current reality.
- Next, connect the present with the past by looking for behavior over time or patterns (e.g., are there other stories that corroborate these events? Are these events a repeated pattern?).
- Describe the systemic structures that are creating the identified behavior patterns. For example, are customer problems resolved by dealing with the symptom rather than by improving or redesigning the process? This type of resolution leads to crisis management and the creation of "heroes" who deal with the symptom in the nick of time to avoid customer complaints or service disaster, rather than encouraging employees to address the agencywide system problems.
- Once a theory is established about what is happening, look at the underlying issues (root causes) to determine future action from the basis of understanding what is happening. For example, What are the mental models (e.g., assumptions, beliefs, or values) that sustain the structure? Or, what is the relationship to the larger system? What is the vision that this pattern is operating under? What is my role in the situation? If a symptom is addressed rather than a root cause, a different symptom will appear somewhere else that has the same root cause.
- The final step is to determine what kinds of changes could be made to prevent this situation from happening in the future. Guiding questions include[24] What is the vision of the future? What assumptions, beliefs, and values will help realize this vision? What systemic structures are required to do this? What

would be the behavior of key indicators if the desired vision became reality? What specific events would illustrate how well the vision is operating on a day-to-day basis?

Cultural System for the Learning Journey

From an individual perspective, one of the most important underpinnings of the practice of systems thinking are attitudes of curiosity (inquiry) and mindfulness. Mindfulness is the heightened awareness of our own thought processes.[25] From an agency perspective, an important underpinning is the ability to delve into the culture and the underlying assumptions, beliefs, and values (mental models) that exist in the culture. Both of these are evolutions, not events. They require an ongoing commitment. Both are difficult if individuals lapse into defensiveness.

Defensiveness is another form of resistance or insecurity. It is one of the main reasons that we focus on external change (internal change is too difficult). So, we focus on government regulation changes (external to the agency) rather than internal agency changes; or management changes (external to the employee) rather than internal employee changes; or patient compliance to a pathway or care plan (external to the caregiver) rather than customer-centered care (internal caregiver changes). Focusing on the external gives the impression of improvement, but until we move forward with internal changes (an inner centeredness), the external lacks substance, becomes boring, and is dehumanized.

Everyone moves to his or her own level of inner centeredness at his or her own rate. A prerequisite for motivating human behavior and development, however, is providing a supportive environment. Key ingredients in a supportive environment include

- clarity about organizational structure
- basic material to accomplish the work at hand
- safety—when people feel safe it is easier for them to express their concerns, desires, and accomplishments, especially when these are below agency expectations
- authentic communication—an open revealing of one person to another in an accepting relationship
- ongoing honest feedback on how well individuals, teams, and the agency are creating and implementing processes and activities
- positive outlook and positive thinking
- respect for each individual
- leadership by example

Another element in dissolving defensiveness is establishing trust and a spirit of collegiality. One of the cornerstones of collegiality is dialogue. Dialogue differs from discussion. Dialogue comes from the Greek term for "through talking" and was used to uncover hidden truths. Currently, it is used as a means to exchange ideas without trying to change the other person's mind. The rules of dialogue include: no arguing, no interrupting, and listen with C.A.R.E. Unfortunately, what usually prevails is discussion. "To discuss" originally meant to "dash to pieces." The underlying purpose of any discussion, no matter how friendly, is to smash the other guy's argument and promote your own.[26] Moving from discussion to dialogue requires practice and is best integrated into an agency culture through practice sessions. Practice sessions using the rules of dialogue can be weekly meetings with no agenda to talk about personal or professional topics.

Team Building (Group Tools)

A team can be defined as an interactive group of people who share a common goal(s) and work together interdependently to achieve that goal(s). There are many types of teams in the home care arena. There are health care teams that provide care with the patient; there are management teams; there are cross-functional work teams to accomplish activities that cross department lines such as introducing a new computer system; and there are CQI project teams. Being a team member is different from working autonomously. Working on one type of team, such as a CQI team, may help one be a better team member on another type of team, such as the caregiving team.

Teams offer greater expertise than any one individual and, therefore, usually provide better total results than would have been accomplished by any or all members acting independently. For a team to be effective, however, it must have the following characteristics:

- clarity of purpose—a mission or goal(s) or a clear vision
- defined activities to accomplish the mission (sometimes called a charter)
- established measurements of progress toward goals
- members who are committed to the team and who possess all the necessary knowledge, skill, and experience to accomplish the activities (diverse talent)
- an identified leader, but a democratic process with open, multidirectional communication and mutual support
- defined roles, responsibilities, accountability, and degrees of authority for each team member
- member involvement that includes a respect for other team members, trust for each other, and sensitivity to each other's needs

- power and incentives to accomplish the mission
- collaboration and cooperation with each other and with nonteam members who can help get the job done
- an inquiring attitude, creativity, and a search for excellence
- optimism, positive thinking, and willingness to take risks

So how does all this relate to meaningful care? Remember, it is a team that gives care. As patients become more active consumers of care, they will rightfully take their place as the leader of their health care team. Clinicians and providers of care need to reexamine their roles and responsibilities on this team. These roles may change from patient to patient depending on the patient's expectations. The need for increased awareness (mindfulness) and for examining systems of care becomes paramount as the care process evolves along with consumer empowerment. Assumptions and beliefs about care and the clinician's role need to be examined.

No longer is there routine care, only perhaps routine team charters that are individualized to meet patient expectations. For example, What activity categories have been established for providing care in your agency? These categories were discussed in Chapter 8 under Clinical Pathways, and again in Chapter 9 in Activity-Based Costing. Now, these categories appear again. This time they are the basis for a team charter for the patient-centered care process. One of these activities could be direct, hands-on care. If so, this would be one of the team's charter activities. Then different types of hands-on care could be defined for each patient by the health care team. How the care would be carried out would be defined in part by guidelines, protocols, and procedures. Defining team membership may be assisted by the use of position descriptions and individual skills and qualities. Conversely, defined team needs may influence position descriptions and required skills and qualities. The interconnectedness of the subprocesses continues to be exposed as the search for meaningful care and performance excellence continues.

CONCLUSION

This chapter has dealt with the essential elements of providing meaningful care. Factors of meaningful care include technical components such as CQI and OBQI and how to get the most out of them to render effective care. They also include people—the empowered consumer and the care provider. As technology advances and the patient becomes the empowered consumer, the provider of care (individual and agency) needs to shift from an external concern for improvement to an internal focus on growth in order to deal with the monumental changes. The secret ingredient to meaningful care becomes the secure care provider who is mindful of his or her activities and is a "perpetual student."

Furthermore, this chapter has continued to examine the interconnectedness of subprocesses within the agency. One of the underpinnings of the consumer-focused care process and its subprocesses is the activities of care. These activities become the basis for clinical pathway development, costing clinical pathways and care, and the health care team charter. These activities may also be pivotal in establishing intensity of care.

NOTES

1. D.A. Peters and J. Pearlson, Clinical Evaluation: Research or Quality Assurance, *Journal of Nursing Quality Assurance* 3, no. 3 (1989): 1–6.

2. D. Christiano, Your Address May Be Hazardous to Your Health, *Good Housekeeping* (January 1998): 62–64.

3. E. Larson, Combining Nursing Quality Assurance and Research Programs, *The Journal of Nursing Administration* (November 1983): 32–38.

4. P. Plsek, *Quality Improvement Projects* (Paul E. Plsek Associates, 1989).

5. R.A. Mueller, Implementing TQM in Health Care Requires Adaptation and Innovation, *Quality Progress* 15, no. 4 (1992): 57–59.

6. D.H. Kim, Service Quality Excellence: Mastering the "Moments of Truth," *The Systems Thinker* 3, no. 7 (1992): 1–7.

7. Mueller, Implementing TQM, 57–59.

8. Mueller, Implementing TQM, 57–59.

9. Kim, Service Quality Excellence, 1–7.

10. P.E. Morrison and J. Heineke, Why Do Health Care Practitioners Resist Quality Management? *Quality Progress* 15, no. 4 (1992): 51–55.

11. *OASIS-B* (Denver, CO: Center for Health Services and Policy Research, 1997).

12. P.W. Shaughnessy and K.S. Crisler, *Outcome Based Quality Improvement* (Denver, CO: Colorado Center for Health Policy and Services Research, 1995), 7.19.

13. D.J. Hulet, Health Status Improvement and Management—The Next Generation of the Healthcare Management Guidelines, located on their Internet site, http://www.milliman.com.

14. R.B. Bruegel, The Increasing Importance of Patient Empowerment and Its Potential Impacts on Home Care Information Systems and Technology, *Home Health Care Management and Practice* 10, no. 2 (1998): 73–79.

15. P.G. Ribnick and V.A. Carrano, Health Care Accountability: Communicating Quality to the Public, *Journal of Nursing Care Quality* 11, no. 6 (1997): 9–13.

16. I. Warner, Telemedicine in Home Care: The Current Status of Practice, *Home Health Care Management and Practice* 10, no. 2 (1998): 66–72.

17. Bruegel, The Increasing Importance of Patient Empowerment, 73–79.

18. Warner, Telemedicine, 66–72.

19. D. Lansky, Foundation for Accountability (FACCT): A Consumer Voice on Health Care Quality, *JCOM* 3, no. 6 (1996): 54–58.

20. R.C. Whiteley, *The Customer Driven Company* (Reading, MA: Addison-Wesley Publishing Company, 1991), 42.

21. Whiteley, *The Customer Driven Company*.

22. M.C. Marill, ed., HEDIS-Based Report Cards Get an F from Consumers, *Patient Satisfaction & Outcomes Management* 2, no. 12 (1996): 135.

23. Lansky, Foundation for Accountability, 54–58.

24. D.H. Kim, From Event Thinking to Systems Thinking, *The Systems Thinker* 7, no. 4 (1996): 6–7.

25. L.B. Sweeney, Life-Long Systems Thinking Practice, *The Systems Thinker* 7, no. 8 (1996): 6–8.

26. R. Poe, The Secret to Teamwork, *Success* (June 1991): 72.

CHAPTER 13

Aligning Stakeholders and Agency Outcomes

Who are stakeholders? Stakeholders are anyone who has an interest in the well-being of the organization. *Stakeholders* is an all-inclusive term for customers that includes the patient, physicians, referral sources, the patient's family, the community, staff, creditors, shareholders, and the board of directors. Stakeholders are concerned about the efficiency and effectiveness of operations and how operations and their results may affect them. Therefore, when identifying an organization's stakeholders one needs to know whom the organization is serving. Who are the agency's customers, both internal and external, and what do they expect in regard to staff, clinical outcomes, and service?

Next comes the reality test. What kind of results will they experience? Does their actual experience exceed both promised and implied expectations? Would current and past experience with your organization cause them to select your agency over a competitor?

Agency staff have the ability to create memorable customer experiences, both good and bad. What are the factors that motivate staff? What inspires staff to give 100 percent effort toward achieving organizational goals? What makes working for this agency better than working for a competitor?

This chapter is about conveying results to stakeholders. Organizations have multiple sets of stakeholders, and understanding what is important to each group of customers is critical. An initial step in understanding whether operations are providing value to stakeholders is to measure what is important to them. To accomplish this task, one must first determine what is important, measure and monitor these criteria, and be willing to make improvements to the underlying processes. Improvements to underlying processes may be necessary for course correction in the event that results are unfavorable, or for providing continual value and enhancement of existing processes.

The chapter

- examines how an agency measures what is important to stakeholders
- reviews the maintenance of a performance measurement system and improvement of results
- discusses the role of management
- concludes with the conveying of results to stakeholders

MEASURE WHAT IS IMPORTANT

Who are an agency's customers? What is important to them? What is important to the agency? What is important to staff? The preceding questions help to create a mindset for looking outside of the traditional thinking box, or at a minimum, outside of our offices for the answers. Stated differently, to understand what is important to measure from the customer's perspective, one of the best places to begin is with the customer. Ask the customers what they expect and want from their interactions with your agency. To begin with a preconceived idea, based upon information you had in your office, could limit the amount of valuable feedback that is gained through customer interaction. There is also a relevance concern. The measurement system that is created should be developed using relevant measures that reflect customer input instead of measures that are only presumed relevant and are basically irrelevant from the customer's perspective. Doing preliminary research to help identify service parameters will help to supplement existing customer knowledge.

There are many ways to find out what your customers expect and want. An inexpensive starting point is doing a literature search to determine what other people have found. Other ways were defined in Chapter 10 and are reviewed here. For example, customer-specific needs can be identified through informal gathering methods such as conversations with patients who have had home health care experiences, conversations with physicians while they are signing orders, or conversations with referral sources or case managers. Formal methods include brainstorming sessions with colleagues, sending written surveys to customers, telephoning customers using script surveys, or holding focus groups. Each approach has a related cost; informal methods are the cheapest, written and telephone surveys are the next most costly, and focus groups are the most expensive vehicle for gathering customer information.

Focus groups are used to gather specific information about a selected customer group, using a sample of the targeted group. They are a tool to gather ideas, solicit feedback, and/or to understand perceptions/feelings of the larger customer group. Members of a focus group usually have a vested interest in the services being offered, and interaction among participants can provide insights that may not appear using another survey method. For instance, asking the question, "Would you recommend this home health agency to your friends?" could be instrumental in gathering additional information about patient expectations and needs. Getting a negative response will require additional investigative work on the part of the facilitator.

Once the agency has a sound understanding of what the patient expects and wants, it will need to move on to the agency's secondary customer groups such as payers, physicians, and referral sources. Where possible, these groups of customers should also be asked to evaluate the patient assessment tool to determine whether they can add valuable input. This second step may seem repetitive, except that payers, physicians, and referral sources also serve the patient. The patient is their primary customer and they need to make sure that the patient's needs are being met.

A process similar to the one identified above can be repeated to gather service parameters for assessing customer satisfaction for the secondary customer group. Payers, physicians, and referral sources are going to be concerned about patient welfare and satisfaction, the agency's ability to consistently demonstrate improvements in ADLs or health status, and their ability to communicate with each other. In the proposed changes to the Medicare Conditions of Participation (COPs), the Health Care Financing Administration (HCFA) has emphasized the development of predictive measures of care. From HCFA's perspective these measures of care include the amount of time for an assessment visit to be completed, medication compliance, effectiveness in training staff, clinical improvements, functional improvements, and patient satisfaction.[1]

The significance of predictive indicators is extremely important. Performance measures fall into two categories: lagging and leading. Lagging indicators are primarily financial and are reflective of events that have already happened. Leading indicators are predictive in nature and act as harbingers of events that have not manifested. For instance, payer and risk mix are the lead indicators in the financial section of a potential agency scorecard. (See Exhibit 4–1 for a listing of possible financial indicators on a scorecard.) They are lead indicators because, if the payer mix would shift to a less profitable mix, the shift would provide a harbinger of financial loss and would precede the reporting of a loss in the financial statements.

From an agency perspective, managers will want to determine how effective they are in pursuing their strategic objectives. Strategic priorities are unique to every agency. One agency may be hospital based, another free-standing, and another part of a large national chain. There are four strategies, however, that were previously presented in Chapter 11 and that apply to all agencies. They are:

1. to demonstrate quality
2. to be as cost-effective as possible

3. to be customer focused and demonstrate stakeholder or customer satisfaction
4. to emphasize organizational learning and growth

Strategies should be supported by the agency's value system and aligned with the agency's measurement system. Strategy development should consider the diverse needs of primary and secondary customer groups. It needs to identify opportunities for meeting customer needs and fulfilling business requirements such as profitability, and it needs to consider the management of the resources that will enable the agency to accomplish its goals. Management of resources should consider both tangible and intangible resources. Staff represent intangible resources that need to be cultivated to meet the ever-changing and evolving needs of the customer and business environment. Strategic measurement systems begin with the development of high-level performance measures to support strategies. Alignment of strategic measures occurs when measures at the strategic level are supported at the process level and then again at the individual, team, and work unit level. Figure 3–3 illustrated the concept of a cascading performance measurement system. Figure 13–1 illustrates alignment between strategy, performance measures, and action plans.

A cascading performance measurement system is critical for the alignment of processes and staff toward common strategies. Figure 13–2 identifies the four generic strategies identified above. Each would use aggregate performance measures to assess whether goals and objectives were being realized. These aggregate measures could then be used for conveying results to stakeholders. In this figure, the strategy illustrated is customer satisfaction. There were five aggregate indicators of customer satisfaction: physician, patient, payer, referral source, and community satisfaction. The outcomes reflected in these aggregate indicators were the result of activities performed in the patient-focused care process—the core process as described earlier in this text.

Therefore, if the goal is to convey ever-improving results to stakeholders there must be alignment between strategic objectives and organizational processes. The concept of cascading performance measurement supports the objective of goal alignment. Rarely is there a one-to-one correlation between strategic indicators and process results. Figure 13–2 is an example of an indicator of customer satisfaction from the patient's perspective that crosses multiple disciplines. Results would be gathered for each of the disciplines and aggregated to determine actual results for conveying patient satisfaction to stakeholders. The importance of a cascading measurement system is that staff can relate to those steps, tasks, and actions that they influence. Figure 13–2 illustrates that aggregate results are derived from six different disciplines. Improvement in aggregate results will occur by addressing individual results. All six disciplines need to be actively involved in the improvement process. Subsequent measurements would deter-

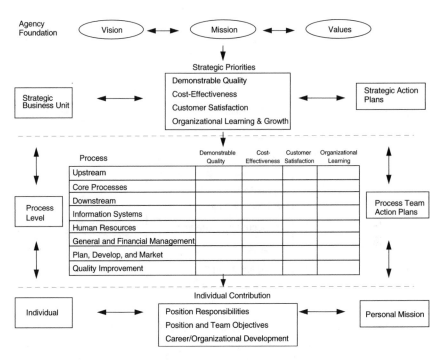

Figure 13–1 Alignment of Strategy, Metrics, and Action Plans

mine whether there was improvement in comparison to baseline results. Discipline-specific results can also be used as an example for other disciplines. For instance, if nursing is achieving a 90 percent satisfaction level and physical therapists are achieving a 60 percent satisfaction level, then the aggregate score is reflective of the respective scores. Improvements in physical therapy scores can be illustrated in contrast to the nursing score. Ultimate improvement may need to address potential root causes such as the use of contracted services. If the goal is to improve aggregate satisfaction, then all of the individual elements will need to bring their respective ratings into the range of excellence. In this case, physical therapy needed to improve to a greater degree than nursing.

Other examples of how the concept of cascading performance measurement could be applied to customer satisfaction would include measuring satisfaction by service line, program, discipline, geographic area, branch office, and team. Measuring satisfaction with suppliers is also very important. Similar to the old saying, "You are judged by the company you keep," a business must make sure that the suppliers it uses are as credible as the business itself. For instance, imagine that an agency's goals are that all staff should be knowledgeable and considerate of patients and their families and belongings, and submit paperwork within 24 hours of visit completion. Then all staff, whether they are independent contractors

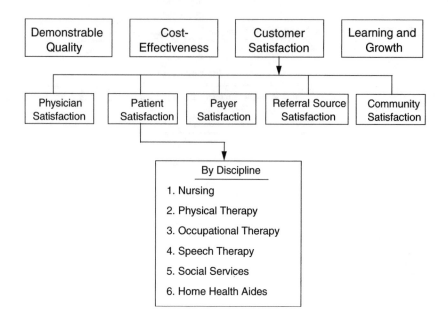

Figure 13–2 Cascading Performance Measurements for Customer Satisfaction

or provided through third-party staffing agencies, should be held to the same high standards.

Another example of a cascading performance measurement system can be applied for the strategy of cost-effectiveness. Figure 13–3 illustrates five categories of cost-effectiveness (payer and risk mix, cash flow to debt ratio, profit by service line, return on equity, and working capital turnover ratio). These categories, originally listed in the financial category of Exhibit 4–1, were deemed to be important to the agency's stakeholders.

In this example the agency may have decided that it wants to achieve, in the aggregate, say a 10 percent profit. This goal has been communicated to internal and external stakeholders. Each service line would contribute to the achievement of this goal. Contributions would be based upon service line cost structure, profitability, and volume. Each service line has activities performed on its behalf with the majority being performed in the patient-focused care processes. Focusing of resources and achieving results will be determined by the agency's process owners and the respective teams that are in place.

Therefore, the basic formula in conveying results to stakeholders is the following:

1. Stakeholders determine what is important to measure.
2. Management determines its strategy by incorporating agency values, customer expectations, agency strengths, and marketplace opportunities. A

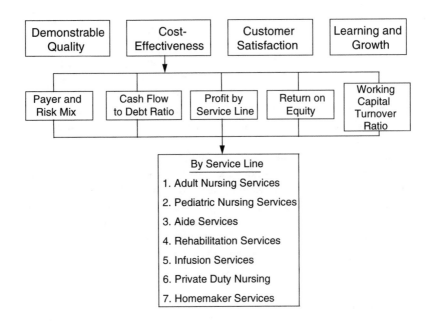

Figure 13–3 Cascading Performance Measurements for Cost-Effectiveness

performance measurement system is developed to support the measurement and management of strategic goals.

3. Management focuses human and organizational resources through the development of action plans (see Chapter 11).
4. Strategic action plans and performance measures are cascaded down to the process level. Cross-fertilization occurs among processes when process-specific goals and objectives are linked to strategic objectives. Process-specific action plans would be developed to identify how each process would contribute to a specific strategic goal. Ideally, process action plans should be reconciled to strategic objectives to verify consistency of approach and alignment of objectives.
5. Alignment of process goals needs to be cascaded down to the team, individual, and work unit level to achieve short- and longer-term success.
6. Initial results will provide a baseline for subsequent measurement. Subsequent results will demonstrate progress or a lack of progress.

Table 13–1 illustrates how cross-fertilization could be put into action using a matrix to align performance measures within each process to one of the strategic priorities. The table depicts the four generic strategies mentioned previously and the processes that occur at every agency. In order to have alignment, every process team and its team leader must be working toward common goals. Therefore, each process would develop metrics to evaluate how it contributes to the achievement of organizational strategies. For example, if an agency's goal is to reduce its cost per visit by 20 percent, then each process team would need to contribute toward this goal. For example, the core process team may set a goal of a 10 percent reduction in cost per visit, the downstream process team may set a goal of 2 percent, and so on. Actual results would determine whether they are making a positive contribution.

Examples of cascading measurements for these strategic priorities can be found in Chapter 9. Table 9–10 illustrates measurements for the strategic goal of cost effectiveness across all agency processes and Table 9–12 illustrates the same concept for internal customer satisfaction. Exhibit 13–1 illustrates metrics that could be used to assess demonstrable quality with respect to each process identified in Table 13–1. Exhibits 13–2 through 13–4 illustrate process-specific metrics to support each remaining strategy identified in Table 13–1.

ROLE OF MANAGEMENT

A basic tenet of management is to demonstrate continuously improving results to stakeholders. This tenet represents a results orientation. If results do not

---

Table 13–1 Cross-Fertilization of Goals and Process-Oriented Measures

	Strategic Priorities			
Process	Demonstratable Quality	Cost-Effectiveness	Customer Satisfaction	Organizational Learning
Upstream				
Core Processes				
Downstream				
Information Systems				
Human Resources				
General and Financial Management				
Plan, Develop, and Marketing				
Quality Improvement				

Exhibit 13–1 Process Metrics To Support Demonstrable Quality

Demonstrable Quality

1. Upstream
   - Percent of patients whose expected outcomes were assessed correctly
   - Percent of insurance information gathered correctly
   - Percent of patients properly admitted
   - Number of data entry errors
2. Core Process
   - Percent of patients who experienced an improvement in ADL
   - Percent of patients who experienced stabilization in ADL
   - Percent of patients whose medical condition improved
   - Percent of patients who managed their medication correctly
   - Number of data entry errors
3. Downstream
   - Percent of patient satisfaction surveys returned
   - Percent of patient records filed correctly
   - Percent of receivables collected
   - Percent of claims submitted correctly
4. Information Systems
   - Percent of system failures/downtime
   - Number of occurrences of unauthorized access or viruses
5. Human Resources
   - Number of job-related injuries
   - Main phone number is answered within three rings
   - Percent of incoming calls routed correctly
   - Payroll errors
6. General and Financial Management
   - Number of corrections to financial statements
   - Number of corrections to cost report
   - Number of corrections from year-end audit
7. Planning, Development, and Marketing
   - Number of contracts awarded
8. Quality Improvement
   - Number of QI projects whose improvement exceeded plan

---

improve, stakeholders question the effectiveness of management. As mentioned above, metrics cannot be assessed in a vacuum. Management needs to measure and manage what provides value to stakeholders. Management also needs to integrate its strategic objectives with customer-focused objectives and the agency's value system. Finally, management needs to align agency resources. Assuming management utilizes a process management orientation, then it would need to cascade strategic measurements down to agency processes to ensure alignment and a common focus. Otherwise, management runs the risk of creating a dysfunc-

Exhibit 13–2 Process Metrics To Support Cost-Effectiveness

Cost-Effectiveness

1. Upstream
   - Cost of upstream process per admission
   - Cost per admission visit
   - Cost per episode
2. Core Process
   - Cost per episode
   - Units per episode
   - Service line profitability—gross profit (revenue less core process cost or unit cost)
3. Downstream
   - Cost of downstream process per admission
   - Cost per patient record
   - Cost per episode
4. Information Systems
   - Number of manual transactions
5. Human Resources
   - Training cost per full-time equivalent (FTE)
   - Effectiveness of training
6. General and Financial Management
   - Working capital turnover
7. Planning, Development, and Marketing
   - Payer mix
   - Risk mix
   - Percent growth by service line
8. Quality Improvement
   - Dollar value of quality improvement (QI) projects exceeds plan

tional organization where everyone does his or her own thing and only gives "lip service" to the attainment of strategic objectives. This orientation supports the saying, "Management begins with measurement." Alignment of goals and objectives can occur through the development of strategic action plans that incorporate each strategic objective. Cross-fertilization across processes occurs when process-specific action plans are developed that support the strategic goals. The development of process-oriented action plans will incorporate each strategic objective and identify how each process team should contribute to the achievement of strategic objectives. Team and individual goals are then aligned to their respective processes.

This alignment of processes with strategic goals also supports the concept of a system. Processes produce results. Results or outcomes are directed toward existing customers, future customers, and the marketplace. Results provide a starting point for organizational learning, continuous improvement, and an en-

Exhibit 13–3 Process Metrics To Support Customer Satisfaction

---

Customer Satisfaction

1. Upstream
   - Intake/information gathering (authorizations and insurance data)
   - Patient transition from hospital to home
   - On-time delivery
   - Staff satisfaction—job, company, team, leadership
2. Core Process
   - Patient satisfaction—service, outcomes, cost, etc.
   - Physician satisfaction—outcomes, communication, cost, etc.
   - Staff satisfaction—job, company, team, leadership
   - Payer—service, outcomes, cost, etc.
3. Downstream
   - Stakeholders satisfied with follow-up
   - Staff satisfaction—job, company, team, leadership
   - Payers satisfied with agency reporting
4. Information Systems
   - Internal customer survey
   - Staff satisfaction—job, company, team, leadership
   - Access to information
5. Human Resources
   - Staff satisfaction—job, company, team, leadership
   - Internal customer survey
6. General and Financial Management
   - Staff satisfaction—job, company, team, leadership
   - Internal customer survey
7. Planning, Development, and Marketing
   - Market share
   - Customer retention/loyalty
   - Staff satisfaction—job, company, team, leadership
   - Internal customer survey
8. Quality Improvement
   - Staff satisfaction—job, company, team, leadership
   - Internal customer survey

---

hancement of stakeholder results. They are a feedback mechanism to foster organizational growth. The principles of organizational learning and growth, continuous improvement, and a results orientation provide an impetus for performance excellence. Performance excellence occurs when the agency exceeds internal goals on a regular basis, exceeds industry benchmarks that are based upon best of class, or exceeds best-of-class benchmarks from outside of the industry. At that point that organization will be eligible for entry into the "Home Health Agency Hall of Fame."

Exhibit 13–4 Process Metrics To Support Organizational Learning and Growth

Organizational Learning and Growth

1. Upstream
   - Decrease cycle time—initial assessment
   - Decrease cycle time—paperwork submission
2. Core Process
   - Decrease cycle time—paperwork submission
   - Decrease cycle time—comprehensive assessment/reassessment
3. Downstream
   - Decrease cycle time—accounts receivable collection
   - Decrease cycle time—record retrieval
4. Information Systems
   - Percent of processes benchmarked
   - Decrease cycle time—project completion time
5. Human Resources
   - Percent of positions targeted for competency-based assessment, development, and training
   - Decrease cycle time—recruitment
   - Improve training retention
   - Percent of training and testing process automated
   - Percent of benefit information automated (earnings to date, paid time off, health coverage, etc.)
   - Percent of job openings posted
   - Percent of policies and procedures on-line
6. General and Financial Management
   - Activities that add value versus those that do not add value
   - Innovation of forecast tools
   - Decrease cycle time—project completion time, budget preparation, statement preparation
   - Supplier performance
7. Planning, Development, and Marketing
   - Percent of employees versus contract staff
   - Decrease cycle time—new contract development
8. Quality Improvement
   - Percent of staff participating on teams
   - Number of quality improvement (QI) projects implemented
   - Number of QI suggestions
   - Percent of staff trained in QI
   - Percent of surveys returned

Organizational learning is inherent in performance excellence. Organizational learning begins with the individual. Individuals contribute to team, process, and organizational growth. Alignment of an individual's growth and performance goals should be consistent with the agency's growth and performance goals. For instance, individual growth could take the form of new work-related opportunities, educational opportunities, or a chance to learn a new technical skill. Organizational performance goals may relate to the individual's ability to streamline his or her job, contribute to the team's success, complete a project, or develop a new skill set. Organizational performance goals also translate to very specific objectives for an individual. For instance, an individual who does data entry in the upstream process would align his or her individual performance goals with an upstream metric for demonstrable quality (e.g., the absence of data entry errors). Monitoring actual results would determine whether the individual was accountable for his or her role in demonstrating quality. If this individual takes responsibility for his or her actions, he or she contributes to the entire system, enabling the downstream team to submit accurate claims and collect receivables in a timely fashion. Educating both teams on system requirements emphasizes the importance of working toward common goals.

The development of goals and performance objectives should be accomplished between the individual and his or her manager. Evaluation of individual annual contributions should include multiple perspectives as illustrated in Figure 13–4.

Not only should supervisors assess individual contributions (assess from above), but individuals should also be assessed by the team with whom they work (peer-level assessment). Peer-level assessment also provides for any self-evaluation. If the goal is for the entire team to contribute to the system, then each team member must carry his or her weight. An analogy can be made using a professional baseball team. When the team is on the field and everyone is working together, then the opposing team has very few opportunities to score runs. If the pitcher is tired, however, or the catcher overthrows first base, or the left fielder misses a fly ball, then the team member is not doing his respective job. The same

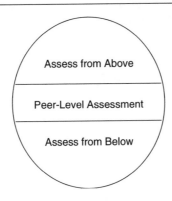

Figure 13–4 Multitiered Assessment To Ensure Alignment of Individual Goals and Efforts with the Business Unit and Team

occurs within process teams. One member not doing his or her respective job drags the whole team down. Each has a responsibility to the team as well as to the team's manager. Therefore, each should be assessed at a peer level, or in this case, at the team level.

If the individual in question is a manager, the bottom section of Figure 13–4 would be included (an assessment from below). The assessment from below would include an upward evaluation of his or her management abilities. Managers are evaluated on their ability to keep staff informed, to lead, and to teach. At a peer level, their contributions would be assessed by themselves and their fellow managers. From above, they would be assessed by their supervisors. If the individual in question was the CEO or other senior manager, then the board of directors would assess his or her respective performance (from above) on the attainment of organizational goals. This approach, illustrated in Figure 13–5, provides for two types of feedback. First, management conveys results to stakeholders. In this example, members of the board of directors are members of the stakeholder group. Utilizing a balanced reporting mechanism similar to the balanced scorecard identified in Exhibit 4–1, the board of directors would be able to evaluate how the organization is performing on multiple levels.

Assessment of senior management would include feedback from the board on organizational results, the second type of feedback. The complete assessment would evaluate how the individual performed from the perspective of peers, from below and from above. The weighting of these factors in relationship to very specific individual and organizational goals determines bonuses or merit increases.

Ideally, all compensation systems should support the attainment of agency goals, be closely linked to organizational performance, and be measurable. Table 13–2 illustrates an approach to the alignment of individual goals to team and organizational goals. Increases or bonuses would be performance based. Increases would be depend upon the achievement of team and organizational goals

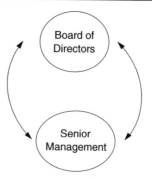

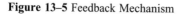

Figure 13–5 Feedback Mechanism

Table 13–2 Illustration of a Performance-Based Weighting System

Criteria	Potential	Assessment	Weight	Increase
Personal goals	10%	60%	.06	.003
Organizational goals	30%	70%	.21	.011
Team goals	60%	80%	.48	.024
			Total Increase	3.8%

instead of 100 percent reliance upon personal goals and objectives. The goal is to create a community of common goals, consistency in incentive systems, and shared vision.

For example, assuming a 5 percent cap on annual increases, an individual has the potential to earn 60 percent of the annual increase cap if his or her respective team attains all goals identified in his or her action plan, 30 percent for the achievement of organizational goals, and 10 percent for the achievement of personal goals. In this example, the team was assessed as meeting 80 percent of its objectives, therefore each team member would receive the same weighting on his or her annual review. The 80 percent assessment should be based upon the team's self-assessment and include input from management. Final scoring may require negotiation between team members and management. Input from other teams may also be considered. The weight is determined by multiplying the potential times the assessment (60% x 80% = .48). The percentage of increase is then calculated by multiplying the weight times the cap, which in this case is 5 percent (80% x 5% = .024 or 2.4%).

Senior management, team leaders, and the board of directors assess the achievement of organizational goals. Their assessment concluded that collectively only 70 percent of the goals were achieved. Everyone in the organization would receive 70 percent of the increase attributable to the achievement of organizational goals. This assessment resulted in a 1.1 percent increase. Finally, each individual, with the help of his or her supervisor, would assess how well he or she achieved personal goals. Differences of opinion would require negotiation. This score incorporates feedback gathered according to the models in Figures 13–4 and 13–5. In this example, this person accomplished 60 percent of his or her goals, resulting in a weighted increase of .003 or .3 percent. The overall total increase for this individual based on the attainment of his or her goals would be 3.8 percent.

At the beginning of this chapter, Figure 13–1 summarized the concept of alignment among the agency's foundation, strategic priorities, the cross-fertilization of objectives with agency processes, and each individual's unique contribution. Figure 13–1 also illustrated the dynamic nature of the relationship among strategy, process objectives, measures, and outcomes, and the individual's role in creating organizational outcomes.

It is the individual who represents the core of any organization. It is the individual who learns and creates organizational learning. It is also the individual who is responsible for making or breaking the organization and its attendent mission and vision. Alignment of values, the development of a shared vision, and the pursuit of performance excellence will provide a catalyst for becoming a recognized leader in a selected field.

METRIC MAINTENANCE

Conveying results to stakeholders is not a static process. Stakeholder perceptions change. Consequently the metrics used to assess whether value is being provided should reflect changing perceptions. Perceptions change because of experiences with other providers, education, the environment, and technology. For instance, a patient who only had one experience with home health may have responded to a patient satisfaction survey with extremely high levels of satisfaction. If the patient has a second experience with a different provider, however, he or she has a baseline to rate the second provider against. This experienced patient may notice things that he or she was not cognizant of in the previous experience. If the third experience occurs with the original provider, the patient will evaluate the current experience based upon two different prior experiences. This patient may be able to identify different facets of customer service that were worse than, better than, different from, or missing from previous experiences. Therefore, the broader one's experiences, the more attentive or aware one will be when assessing current experiences.

For example, someone who flies infrequently usually rates satisfaction based upon obvious factors such as whether luggage arrived at the same destination as the individual, whether the crew was friendly, and whether the flight was relatively comfortable. Frequent travelers would expand this rating system into the availability of storage for carry-on luggage, whether the flight departed and arrived on time, the ability to get connecting flights, and the airline's communication process for flight cancellation and holding a connecting flight.

Customers/stakeholders have different levels of expectations regarding service, organizational results, and personal opportunities. Expectations are based upon their education, prior experiences, and objectives. Agency management must pay attention to the changing voice of the customer and track the metrics that reflect changing attitudes and perceptions. Reassessing customer perceptions should be tied into the annual strategic planning process. During this process a review can be made of current metrics, improvements in technology, environmental changes that lend themselves to updating the assessment system, and evaluation results. This process also needs to evaluate whether the right things are being measured. For instance, an agency that has recently implemented an ABCM system and gathered data (e.g., how much time was being spent on travel, documentation, providing hands-on care, and case conferences) would be able to assess changing metrics regarding productivity. Adopting a new metric, using activities, could look at the percent of time field staff spent doing value-adding activities (e.g., hands-on care and case conferencing versus time spent on activities that add cost such as travel). Improving an agency's information infrastructure will produce metrics that have meaning to shareholders, instead of using metrics based on system limitations such as visits per day.

Conveying results to stakeholders should be approached from the same perspective as continuously improving organizational results. Metrics need to be improved, results need to be improved, and the forum for communicating results will always need to be improved. Management will need to be aware of results generated by the OASIS project, the Joint Commission's ORYX initiative, the CHAP benchmarking study, and state association results. These sources will identify what to measure and what kind of results are being achieved. They will provide opportunities for gathering benchmark data. Benchmarks provide a valuable tool for demonstrating results to stakeholders. Care should be taken to identify "best of class" benchmarks where possible instead of relying solely upon averages. If an agency relies upon demonstrating its results in comparison to averages, then it is aspiring to be average, and not the best.

IMPROVEMENT OF OUTCOMES

Conveying results to stakeholders needs to consider improvement of outcomes. The Joint Commission includes improvement of performance objectives in its accreditation guidelines.[2] HCFA's expected revision to the Medicare COPs for home health agencies illustrates its interest in continuous improvement of outcomes and organizational efficiencies.[3] The National Committee for Quality Assurance (NCQA) accreditation standards fall into six broad categories listed previously in this book. Each category is weighted. Quality improvement is the largest category and accounts for 40 percent of a health plan's score. This category addresses quality of care, consistency across all aspects of its delivery system, patient access, and whether the plan can demonstrate improvements in care and services.[4]

Improvement in results is the concern of accreditation and regulatory bodies, which are stakeholders in an agency's results. Although these stakeholders do not pay the bills, they can certainly influence whether the bills get paid. Improvement has been addressed in previous chapters from an internal perspective. Demonstrating continuous improvement to stakeholders requires "walking the walk." This is similar to the way the individual is accountable within the organization.

Continuous improvement illustrates how the organization is accountable to those it serves. Accountability is illustrated by showing ever-improving results to all stakeholder groups. Improvement becomes the external exemplification of a continuous improvement philosophy and a results orientation.

Demonstrating results externally requires looking inward to where the processes (activities) take place. It requires the efforts of individuals, teams, and work units to accomplish improvements, an understanding of what is important to measure from the stakeholder's perspective, and the acquisition or development of an information infrastructure that facilitates the collection and management of data. Demonstrating results also requires a shift to a process orientation and the development of an organizational culture that values continuous improvement, manages by fact, and is willing to work at eliminating root causes instead of merely treating symptoms.

The following improvement example demonstrates a willingness to examine the underlying causes of a problem that reflected an outcome result much lower than results from other agencies.

A particular HHA [home health agency] receives an outcome report that shows that 20 percent of its orthopedic patients improved in ability to ambulate by either the 60th day of treatment or the date of discharge, depending upon which came first. The HHA's 20–percent outcome compares with a 40–percent aggregated outcome of the orthopedic patients from all demonstration agencies. Because this 20–percent outcome finding is significantly less than the 40–percent aggregated outcome, the staff makes a determination that this is an outcome that should be investigated further. Using record review, team evaluation and other quality improvement techniques, the HHA staff determines that a potential reason for the low rate of improvement is lack of coordination between physical therapists and other care providers. This lack of coordination in turn, results in minimal reinforcement of patient exercise programs by others on the care delivery team. The agency staff, therefore, develops and implements a precise action plan or performance improvement plan that strengthens team coordination of specific and relevant caregiving actions. The next outcome report indicates that the number of orthopedic patients improving in ability to ambulate is 35–percent, suggesting that the performance improvement activities resulted in better patient care, thereby producing improved outcomes.[5] (p.11039)

This example demonstrates how comparative data can be used to assess results and how staff can be brought together to analyze and solve problems. Once results are adjusted for risk, there is an opportunity to utilize results for marketing purposes, setting goals and objectives, and being recognized for performance excellence.

The challenge with any measurement system is to identify milestones or intermediate points where progress is assessed. These intermediate points may be on a visit-by-visit basis if one is using an expected outcome system. (See Chapter 6 on Outcomes.) An expected outcome is set at the beginning of care and intermediate milestones are identified at critical points in the care process. The intermediate milestones identify patient progress on a care plan that has been customized for the patient's specific problems. Assessing progress against milestones enables care providers to determine whether the care plan is on target or whether it needs to be revised. This is similar to an airplane that flies between two cities. The pilot sets the airplane's direction once it has achieved a proper elevation. Periodically, the pilot assesses whether the flight is on course. Course assessment can require either an adjustment in direction, speed, or altitude, or no change at all. The assessment of direction occurs frequently so that timely adjustments can be made, thus ensuring that passengers arrive at the correct destination and on time. So it is with achieving expected outcomes. Assessment on a regular basis requires timely interventions so that outcomes can be ensured. There are many variables that are beyond management's control; however, the evaluation of milestones and the corresponding adjustments are within management's control.

Assessing progress against milestones also occurs with organizational outcomes, whether results are clinical, financial, process oriented, or customer related. There is a cost associated with this data collection, compiling of results, and analysis. There is a cost to improving outcomes; however, benefits should outweigh the cost of improvements.

Sometimes benefits are difficult to quantify. For instance, does a 5 percent improvement in customer satisfaction warrant an expenditure today? This poses a dilemma for the organization because financial expenditures tend to have short time horizons and customer satisfaction has an indefinite time horizon with intangible results. There is a fundamental truth, however, that is difficult to factor into the improvement equation—namely, it is less costly to maintain existing customers than it is to obtain new customers. This fundamental truth can be illustrated by thinking about the amount of revenue and profits that would be lost over the course of time, say 5 to 10 years, compared to the resource or cash outflow related to a customer satisfaction enhancement.

Acquiring new customers requires time, marketing dollars, and potential organizational changes. It takes time to find customers, court customers, and convince them that your services are superior to those they are currently receiving. They may ask for results that support your claims. This scenario comes full circle to a similar point except that now it is a potential customer who is pointing out that your patient satisfaction scores are 5 percent lower than those produced by their existing provider. Unfortunately, not only is there the potential to lose an existing customer, but it is difficult to attract new customers with less than stellar scores.

Continuous improvement is a cost of doing business. There are four costs related to quality: (1) prevention cost, (2) appraisal cost, (3) internal failure cost, and (4) external failure cost.[6] Examples of these costs are listed in Table 13–3.

Continuous improvement should emphasize prevention, reducing internal and external failures, and resolving problems at the source or root cause. For instance, how many customer complaints did an agency receive during the past quarter? Were those complaints attributable to a particular problem such as poor service delivery of equipment and supplies, or were they attributable to a specific nurse, therapist, or aide? Investigating beyond the symptom will facilitate problem resolution. The goal is to use the agency's performance measurement system to identify when problems are significant and take action before they manifest in external failure costs. External failure costs have the potential to foreshadow the lack of economic viability. Internal failure costs create unnecessary expenses and prohibit the achievement of cost-effectiveness. Appraisal cost is associated with keeping the agency on course. Prevention and appraisal costs are critical to long-term survival. They are also the cornerstone of continuous improvement.

Table 13–3 Costs of Quality

Costs of Quality	Examples
Prevention	Assessment of staff/vendor abilities before hiring/using
	Policies, procedures, and position descriptions
	The planning function, forecasting, and market analysis
	New service or program design and testing
	Training
	Background checks
Appraisal	Compliance audits, Joint Commission surveys, state surveys
	The quality assurance/improvement function
	Equipment recalibration
	In-process, milestone, and strategic review
Internal failure	Rework, rekeying, duplicate data entry
	Work-related accidents
	Staff turnover
	Excess inventory, poor cash flow, and excessive interest expense
	Internal reporting errors and corrections
External failure	Bad debt
	Loss of contracts, market share, and referral sources
	Stakeholder dissatisfaction
	Pricing errors

CONVEYING RESULTS TO STAKEHOLDERS

Conveying results to stakeholders occurs through the production and distribution of annual reports, regularly scheduled meetings, or one-on-one communication. The selected communication methodology depends upon whether the communication goal is directed toward internal or external customers. The distribution of annual reports has been the traditional means for sharing financial reports with external customers. Typically results are validated by an independent auditor before distribution. Some organizations are beginning to supplement traditional financial statement data with information regarding the organization's vision and mission, customer and staff satisfaction, process improvements, and organizational growth.

The communication of data to external customers has always been important for attracting new customers or investors, for retaining current customers and investors, and for supporting the requirements of third parties such as regulatory agencies, creditors, and partners. The investment community recognizes the importance of assessing both financial and nonfinancial indicators. The following is a list of eight categories of nonfinancial criteria used by analysts when determining whether to divest the stock of an organization from their investment portfolios.[7]

1. *Quality Management:* Criteria assess the quality of organizational vision, leadership style, management experience, and the execution and quality of corporate strategy.
2. *Effectiveness of New Product Development:* Criteria address how the organization approaches research, the amount of revenue derived from new product offerings, the cycle time associated with new product development, and the efficiency of the development process.
3. *Strength of Market Position:* Criteria address the organization's market share, capabilities, image, and ability to innovate.
4. *Strength of Corporate Culture:* Criteria address the organization's ability to attract and retain talented staff, staff turnover, the use of teams, the quality of the workforce, and the use of performance-based incentive systems.
5. *Effectiveness of Executive Compensation Policies:* Criteria assess the alignment of compensation policies among all levels of staff and organizational objectives.
6. *Quality of Investor Communications:* Criteria address management credibility, ease of access to management, the quality of published materials, and the organization's approach to customer relations.
7. *Quality of Product and Services:* Criteria address the quality of processes, customer-perceived quality, external failure rates, and whether the organization has won any quality awards.

8. *Level of Customer Satisfaction:* Criteria address customer satisfaction, repeat sales, customer retention, the level of complaints, and the adequacy of the responses to complaints.

Another example of communicating data to external customers is the Health Plan Employer Data and Information Set (HEDIS) report card developed by the NCQA to share health plan results with potential and existing stakeholders. The report card consists of eight categories that convey information important to potential and existing stakeholders: (1) the effectiveness of care, (2) access to care, (3) member satisfaction, (4) health plan stability (provider turnover and financial stability), (5) use of services, (6) cost of care, (7) informed choices, and (8) health plan descriptive information. These eight categories provide a wide range of indicators to help stakeholders make informed decisions regarding the purchase of health plans.

Results should also be shared with the employees of an organization. Sharing results with staff can be accomplished through monthly, quarterly, and annual meetings, use of electronic mail (e-mail), voice mail, newsletters, formalized reports, and face-to-face communication. The selection of a communication methodology will be determined by the objective of the communication. For instance, electronic or voice mail are appropriate for providing late-breaking news updates. Face-to-face communication is appropriate when there is a need for interaction.

Another vehicle for communicating with employees and other stakeholders is the storyboard. The storyboard is an excellent visual tool to illustrate how decisions were made and provide a living document of a journey. A storyboard can be constructed on a piece of paper, a poster, or on a bulletin board. The key point is that the storyboard needs to be visible in order to convey its story.

In essence, the storyboard becomes a testimonial to a team's progress with a given task. Figure 13–6 illustrates how a storyboard can be designed to convey results to stakeholders. In this example the storyboard begins with a mission statement developed for the task at hand. The next section identifies the problem to be resolved or the desired outcome to be achieved. The third box identifies the agency's current situation. The fourth box identifies an improvement strategy, and the last box identifies how the organization, team, or work unit intends to follow up on initial improvements and may identify what their future may be.

The following is an example of how the storyboard could be used to convey results to stakeholders. It illustrates how a clinical pathway development project was identified, what steps supported the creation of the clinical pathway, and the agency's plans for subsequent monitoring and improvement of the clinical pathway. In this example, a cross-functional multidisciplinary team was formed that consisted of nurses, therapists, aides, a representative from the information

1. Mission statement	2. Desired outcome to be achieved	3. Current situation and statement of problem
4. Process improvement strategy		5. Results and follow-up

Figure 13–6 Potential Storyboard Format

services and financial management teams, and the clinical team leader. This group drafted a straightforward mission statement (box 1), "To develop a clinical pathway for the most common medical problem experienced by our agency." The problem being addressed was the need to develop one clinical pathway. This box (2) could also include the time frame in which the implementation team planned to complete the development of the clinical pathway. Both the mission and problem would be written on the storyboard.

The team members gathered data on all patient diagnoses the agency had treated during the past year. They utilized a Pareto chart (see Figure 11–5) to identify what patient conditions occurred most frequently. Their analysis indicated that chronic heart failure (CHF) was the most frequently occuring problem. This process led to subsequent analysis and development of a critical pathway. The Pareto chart indicating patient problems was placed in the number three box of the storyboard depicting the current situation.

The team members' next step was to produce a flowchart of existing processes (see Figure 7–1), utilize a cause and effect analysis (see Figure 12–1) to identify the elements that needed to be included on the critical pathway, and look at integrating cost data from the ABCM system, so they would be able to cost and quantify clinical results. The team also identified milestones and appropriate performance measures. Flowcharts were displayed on the storyboard (box 4) along with the cause and effect diagrams. The team members also decided to illustrate initial baselines they had developed on cost and results.

The final square, results and follow-up, mentioned that the team will collect data for six months before looking at the next step in fine-tuning the initial critical pathway. The completed storyboard can be used for education of other staff, teams, stakeholders, and Joint Commission surveyors.

The storyboard provides a visual tool to illustrate results and is useful for internally communicating to stakeholders. Another visual tool is the trending of data. Trending data allows stakeholders to visualize progress over time.

Assuming an agency would aggregate its customer satisfaction scores to arrive at one value, Figure 13–7 illustrates the results of an annual assessment and subsequent trended results. Figure 13–7 also illustrates where actual results are in relation to a specific benchmark and stretch targets (targets yet to be accomplished). The significance of this illustration is that it conveys to stakeholders that this organization is serious about customer satisfaction. Negative results were experienced in 1995. These results may have been attributable to changes in the measurement system or some other reason. Legitimate reasons should be footnoted to add additional value to the illustration. Both 1996 and 1997 show progressive improvement over 1995 results, with 1997 results exceeding benchmarked results. The illustration also shows the agency's expectations for future customer satisfaction results given a two-year and five-year time frame.

CONCLUSION

Conveying results to stakeholders is a serious process—stakeholders have a vested interest in the well-being of an organization. Successful communication of results begins with understanding what is important to the various stakeholder groups. Once management understands how stakeholders measure organizational success, they can set up the system to gather, measure, and manage the data that are important from stakeholder perspectives.

Conveying results to stakeholders is about listening to the customer voice, focusing on the diverse needs of various stakeholder groups, and developing strategies to meet their respective needs. Listening to the voice of stakeholders is a never-ending process. It is also an evolutionary process. Stakeholder require-

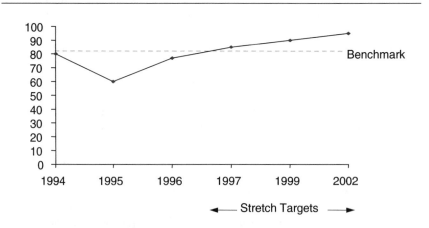

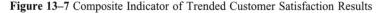

Figure 13–7 Composite Indicator of Trended Customer Satisfaction Results

ments and perceptions change over time. Listening to evolving needs and requirements provides an early warning system for opportunity identification. Concurrently, early warning systems also foretell of changes that may be necessary in the agency's performance measurement system.

Conveying results can also be thought of as a business philosophy. If one views stakeholders as partners, then the organization has a vested interest in achieving continuously improving results. This vested interest may stimulate the pursuit of performance excellence. Performance excellence is an internal drive to be the best. It is a philosophy that is not content with mediocre or average results. It requires working in conjunction with stakeholders, understanding their needs, and mutually developing strategies that create a win-win situation for both stakeholder and provider organization. Long-term viability does not happen accidentally. It requires planning; the development of partnerships with stakeholders; the development of organizations that are strategically aligned with their vision, processes, and staff; and a willingness on the part of everyone to make results happen.

NOTES

1. HCFA, Medicare and Medicaid Programs: Use of the OASIS as Part of the Conditions of Participation for Home Health Agencies, *Federal Register* 62, no. 46 (10 March 1997): 11039.
2. Joint Commission, *1997–98 Comprehensive Accreditation for Home Care*, 1st ed., Section 6, 1996.
3. HCFA, Conditions of Participation, 11039.
4. NCQA Accreditation Guidelines, located at NCQA Internet website at http://www.ncqa.org/acred.htm.
5. HCFA, Conditions of Participation, 11039.
6. J. Campanella, *Principles of Quality Cost*, 2nd ed. (Milwaukee, WI: ASQC Quality Press, 1990).
7. P. Bierbusse and T. Siesfeld, Measures That Matter, *Strategic Performance Measurement* 1, no. 2 (April/May 1997): 6–11.

PART IV

Controlling Your Destiny

CHAPTER 14

The Capstone: What Is It All About?

> The world that we have made as a result of the level of thinking we have done thus far creates problems that we cannot solve at the same level as they were created.
>
> —Albert Einstein, 1946

The preceding quote is the foundation for a paradigm shift. The entire health care delivery system is in the process of a metamorphosis. Its eventual shape, complexion, and composition will not be known for some time. Several facts, however, are very clear. First, the old health care system is changing because of evolving societal conditions; increased use of sophisticated technology; rising health care costs; changes in health care financing, reimbursement, and regulation; and unchecked growth in utilization. Today the patient is confused about how, when, or where to receive care.

Second, the former health care system enabled home health care entrepreneurs to start their own businesses in a relatively risk-free environment. Cost reimbursement created a safety net that protected home health care providers by reimbursing them for reasonable costs associated with providing care to homebound patients. Cost reimbursement contained some elements of risk such as having cost denied, incurring costs that were outside of the reimbursement formula, providing services that were deemed inappropriate, or experiencing cash flow problems. But following the rules and regulations associated with cost reimbursement and the conditions of participation enabled home health care managers to develop organizations that served their respective communities and met patient needs.

Third, these rules are changing because of the broader restructuring that is occurring as part of the health care delivery system's metamorphosis. The home health care organizations that were built during the decades of cost reimbursement are being forced to rethink the way they provide care. They are being forced to reconsider the way they hire, compensate, retain, educate, and interact with staff.

359

They are also being forced to reevaluate what is important from the perspective of both the internal and external customer. Home care organizations also are being forced to redesign processes for efficiency, effectiveness, and the provision of value.

In a sense, home health care providers are fortunate in that they still have a window of cost reimbursement opportunity available to create organizations that will survive in a health care delivery system characterized by managed care and provider risk. This book contains concepts, tools, and strategies for developing organizations that are customer focused, values driven, and process oriented. Ideas for managing cost, demonstrating quality, measuring results, and aligning staff toward common goals are presented.

This book has built upon Einstein's quote above, and recognized that home health administrators will need to develop a new way of thinking if they are interested in moving their agencies through the twenty-first century. This new way of thinking will require relinquishing some control, transferring ownership and responsibility to staff, and developing organizations that own a shared vision of their collective destiny to work toward common goals. To accomplish these objectives, managers, administrators, and staff will need to look at the organization as a whole to determine how each individual contributes. They will also need to appreciate that organizational survival depends on the actions of all staff, not a select few.

This chapter has been named the capstone—a crowning event. The purpose of this chapter is to

- Synthesize key concepts presented throughout the book
- Discuss the process of agency transformation
- Enumerate critical steps for agency survival in moving through the twenty-first century

From a system's perspective, the crowning event is the outcome(s) that an effective organization demonstrates as illustrated in Figure 14–1. The level of the outcome(s) is determined through continuous quality improvement (CQI) and organizational learning; the relevancy of the outcome(s) is determined by leadership following the customer and market focus.

Positive outcomes, however, are only one indicator of quality, and quality is only one indicator of effectiveness. Therefore, quality cannot exist without positive outcomes, and effectiveness cannot exist without quality. The converse is not true, however; one cannot conclude that because there are positive outcomes, quality exists, or because quality exists the organization is deemed effective.[1] Performance excellence is more than quality and effectiveness. It is the byproduct of organizational alignment, a long-term commitment to continuous improve-

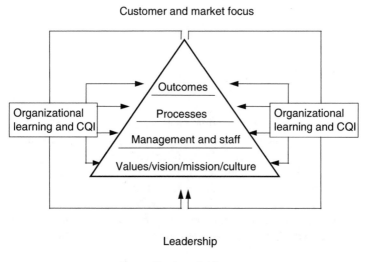

Customer and market focus

Outcomes

Organizational learning and CQI

Processes

Organizational learning and CQI

Management and staff

Values/vision/mission/culture

Leadership

Organizational Alignment

Figure 14–1 Systems Model

ment, and an investment in personal and organizational growth. To achieve performance excellence requires practice, an investment in people, a willingness to replace control with trust, and the strength and commitment to eliminate patterns and practices that no longer serve the organization's customers.

SURVIVING TODAY

The first step to success is survival. The biggest question that agencies are asking right now is, What do I have to do today to stay alive? Marked hazards to this survival include the interim payment system (IPS), prospective payment, new conditions of participation (COPs), surety bonds, ORYX, and OASIS. Some agencies are addressing these concerns by putting compliance programs into place to ensure they meet all the required criteria. Authorities tell us that forward-thinking agencies are becoming proactive by incorporating the following tasks into their agency management:[2]

- obtaining agency accreditation by the Joint Commission or CHAP
- integrating OASIS into their data collection now
- tracking outcomes for clinical status, patient and referral satisfaction, and financial status

- implementing outcomes-based quality improvement (OBQI)
- offering disease management programs
- using clinical pathways
- tracking rehospitalization rates
- automating information systems to integrate services, data, and outcomes

Staying alive also requires proactively managing the agency's cost situation. If the agency's cost per patient is lower than the agency's census division average, it receives a higher per beneficiary limit under IPS. If its costs are higher than the average, it faces a lower per beneficiary limit.[3]

Many of these actions have been discussed in preceding chapters and will indeed be helpful. The question is, are these enough? The old methods of reimbursement, accountability, and providing care are coming to an end, and home care is moving into uncharted territory. How can agencies assure themselves of success?

Hazards exist that are not marked.

—Sign on a ski slope

INTERDEPENDENCE

As a society we are interdependent. When driving down the highway at 65 miles an hour we need to pay attention, stay in our lane, and operate vehicles safely, and we depend on others to do the same. We are dependent upon the utility companies to provide energy, on farmers to produce crops and raise cattle, and on trucking companies to bring crops and cattle to the market, and they are dependent upon us to pay for these products. We depend on the media to keep us up to date with current events, and they depend on us to provide accurate facts. And so it is with a home health care agency. Home care is dependent on the decisions of regulators and the loyalty of staff and customers, and they are dependent upon us to provide care and a place of employment.

A home health care agency has various interdependent processes that, when viewed together, create a system. Processes are composed of activities performed by people. People collectively contribute to process goals. When any one of an agency's processes (or the person performing the activity) becomes misaligned and forgets its purpose, or loses sight of the collective vision, or does not follow up or follow through on promises, then the entire system suffers. Perhaps this point is best illustrated through the use of a fable by Aesop entitled, *The Rebellion against the Stomach.*

Once a man had a dream in which his hands and feet and mouth and brain all began to rebel against his stomach.

"You good for nothing sluggard!" the hands said. "We work all day long, sawing and hammering and lifting and carrying. By evening we're covered with blisters and scratches, and our joints ache, and we're covered with dirt. And meanwhile you just sit there, hogging all the food."

"We agree!" cried the feet. "Think how sore we get, walking back and forth all day long. And you just stuff yourself full, you greedy pig, so that you're that much heavier to carry about."

"That's right!" whined the mouth. "Where do you think all that food you love comes from? I'm the one who has to chew it all up, and as soon as I'm finished you suck it all down for yourself. Do you call that fair?"

"And what about me?" called the brain. "Do you think it's easy being up here, having to think about where your next meal is going to come from? And yet I get nothing at all for my pains."

And one by one the parts of the body joined the complaint against the stomach, which didn't say anything at all.

"I have an idea," the brain finally announced. "Let's all rebel against this lazy belly, and stop working for it."

"Superb idea!" all the other members and organs agreed. "We'll teach you how important we are, you pig. Then maybe you'll do a little work of your own."

So they all stopped working. The hands refused to do any lifting or carrying. The feet refused to walk. The mouth promised not to chew or swallow a single bite. And the brain swore it wouldn't come up with any more bright ideas. At first the stomach growled a bit, as it always did when it was hungry. But after a while it was quiet.

Then, to the dreaming man's surprise, he found he could not walk. He could not grasp anything in his hands. He could not even open his mouth. And he suddenly began to feel rather ill.

The dream seemed to go on for several days. As each day passed, the man felt worse and worse. "This rebellion had better not last much longer," he thought to himself, "or I'll starve."

Meanwhile, the hands and feet and mouth and brain just lay there, getting weaker and weaker. At first they roused themselves just enough to taunt the stomach every once in a while, but before long they didn't even have the energy for that.

Finally the man heard a faint voice coming from the direction of his feet.

"It could be that we were wrong," they were saying. "We suppose the stomach might have been working in his own way all along."

"I was just thinking the same thing," murmured the brain. "It's true he's been getting all the food. But it seems he's been sending most of it right back to us."

"We might as well admit our error," the mouth said. "The stomach has just as much work to do as the hands and feet and brain and teeth."

"Then let's all get back to work," they cried together. And at that the man woke up.

To his relief, he discovered his feet could walk again. His hands could grasp, his mouth could chew, and his brain could now think clearly. He began to feel much better.

"Well, there's a lesson for me," he thought as he filled his stomach at breakfast. "Either we all work together, or nothing works at all."*

When any process becomes dysfunctional, the entire system will suffer. As exemplified by Aesop's Fable, all processes within an organization need to work toward a common goal. Figure 14–1 illustrates that system output (results or outcomes) is the result of a strong foundation (vision, mission, values, and culture). It is the organizational foundation and committed leadership that guide management and staff in the development of processes and the subsequent realization of results.

As home care providers we are interdependent. We depend on our employees and on our customers. Understanding agency requirements will occur through listening to the voice of the customer, whether the customer is outside or inside the agency. It is the alignment between the environment or marketplace—listening to the needs, expectations, and desires of customers—and the design of processes to meet consumer needs that will ensure long-term survival. Without ongoing communication, respect, and a willingness to gather and act upon feedback, the system will create its own reality, and this reality could be quite different from what is necessary to survive.

Figure 14–1 illustrates that the system gets feedback on the results that it produces from its customers and the marketplace. This feedback provides the basis for organizational learning and continuous improvement. The combination of organizational learning and continuous improvement has the ability to create an

---

Source: Reprinted with the permission of Simon & Schuster from THE BOOK OF VIRTUES by William J. Bennett. Copyright © 1993, by William J. Bennett.

environment that is vision driven and values based, and strives for the achievement of ever-improving results, or performance excellence.

ORGANIZATIONAL LEARNING AND CONTINUOUS IMPROVEMENT

The Chinese understood the concepts of organizational learning and continuous improvement long before these topics became popular in American business culture. An old Chinese proverb tells us:

If you want 1 year of prosperity, grow grain.

If you want 10 years of prosperity, grow trees.

If you want 100 years of prosperity, grow people.

A more contemporary version can be found in the results of the 1997 football season. Dan Reeves returned to his hometown to coach the Atlanta Falcons. They lost their first five games and seven of their first eight. But after this midseason crisis, they turned around and won five of their next six games. The reason? Reeves changed his strategy to increase the teaching part of his job. Instead of blaming the players for poor performance, he explained why they were losing. He urged patience and dedication to the team's goals. The players responded by learning how to win.[4]

Both of these examples help to demonstrate the concept of organizational learning. Organizational learning occurs when knowledge is acquired, shared, and put into operation.[5] Knowledge is the collective experience of the organization, which consists of the interaction of explicit and tacit knowledge. Explicit knowledge consists of the information that can be expressed or codified into knowledge repositories such as standards and guidelines. Tacit knowledge includes what the organization knows, including things it knows how to do, but cannot codify. Much of the clinical care in home care is still tacit knowledge. Learning through experience increases tacit knowledge, and codifying the experience increases explicit knowledge.[6]

The acquisition of knowledge is a multivariate. One essential element for a knowledge-creating organization is diversity in the talent pool available within the agency. Diversity nurtures a variety of viewpoints and insights upon which knowledge thrives. Knowledge is based on intuition and information. Intuition assists in the formation of tacit knowledge. Information is based on data. Explicit knowledge can be increased by codifying, as much as possible, what the agency knows how to do—processes, procedures, policies, and so on. Explicit knowledge also is acquired by recognizing a need to change, or improve, or taking advantage of a window of opportunity. A window of opportunity exists when a gap is recognized between organizational vision and actual results (originally depicted in Figure 3–2). The assumption is that an agency knows how to measure performance (i.e., has a codified performance measurement system) and knows how to assess variances.

Once a gap is recognized and the need for further information is identified, the process of acquiring data begins. Data acquisition occurs through formally or informally gathering feedback from customers, collecting clinical data from the field, collecting data from internal processes, or gathering data from outside of the agency via conferences, literature search, or through the use of consultants. Data acquisition can be the responsibility of one person, a team, multiple teams, or everyone in the organization. The challenge is to gather data in an organized fashion, analyze the data, reflect upon resulting information, determine a course of action, and share results and strategies with the entire organization.

Sharing of results will depend upon how the agency views information. The important consideration is that information is power. The alignment of organizational resources requires providing access to information. Information can be distributed by making copies of reports, placing results on the agency's intranet, or holding meetings and presentations. Access to information can be as simple as sharing quarterly results of customer satisfaction, employee satisfaction, process improvement initiatives, cycle time reductions, financial results, and clinical results. Sharing information is a way of empowering staff. It is a vehicle to assist them in making informed decisions. Moreover, the approach to sharing of information, similar to the gathering of data, should be consistent with strategic intent and objectives. For instance, gathering data and sharing information that has no relevance to the provision of customer value is a waste of time. But gathering data and sharing information that enhances staff competency, improves decision-making capabilities, and promotes a better understanding of organizational opportunities (i.e., to become more cost-effective or to demonstrate quality) will provide value. This information increases the knowledge level of both the organization and staff.

The next step is placing the knowledge into operation, which is how organizational learning occurs. Organizational learning develops when staff acquire knowledge, share it with peers, and then determine a course of action to correct a current condition or forge a new path. Organizational learning is action oriented. It also provides the framework for continuous improvement. Taking action produces results. Sharing results forms the foundation for more new actions that can enhance results even further. This continual learning underscores the importance of supporting organizational learning as an alternative to "managing." Managing may not even apply as new approaches are utilized to unleash the creative capability of all members of an organization. It is no longer the role of leaders to provide the answers, but instead to provide others with the opportunity to continually make the organization better. As the Chinese proverb says, "If you want 100 years of prosperity, grow people." As staff grow and evolve, they will develop better ways of assessing performance, understanding the customer, and exceeding internal and external expectations.

Organizational learning perpetuates an environment of continuous improvement, of which CQI is but one element. Not all learning is for quality improvement, although many agencies focus on quality or put all learning under that umbrella. There is also learning for improvement in profitability, agency mission, caring, well-being, morale, partnerships, community involvement, shared values, and so on. The same principles apply for managing any of these processes, as was discussed in Chapter 11. The key is to focus on a process and proceed from there. This understanding of continuous improvement is important because too often agencies limit learning to quality improvement, and there are other important dimensions within an agency that are overlooked as a result.

COST AND QUALITY

Systems thinking, organizational learning, and continuous improvement represent methodologies for understanding organizational interdependence and provide a framework for pursuing performance excellence. Cost and quality are two measures of the fitness of the agency, similar to weight and muscle mass being two measures of the fitness of the human body. Thus, managing cost and quality is essential to maintaining the fitness of the agency. Fitness is a prerequisite for long-term survival as the health care delivery system goes through its metamorphosis; this is similar to the need for maintaining body fitness as a person goes through the metamorphosis of a midlife crisis. The earlier chapters of this text discussed the achievement of ever-improving levels of cost-effectiveness and demonstrable quality. Key elements are extracted here to present a formula for maintaining a "fit" agency. These elements are depicted in Figure 14–2.

Essentially Figure 14–2 illustrates that the degree of cost-effectiveness and level of quality within an organization depend on the alignment of human resources to strategic and process-oriented goals, the optimization of customer-focused processes, and the ongoing accessibility of information to all for organization learning and management. To the degree that any of these components are dysfunctional, the organization's ability to maintain performance excellence levels of cost-effectiveness and quality will be hampered. The analogy to the human body would be that the amount of muscle tone and the level of weight (number of pounds) on a person depend on the alignment of the personal resources, the optimization of fitness-focused processes, and the accessibility of diet and exercise information. In other words, the fitness of the individual depends

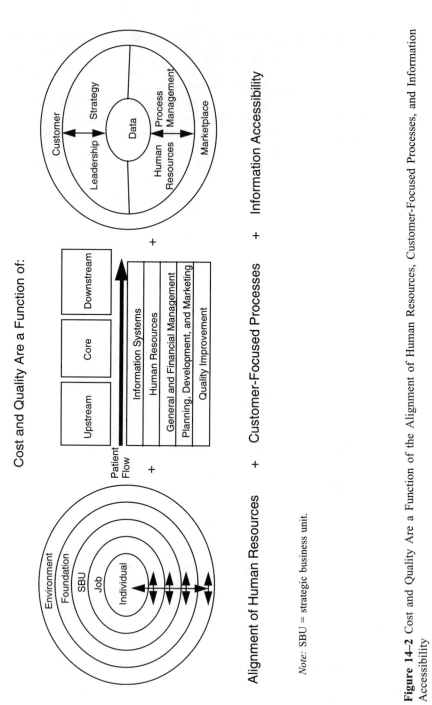

Figure 14-2 Cost and Quality Are a Function of the Alignment of Human Resources, Customer-Focused Processes, and Information Accessibility

on how aligned he or she is physically, emotionally, and financially to meet the goal of physical fitness; how well he or she exercises and eats (fitness processes); and how accessible information is regarding fitness. As challenging as fitness may be for an individual, it is even more complicated for an entire organization. Each of the organizational components depicted in Figure 14–2 are discussed below.

Alignment of Human Resources. Alignment of human resources was discussed in Chapter 5. What is important is that an individual's personal values, professional or occupational mission, and vision be in concert with the mission, vision, values of his or her job, strategic business unit (SBU), the agency (labeled foundation in Figure 14–2), and the community (environment) of the agency. The greater the alignment, the easier it is to attain cost-effectiveness and quality. For instance, if there is no alignment between the individual and his or her team, SBU, or workplace, there is the potential for the wasting of resources. Wasted resources result when work is not completed in a timely and proper fashion. Wasted resources will occur through turf wars, bickering and squabbling between co-workers, the pursuit of hidden agendas, and emphasizing personal pursuits rather than organizational objectives. Lack of alignment could be attributable to the organization's culture, its incentive systems, or inconsistent values between staff and the organization. Lack of alignment between the individual and the organization will increase cost and lower quality, both of which will become visible to the agency's customers.

This wasting of resources can be further exemplified in the analogy with the human body. If a person is not aligned emotionally to increase muscle mass or to release weight, he or she will debate internally about what foods to eat or how much to exercise. Lack of alignment results in buying health food that goes uneaten or joining a gym and never going. These are wasted resources, not to mention the time wasted debating with oneself and others about what to do.

Customer-Focused Processes. The second element of the equation, customer-focused processes, was introduced in Chapter 9. Customer-focused processes describe an agency as composed of two major groups of interdependent processes. As depicted in Figure 14–2, these are (1) patient-focused care processes depicted as upstream, core, and downstream; and (2) support processes depicted as information systems; human resources; general and financial management; planning, development and marketing; and quality improvement. The development of a process orientation enables the agency to identify process customers, measure cost and quality, and identify process-specific goals and objectives that are aligned to an organizational strategy. It is the shift away from a departmental (or task) orientation to one of process and activity management that provides a framework for assessing the elements of a process, identifying opportunities for learning and improvement, and facilitating the measurement of results that makes the management of cost and quality a reality.

These same opportunities occur when one looks at exercise and diet as interdependent activities rather as isolated tasks. As tasks, one can consider preparing a meal a task (or burden), or walking as a task that must be completed. When these are viewed as activities within a larger process, however, the opportunities for learning and measurement multiply. For example, when preparing a meal is seen as an activity that contributes to the process of weight control, different methods of meal preparation can be tried and the weight gain or loss can be monitored to determine the effectiveness of broiling instead of frying, for example.

Information Accessibility. Information accessibility helps staff develop a culture that supports a management-by-fact philosophy. Information accessibility was introduced in Chapter 12. It begins with data collection. Data are then formatted into four domains of information, represented in Figure 14–2 as strategy, process management, human resources, and leadership. The resulting information is made accessible to internal customers, secondary or intermediate customers, and end users in the marketplace. Data and their subsequent transition into information provides properly trained staff with the clues to solve problems, forge new directions, and eliminate old patterns that no longer serve them or the agency. Each element of data offers the opportunity for subsequent learning and improvement, providing there is a willingness to move beyond the status quo.

The same is true in the quest for physical fitness in the human body. The availability of data about diet, exercise, digestion, and nutritional needs contributes to the ability to maintain fitness. For example, knowing the caloric value, fat content, and other nutritional components of a given food aids in the decision-making process regarding whether that food contributes positively to the individual's fitness plan. The individual can then decide whether he or she is willing to omit foods that will prevent him or her from attaining a new level of fitness. Customers have found this information so valuable that, recently, the regulations regarding nutritional labels on foods were changed to provide better information. Customers of home care are also beginning to demand better information.

Another important aspect to the cost and quality formula depicted in Figure 14–2 is the blending of the external and internal perspectives. The external element is evident in alignment of human resources and information accessibility. Under alignment of human resources, it can be seen that the individual interacts with the external world—with customers, coworkers, consultants, educators, and the community as a whole. Staff are a conduit for gathering and sharing information. They become emissaries of goodwill in sharing the agency's mission and values. They become listening posts to gather information about the needs of the customer and the community and have the potential to identify new organizational opportunities that may be created because of the changing health care delivery system.

Information accessibility also has an external perspective. Information is potentially made available to all customers: internal, external, and the marketplace. Information is formatted for agency leadership, strategic planning efforts, human resource requirements, and process management expectations. Formatting the data is an important element because it makes information available to the customer; it is also critical to format it in a way that promotes relevance and ultimately knowledge. Agencies have been fearful of sharing data with competitors and regulators since data have previously been used for punishment. In the new paradigm, data are for learning. The proper formatting of data is key in the transition.

Data are also gathered from the external environment and combined with internal results to provide a core for future decisions and analysis. It is the data core (data set) that creates power and competitive advantage for organizations. When analyzed, the data set provides management and staff with the feedback (information) to create efficient and effective processes. Unfortunately, defining a data set (especially a clinical data set) within an agency has been an impediment to defining and measuring an agency's contribution to the health care of the community. This scenario is repeated on the national level, where defining home care's contribution is hindered by the diversity and diffusion of its collective data set.

The internal component of Figure 14–2 seems to be the customer-focused process since it focuses on agency operations. It is also external, however; customer-focused processes are designed to meet the needs of the organization and customers (internal and external). Management and staff collectively produce goods and services to meet the needs of customers and to satisfy the mission of the organization. Data from the environment are gathered through staff interaction or formal data collection activities. Once in the agency, data are used to refine processes.

Individually, these three components—aligned human resources, customer-focused processes, and information accessibility—make up the agency's infrastructure. Together, they provide a tool to manage cost and quality and keep an agency "fit."

ORGANIZATIONAL GLUE

One of the most powerful observations that can be made about Figure 14–2 is that the formula begins with human resources (individuals), and human resources can be found in each of the other two elements. This observation indicates that individuals are the glue that hold together the agency's infrastructure. It is the assessment of the values of these individuals (the collective assessment being the agency's values if there is alignment) that is a measure of the organization's well-being. Well-being is another important element of success. To use the analogy of fitness once more, a person may be physically fit as determined by body measurements, but may have cancer, be depressed, or have his or her well-being compromised in other ways.

To continue further with this analogy, many persons have attempted physical fitness, or weight loss, and have found that the fitness plan did not work. This failure is especially predominant with get-thin-fast plans. One result of the failure is that the individual learns that there is more to life than just being fit. So it is with an agency's fitness program (cost and quality). There is more to agency success than just fitness—there is also well-being.

Although more difficult than measuring cost and quality, assessing an agency's level of well-being is also possible. In fact, in a review of visionary companies such as Nordstrom, Sony, Walt Disney, Hewlett-Packard, and IBM, it was found that 44 percent of these companies had words in their mission statements that reflected well-being and only 26 percent had words that focused on organizational fitness.[7] Richard Barrett[8] enumerates indicators of organizational well-being such as creativity, innovation, learning, personal fulfillment, trust, cohesion, and morale. An example of how these indicators are incorporated into an organization's strategic goals and measurement process comes from 3M. One of its corporate targets was for 25 percent of its income to come from innovations. The result of this target was the now-famous Post-it notes that are used everywhere.

Because the organizational assessment is the collective assessment of all the individuals working there, including the leadership, agency transformation or change will be only as great as the collective individual change. Overall organizational change will not advance further than the level of growth of the leadership (i.e., the corporate culture cannot go beyond the level of growth of the leader). Workers change as they move through an evolution of consciousness over the course of their career. Their first need is to make money; second, a need to belong; and third, a need for status or power. Once the third level is reached and an individual finds that things aren't working, he or she begins to go through a transformation. At this point, the worker moves into being of service, making a difference, or becoming a change agent. Whatever the stage of growth of a worker, he or she will find a company with a similar attitude.[9] Thus, if the leader of a company establishes a corporate culture around making money, that is the type of worker who will work there; if the culture is one of service, that's the type of the worker who will migrate to that organization.

Change does not occur without effort. Change requires a commitment to follow one's dreams. How many times does one look in the mirror and decide to lose 15, or so, pounds? Everyone begins a diet with good intentions, and some realize their goal. Others, however, give up because it is too difficult to break old patterns of poor eating, snacking, or stopping at a fast-food restaurant instead of the salad bar.

How much easier it is to look for the quick fixes to weight loss—the magic pill, liquid diets, or cosmetic surgery. Unfortunately, many give up because there is no easy solution or quick fix.

"The quick-fix mentality also makes us 'system blind.' Many of today's problems come from yesterday's solutions, and many of today's solutions will be tomorrow's problems. What is most perplexing is that many quick fixes, from cost cutting to marketing promotions, are implemented even though no one believes they address underlying problems. But people still feel compelled to implement these 'solutions.' The need is to show results, and fast, regardless of the long-term, systemwide consequences."[10 (p.21)] This mandate to show fast results is a problem when addressing symptoms such as being overweight, having a high cost per visit, or poor staff morale. There needs to be a willingness to go below the events or symptoms and address the underlying patterns. It is only through root cause analysis that organizations will change their "mental models" in how they serve the customer and design their organization.

Real learning occurs when change is motivated from an intrinsic desire. It occurs when an individual is excited about creating a future that is different from the reality of today and when that individual feels like an important, respected part of the organization that is being created. To create organizations that will transition through the twenty-first century requires an intrinsic desire to make a difference in home care. Management can adopt the tools mentioned in this book especially for improving cost and quality, but more important, management can involve staff. As mentioned above, staff are the most important element of the organizational infrastructure. It is the alignment of staff and agency values that is the key to agency well-being.

Alignment of values, however, does not eliminate the diversity of views, cultures, approaches, styles, and levels of understanding. Diversity presents a challenge and an opportunity for managers. As a challenge, it requires effort and patience to develop a common understanding and a platform for organizational change, learning, and improvement. Diversity also presents a challenge because different groups of staff will require different incentives and opportunities to spark their interest and inspire them to grow within the organization. As an opportunity, however, diversity means that everyone has different perspectives, and collectively, this uniqueness has the potential of creating something that is richer and fuller than if everyone thought and acted the same and viewed life through the same set of lenses.

The key to dealing with both alignment and diversity is the concept of the learning organization. The following quote states it best:

> We believe a learning organization must be grounded in three foundations: (1) a culture based on transcendent human values of love, wonder, humility, and compassion; (2) a set of practices for generative conversa-

tion and coordinated action; and (3) a capacity to see and work with the flow of life as a system.

In learning organizations, cultural norms defy our business tradition. Acceptance of the other as a legitimate being—a Thou—(our meaning of love) replaces the traditional will to homogeneity. The ever-surprising manifestations of the world show up as opportunities to grow, as opposed to frustrating breakdowns for which somebody must take the blame (wonder). People understand that life is not condensable, that any model is an operational simplification always ready for improvement (humility). And when they encounter behaviors that they neither understand nor condone, people are able to appreciate that such actions arise from viewpoints and forces that are, in some sense, as valid as the viewpoints and forces that influence their own behaviors (compassion).

Learning organizations are a space for generative conversations and concerted action. In them, language functions as a device for connection, invention, and coordination. People can talk from their hearts and connect with one another in the spirit of dialogue (from the Greek dia+logos—moving through). Their dialogue weaves a common ongoing fabric and connects them at a deep level of being. When people talk and listen to each other this way, they create a field of alignment that produces tremendous power to invent new realities in conversation, and to bring about these new realities in action.

In learning organizations, people are always inquiring into the systemic consequences of their actions, rather than just focusing on the local consequences. They can understand the interdependencies underlying complex issues and act with perceptiveness and leverage. They are patient in seeking deeper understanding rather than striking out to "fix" problem symptoms—because they know that most fixes are temporary at best, and often result in more severe problems in the future.

As a result of these capabilities, learning organizations are both more generative and more adaptive than traditional organizations. Because of their commitment, openness, and ability to deal with complexity, people find security not in stability but in the dynamic equilibrium between holding on and letting go—holding on and letting go of beliefs, assumptions, and certainties. What they know takes a second place to what they can learn, and simplistic answers are always less important than penetrating questions."*

Source: Reprinted by permission of the publisher from ORGANIZATIONAL DYNAMICS AUTUMN 1993 © 1993. American Management Association, New York. http://www.amanet.org. All rights reserved.

To develop this type of organization, foster intrinsic motivation in staff, and create a culture that is based upon trust instead of fear, requires giving up many old mental models such as that staff are lazy, can't make appropriate decisions, or are not accountable. Inherent in such mental models is the need to create layers of management. What is created is a police environment, with regulatory agencies and managers acting as police instead of mentors, coaches, or teachers. The shift in thinking inherent in the new paradigm is to erase the hierarchical layers and work as partners. In a sense, it is a revolution. "The revolution is for organizations to become the place where our personal values intersect. Reforming our organizations so that our spirit is answered and our ability to serve customers, in the broadest sense, is guaranteed. Stewardship is the strategy that embodies this goal. Stewardship enables the use of power with grace."[11] (p.45)

Stewardship is creating a workplace of equals. A workplace where workers are not protected by managers and managers do not have rights and privileges over and above those of staff. It is about shared governance, ownership in the economic results of the organization, and an overriding need to be of service to the customer and the community instead of focusing on what is in it for me. "Me" wins when the customer wins. Stewardship requires discontinuing the blame game and replacing it with mutual respect, ownership, and a willingness to make difficult decisions. Stewardship is about partnership and joint accountability; it does not require an abdication of leadership. It does, however, require giving up control, rewards, and punishments in exchange for honest communication, trust, and faith in co-workers.

COMMUNITY

In the beginning was the environment (see Chapter 4) and in the end there is a community. There are two types of community: community the place and community the process. Community the place encompasses several different levels. At a macro level, it is the area in which we live. This community is made up of many businesses, homes, streets, and activities. Another level of community within the macro level is the health care community. This community is made up of hospitals, physicians, home care agencies, and various other medical practitioners. This community works in partnership with employers, third-party insurers, and individuals to prevent and cure disease and maintain wellness within the community. Within the medical community are the various providers of health care services. Each provider can be thought of as a subcommunity.

Figure 14–3 illustrates the place of community as a place for health.

People reside in the community as individuals and families. These same people may be also be employees in various subcommunities. Regardless, they represent inputs (I) into the various activities (A) for their respective subcommunities

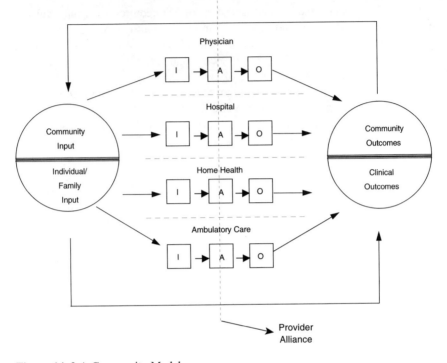

Figure 14–3 A Community Model

(physician, hospital, home health, ambulatory care). Each respective subcommunity contributes outputs (O) to the goals of the larger community to demonstrate outcomes as indicated in Figure 14–3. When viewed as a whole, or system, there is an opportunity to see how each microcommunity (provider) contributes to the larger whole. For instance, do all providers work toward the achievement of common outcomes with respect to the individuals within their community? Do they provide care in the most logical location to maximize return and minimize resource consumption? Do they communicate with one another in an efficient and effective manner? Do they understand which activities add value or merely add cost because they are duplicative?

Besides being a place, community is also a process. As a process, community occurs when the people connected by geography, common goals, or employer feel secure and trusted and consider themselves partners in creating a learning environment. Community the process is based on authentic communication and is characterized by mutual service, encouragement, and support.[12] Also, community as a process can be developed like any other process, although it is more than simply managing a process (i.e., learning the concepts, teaching the concepts to others, and monitoring the impact of the education on performance to determine success). Community the process is a journey that requires commitment to interacting with people in a way that promotes respect, tolerance, and growth; working a process that never ends; and developing relationships that go deeper than surface appearances.[13]

The opposite of community the process is *dis-society*.[14] Many neighborhoods experience dis-society with gang wars, drugs, and robberies. Home care agencies experience dis-society when clinicians exaggerate patient acuity or complexity to get extra time or resources, or when staff lie about results or abilities in order to look good. No level of community (the place) ever experiences community (the process) or dis-society all of the time, but rather will fall along different points on the continuum at different times. Moving toward more community (the process) does entail challenging the following existing myths:[15]

1. MYTH: "If we build community, money will follow."
   TRUTH: It is possible to do all the right things to build community and not be profitable. Organizations with employees committed to a common vision, teamwork, and authentic communication, however, often have a healthier and more profitable environment in the long term.
2. MYTH: "Community and hierarchy are incompatible."
   TRUTH: The presence and practice of community-building disciplines such as listening with C.A.R.E., showing respect, and serving employees is more critical than the presence or absence of a hierarchy.
3. MYTH: "Building community is the responsibility of top management."
   TRUTH: The idea may start at the top, but how far it spreads depends on the commitment of people at all levels. The more mutual the endeavor, the better the results.
4. MYTH: "A community-building program will create community."
   TRUTH: Programs do not create community, people do. Developing healthier relationships takes time, energy, and commitment.

Figure 14–4 illustrates a model that facilitates the ongoing process toward community. This model begins with the empowered individual (consumer, resident, person), who is becoming more prevalent in society. As this person becomes more knowledgeable and relates better with all aspects of his or her life, this person will become more involved in maintaining wellness. This process can already be seen as people become more informed consumers regarding food, safety, and health care. The increased consumer involvement in home care has been discussed earlier in this book. As these consumers relate more with their local health care providers, partnerships will develop and providers will see the need for providing services to the community. Local wellness communities will begin to form and as more of these do, global wellness will develop regionally, then at the state level, and someday progress to a national philosophy. Because of

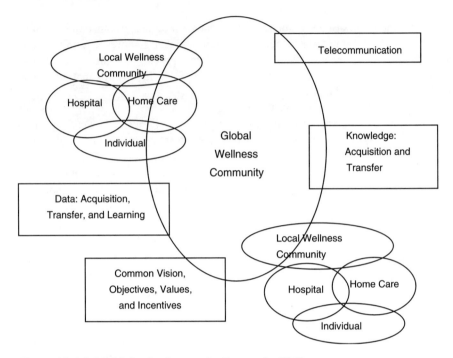

Figure 14–4 A Model for the Community Process for Wellness

the heterogeneity of consumers, it may very well be that multiple local wellness communities develop around shared values. The global wellness community will provide the cornerstones that link these communities.

Figure 14–4 identifies four of these cornerstones for the global wellness community. These are (1) a common vision, (2) communication, (3) data acquisition and transformation, and (4) knowledge. A common vision of a healthy community is the key to making it happen. Communication with each other for support, coaching, and learning is also important. Communication can be face to face and, as communities grow, it can be through various means of telecommunication. Collecting data to aid in learning is key to monitoring growth and change. Finally, understanding what is happening by acquiring knowledge is the basis for the next step of growth (different for different communities) that will always be there in this lifelong process. Besides consumer empowerment and access to health information, other changes would take place in these wellness communities, such as

1. more evidenced-based medicine and alternate ways of healing as education replaced the "cure" of symptoms

2. an increase in consumer and provider decision and support information
3. greater emphasis on quality of life rather than simply the absence of disease

The two community models presented in Figures 14–3 and 14–4 have many similarities. Figure 14–4 is more encompassing and holistic. What is primarily different, however, is the perspective or focus. Figure 14–3 represents community as a place with a process for improving the health outcomes within that place. Figure 14–4 represents community as a process for global wellness, which then becomes a place to reside. Neither is right nor wrong; they are simply different viewpoints.

Community is a process and a place, a journey and a destination. Viewing community in this way supports the growth of stewardship, serving others while serving ourselves. If individuals within the community take ownership for their lifestyles to maintain health and promote safety, the focus of health care would shift away from being primarily "back-end" and expensive, to being preventive and resource efficient. Then, by partnering with each other and with health care providers, we could begin to shift our health care model away from one of crisis management to one that is based upon holism and prevention—a global wellness community in which to live. The process has already begun.

THE KEYS TO SUCCESS

As a home care provider in this evolving community, how does one succeed? Everyone is looking for the "how to" or wondering what do to. The solution is not so easy in this complex, turbulent world of home care. It is the authors' belief that it is easier to find a boat and try to ride down this turbulent river than it is to stop the river from flowing. So, given the parameters of the new paradigm that is unfolding, the authors offer the following list as clues for how to proceed, in addition to the tasks that were mentioned earlier in the chapter. Each of these keys has been discussed more fully earlier in the book. Each of these is a journey, not a single task or event. Success lies not in how many are done, but rather in the genuineness of the commitment.

- Create an environment in which people feel safe and secure.
- Create an agency environment of teamwork and exploration.
- Develop a strategic planning process that includes internal and external customers.
- Clearly define agency mission and vision.
- Elicit the values that are encapsulated in the mission and vision and live by them or change them.
- Standardize work operations (e.g., agency and staff standards, policies, position descriptions, and so on).

- Design work flowcharts for support processes and subprocesses, track variations, and modify as indicated.
- Define a clinical data set that describes the scope and depth of agency services (e.g., OASIS + + + +) in concert with agency mission and vision.
- Establish a means for gathering (electronic or manual), aggregating, and analyzing sound data (e.g., data with integrity).
- Pursue performance excellence.
- Create an expectation and process for open communication (accessing and disseminating information) to and from leadership, management, staff, customers, and the community (e.g., surveys, focus groups, letters, reports, scorecards).
- Anticipate customer expectations.
- Respect, trust, and acknowledge and hold accountable all who work in the agency. People are an agency's most important resource.
- Orient all new staff to the agency mission, vision, and values and evaluate their commitment and alignment to the mission, vision, and values.
- Define agency clinical guidelines (procedures, protocols, and pathways) for diagnoses or patient conditions treated by the agency (core process).
- Track variations to the clinical guidelines and modify as indicated.
- Acknowledge the contribution of the upstream and downstream processes to the core process. Prepare flowcharts for these processes and track for variations.
- Define measurement indicators (e.g., metrics, outcomes) that capture cost, quality, and agency well-being and establish a continuous improvement program that measures improvement and organizational growth.
- Seek out and address root causes, not symptoms.
- Cost out the activities that support all defined processes.
- Create a learning environment and educate, educate, educate.
- Create a corporate culture that rewards good behavior; celebrate successes.
- Take risks and make the difficult decisions.
- As an individual and as an agency, be a steward and be of service to all the communities of which you are a member.

CONCLUSION

It is true that "we must continually challenge the past so that we can renew ourselves each day."[16] If long-term survival, growth, and success are aspirations for your agency, then there must be a willingness to challenge the patterns that currently exist within your organization. These patterns were created in an environment that was cost reimbursed and made sense at the time they were created, but may no longer provide value in an environment that is dominated by managed care and shrinking health care dollars. Furthermore, blindly following the path that others have created without reflecting and questioning whether this path is consistent with your vision, whether it is meeting the needs of your customers, or whether it is consistent with organizational values is the hallmark of ineffective leadership.

The tools and concepts in this text dealt with quality, measurement, processes, and the management of cost and activities. We believe that an organization needs to be built upon values, have a mission that inspires staff, and be consistent with values and daily actions, and that organizational values and mission are inspired by a vision of a desired future state. Tools and concepts are not enough, however.

Of greater importance is the harnessing of the latent potential in all staff through investing in them and creating a win-win environment where both the individual and organization can flourish. There needs to be an underlying philosophy that values staff and demonstrates that their contributions are valued. Believing in individuals and providing them with the resources to do the job will be critical to creating organizations that will survive through the twenty-first century.

We all have a tendency to believe that somewhere *out there* lies *the* answer to how to successfully run our agency. Once we find that answer, all we have to do is follow the steps, like a recipe, and our job will become easy. Meanwhile, as we keep looking, we uncover more and sometimes deeper problems. Unfortunately, there is no one simple answer. If we view these problems as a series of tasks that have to be done, learning becomes limited and the journey becomes a treadmill going nowhere. The result is frustration and burnout.

> Many organizations will fail in their quest for total quality service, not because their leaders don't understand the concept or technical require-ments for achieving it, but because they don't realize that the heart of the service journey is spiritual rather than mechanical.[17]
>
> —Karl Albrecht

The answer to the problems lies elsewhere. The answer is, in fact, the quest: the discovery of the problem and the greater understanding (knowledge) that is gained as we delve into the underlying issues. Such is the value of the systems approach. Viewing things as a system allows us to look beyond the individual tasks to the process of which they are a part, to the system of which the process is a part, and so on. The result is an increasing level of knowledge. The more we know, the more conscious choices (or informed decisions) we can make, and the more we can direct our boat down the river on a course that will get us successfully to our destination.

So the solution becomes rather straightforward. We need to align our intent with our values, balance our actions within our hearts and minds, and develop organizational alignment using values, vision, and partnership to foster accountability. We need to manage cost and demonstrate quality that occurs through the alignment of human resources, the development of a process orientation, and the use of data to create organizational learning. And above all, we need to listen to what our customers are saying, because they will provide us with the clues and opportunities for long-term survival.

NOTES

1. B.A. Mark, The Black Box of Patient Outcomes Research, *Image* 27, no. 1 (1995): 42.
2. *Continuing Care*, Facing the Upcoming Challenges in Home Health Care, *Continuing Care* (July/August 1997), as reported in *Home Health Digest* 3, no. 4 (1997): 1.
3. J. Marcus, Staying Alive: New Payment System Can Ring Death Knell for Agencies That Fail To Act, *Home Health Digest* 3, no. 6 (1997): 1–2.
4. G. Miles, Back Home Near Rome, *The Philadelphia Inquirer,* 13 December 1997: D1–D2.
5. E.C. Nevis et al., Understanding Organizations as Learning Systems, MIT, Copyright 1997, Found on the Internet.
6. R.M. Gorey and D.R. Dobat, Managing the Knowledge Era, *The Systems Thinker* 7, no. 8 (1996): 1–5.
7. R. Barrett, Spirituality in Business Life: A Values Driven Approach to Organizational Transformation (Presentation at the University of Santa Monica, Santa Monica, CA, March 1997).
8. Barrett, Spirituality in Business Life.
9. Barrett, Spirituality in Business Life.
10. S. Chawla and J. Renesch, eds., *Learning Organizations: Developing Cultures for Tomorrow's Workplace* (Portland, OR: Productivity Press, 1995), 21.
11. P. Block, *Stewardship* (San Francisco: Berrett-Koehler Publishers, 1996), 45.
12. G. Zlevor, Creating a New Workplace: Making a Commitment to Community, *The Systems Thinker* 5, no. 7 (1994): 1–4.
13. Zlevor, Creating a New Workplace, 1–4.
14. Zlevor, Creating a New Workplace, 1–4.
15. Zlevor, Creating a New Workplace, 1–4.
16. S. Ghoshal and C.A. Bartlett, Rebuilding Behavioral Context: A Blueprint for Corporate Renewal, *Sloan Management Review* 37, no. 2 (Winter 1996): 23–36.
17. K. Albrecht, The Only Thing That Matters, listed as a source on the Internet, 271.

GLOSSARY

AARP	American Association of Retired Persons.
ABCM	Activity-based cost management.
ADL	Activity of daily living.
AHCPR	Agency for Health Care Policy and Research.
ANA	American Nurses Association.
Activities	An accumulation of steps, tasks, and actions. Activities usually denote action.
BSC	Balanced scorecard.
CEO	Chief executive officer.
CFO	Chief financial officer.
CHAP	Community Health Accreditation Program.
CHF	Chronic heart failure.
CHIRS	Community Health Intensity Rating Scale.
COBRA	Consolidated Omnibus Budget Reconciliation Act.
COPs	Conditions of participation.
CPA	Certified public accountant.
CPR	Computerized patient record.
CQI	Continuous quality improvement.
CVA	Cardiovascular accident.

Care Map®	One of several proprietary names given to a form of clinical pathway.
Clinical pathway	A predetermined, optimal sequencing and timing of clinical activities by the health care team that guides a patient with a defined health problem(s) through a course of care toward expected outcomes.
Community	A place where people are connected by geography, common goals, managed care plan, employer. Also the process of interacting with people in an authentic manner that is characterized by mutual service, encouragement, and support.
Consumer	Same as customer.
Core process	The heart of the patient-focused care process, where the defined activities (e.g., hands-on care, scheduling, case management, patient education, and traveling) are performed.
Customer	An internal or external consumer of the product or service. Everyone whose decisions determine the success of the agency. The term *customer* is used to identify staff (internal customers), payers, patients, families of patients, physicians, institutional referral sources, suppliers, and others.
DRG	Diagnosis-related group.
Data	Elements; fundamental facts.
Downstream process	The last segment of the patient-focused care process. The downstream process is responsible for the activities associated with billing, records management, and patient follow-up.
Drivers	Defines a relationship between events and activities, resources and activities, and activities and objectives.
Expected outcome	What the process is predetermined to look like once it is complete. For example, the picture on the jigsaw puzzle box is what the puzzle will look like once the process of putting it together is complete. Outcomes include a measurable behavior and a time frame for a given entity (patient, agency, team, and so on).

FACCT	Foundation for Accountability.
Forum	Forum for Quality and Effectiveness in Health Care (an office within AHCPR).
FTE	Full-time equivalent. Calculation in home care is usually based upon 2,080 hours per year.
GAAP	Generally accepted accounting principles.
Goal	Something to be attained. Sometimes referred to as a budgeted objective or a stretch target. A goal represents a change from a baseline. Goals can reflect gains and losses.
HCFA	Health Care Financing Administration.
HEDIS	Health Plan Employer Data and Information Set.
HHCC	Home Health Care Clarifications.
HHUG	Home Health Utilization Group.
HIM II	Health Insurance Manual, Section II.
HIV/AIDS	Human immunodeficiency virus/acquired immune deficiency syndrome.
HL7	Health language 7.
HMO	Health maintenance organization.
IADL	Instrumental activity of daily living.
IANS	Institute for Ancillary Network Standards.
IPS	Interim payment system.
IRS	Internal Revenue Service.
Individual's chart	Graph of data using statistical methodology for calculating upper and lower control limits when data is variable and frequency is unknown.
Information	A summary of relevant data that is useful for understanding; the acquisition of knowledge.
Input	Resources used in a process. Resources consist of labor and benefits, supplies, materials, capital, and technology. Management can influence input through training, defining supply and material requirements,

and investing in an organizations infrastructure; information technology.

Joint Commission

Joint Commission on Accreditation of Healthcare Organizations.

LANs

Local area networks.

LCL

Lower control limits. Statistically determined lower boundary that determine, along with the UCL, whether a process is in or out of control.

Lagging indicators

Lagging indicators are performance measures that provide information about events that have already taken place. An excellent example of lagging indicators is the financial results of operation. Financial results reflect contracts and decisions that have been put into action months and years before the financial reports are produced.

Leading indicators

Leading indicators provide a foreshadowing of events. For instance, a shift in payer mix will indicate changes in revenues and income; decreases in customer satisfaction have the potential to prevent contracts from being renewed; and decreases in staff satisfaction have the potential to foreshadow turnover.

MCO

Managed care organization.

Management

With respect to performance measurement, management is the identification of performance measures that convey value to stakeholders and the alignment of organizational resources toward continuous improvement of outcomes.

Measurement

Measurement is the quantification of an indicator. The time frame of a measurement is metric dependent. A temperature reading could be noted hourly, a sphgmometer reading every several minutes, patient satisfaction on an episode-by-episode basis, and physician satisfaction quarterly, semiannually, or annually.

Metrics

An all-inclusive term for multiple performance measures. See *Performance measure*.

Moving range	A supporting calculation for an individual's chart. The calculation is based upon the difference in resource requirements from preceding calculations.
NAHC	National Association for Home Care.
NAMES	National Association of Medical Equipment Suppliers.
NANDA	North American Nursing Diagnosis Association.
NCCNHR	National Citizens Coalition for Nursing Home Reform.
NCQA	National Committee for Quality Assurance.
NIC	Nursing Interventions Classification.
NMDS	Nursing Minimum Data Set.
NOC	Nursing-Sensitive Outcome Classification.
NOLF	National Organization Liaison Forum.
NPV	Net present value.
OASIS	Outcome and Assessment Information Set.
OBQI	Outcome-based quality improvement.
ORT	Operation Restore Trust.
Outcome	Outcome is a result. It is the end result of a process or activity.
Output	The end result of a process. Output can be what an external consumer will see (a completed product or activity), or output can result in the completion of the first of a series of steps. In the latter case, output is seen by an internal customer. All output can be influenced by management intervention to affect its cost, the time it takes to produce or complete, and whether the output satisfies the external or internal customer.
P & L	Profit and loss (statement).
PDCA	Plan-Do-Check-Act (cycle).
Paradigm	A model or pattern used to explain fundamental change.

Patient-focused care process	An agency's reason for being. This process is where value is provided to patients. The patient-focused care process includes three elements: the upstream, core, and downstream processes.
Payer mix	Summarization of revenues based upon payer source.
Performance measure	Performance measures are indices or metrics that have been calculated to assess performance or output. Performance measures can include indicators of time, clinical quality, customer satisfaction, financial performance, and organizational growth. Performance measures apply to processes, activities, and end results. Performance measures can be predictive or lagging indicators.
Primary customers	The end users of a service or product. In home care it is patients and their family. Value is created by providing services to support the patient's healing process. Physicians, payers, and referral sources are secondary customers. They are concerned about the results that are achieved and the agency's ability to keep them informed of progress.
Process	Processes are made up of three elements: input, process, and output. Input represents the ingredients that go into a process. Typically, input consists of labor and benefits, supplies, materials, capital, and technology. Process type and sequence will determine input requirements. Process represents the activities, steps, tasks, actions, and protocols that occur to create a product or service. Output is the result of the process; it is the service that has been created or the activities that have been completed. Output can be assessed through performance measures such as cost, quality, and time.
Pure outcome	A change in a patient's health status (physiologic, functional, cognitive, emotional, and/or behavioral) between two or more points in time.
QA	Quality assurance.
ROI	Return on investment.

Result	Results are outcomes. They are the effect of a process or activity.
Risk mix	Summary of revenue, in percent format, by payment methodology. Examples would include percent of revenues attributable to cost reimbursement, per visit, discounted per visit, episodic, and capitated. The shift away from cost reimbursement to payment methodologies with a higher degree of risk indicates the potential for profit and losses. Increasing risk needs to be conveyed to the board and management.
SBU	Strategic business unit. SBUs include branches or divisions within the agency umbrella. A stand-alone agency would have one strategic business plan. If an agency were large and had multiple divisions, service segments, and branches, it might have separate strategic business plans to accommodate the difference between divisions, service lines, and branches. Each SBU would have its own specific goals and objectives as well as goals and objectives that are common to all SBUs.
SD	Standard deviation.
SE	Standard error.
SHIRS	School Health Intensity Rating Scale.
SWOT analysis	Consideration of strengths, weaknesses, opportunities, and threats.
Secondary or intermediate customers	These are the physicians, payers, and various sources that refer patients to the agency. They are concerned about how effective service provision is in assisting patients with their healing process. The goal is to keep this group of customers informed and to exceed promises and expectations regarding service delivery, the demonstration of clinical outcomes, and patient satisfaction.
Stakeholder	Anyone who has an interest in the well-being of the organization. Stakeholders is also an all-inclusive term for customers that includes the patient, physicians, referral sources, the patient's family, the com-

munity, staff, creditors, shareholders, and the board of directors.

Strategy

Strategy is the development of a plan, the setting of goals or objectives. Goals and objectives are measurable. Strategy is the sequence of activities that must be completed to accomplish short- and long-term goals and objectives.

Stretch target

A goal or objective that is future oriented and requires improvement of existing results in order to be achieved.

Suboptimization

The greater potential of the system is not realized because one of the supporting elements is out of sync with the system's larger mission. Optimization occurs when there is a balance among the multiple needs of stakeholders. Suboptimization could occur because of an imbalance between strategies. For instance, if an agency focuses on cost-effectiveness without regard for clinical outcomes and patient satisfaction, then the organization is emphasizing short-term results. An imbalance has occurred between the needs of multiple stakeholders. Conversely, an emphasis on clinical outcomes without regard for cost-effectiveness could create economic problems, thus creating an imbalance between stakeholders.

Support processes

Support processes support the patient-focused care processes. Support processes include human resources, information systems, general and financial management, quality improvement, and the planning and marketing functions.

System

A series of interrelated processes working toward a shared goal or vision.

TQM

Total quality management.

UCL

Upper control limit. Statistically determined upper boundary that determines, along with the LCL, whether a process is in or out of control.

UNLS

Unified Nursing Language System.

Upstream process

The first segment of the patient-focused care process. The job of the upstream process in home care is to determine whether the patient should be admitted onto service and to gather appropriate data to begin the care planning process. Activities that are performed as part of this process relate to intake, the initial assessment visit, and the gathering and processing of patient data.

Value   Something of importance, benefit, or usefulness from a consumer's perspective.

Values   Personal and organizational principles that provide the foundation for decision making.

Working capital T/O   Working capital turnover ratio. Net patient revenue divided by working capital. An indicator of how well management is utilizing agency resources.

INDEX

ABOUT THE AUTHORS

Donna Ambler Peters, PhD, RN, FAAN, is currently senior product consultant for Delta Health Systems in Altoona, Pennsylvania. Her responsibilities include articulating product lines from a clinical perspective and setting and identifying product vision. In addition, she is an associate of the Corridor Group.

Dr. Peters' extensive background and experience in home care, quality assurance, outcomes, and documentation systems provides the focus of her home care clinical and administrative expertise. She is a graduate of the University of Pennsylvania for both her baccalaureate and doctorate degrees, and of the University of Iowa for her master's degree in nursing administration. She has held positions with the Johns Hopkins Hospital, the Robert Wood Johnson Foundation, and the Community Health Accreditation Program (CHAP), where she was the principal investigator for In Search of Excellence, a $1.2 million project funded by Kellogg to develop outcomes for home care.

Dr. Peters is a favored speaker throughout the country on home care topics, particularly on quality, outcomes, and data management. She has represented home care at several invitational conferences and has spoken at numerous state and national conferences. Dr. Peters has written numerous journal articles and book chapters, and serves on the editorial boards of several journals.

Tad McKeon, CPA, MBA, CQM, is the principal consultant in the firm of McKeon & Associates, a home health consulting firm in Jeffersonville, Pennsylvania. Mr. McKeon has an MBA in financial management from Temple University, is an adjunct professor at The Pennsylvania State University, and is certified by the American Society of Quality Control as a quality manager. He is a nationally recognized speaker on activity-based cost management and process improvement as well as the author of *Home Health Financial Management* and a contributing author to *Clinical Pathways for the Multidisciplinary Home Care*

Team. Mr. McKeon serves as a senior board examiner for the Malcolm Baldrige National Quality Award and was asked to be the team leader in creating a case study using a fictitious home health care agency, which applied for the National Quality Award, to exemplify how the concepts of performance excellence would apply to the home health industry. Mr. McKeon also serves on the editorial board for the *Journal of Home Health Care Management and Practice, Home Health Care Data Quarterly*, and *Home Health Care Revenue Report*.